Bile Acids in Hepatobiliary Disease

Bile Acids in Hepatobiliary Disease

Edited by

T.C. Northfield
H.A. Ahmed
R.P. Jazrawi
Department of Gastroenterology, Endocrinology and Metabolism
St George's Hospital Medical School
London, UK

P.L. Zentler-Munro
Raigmore Hospital
Inverness, UK

Proceedings of the Falk Workshop held in London, UK, 29–30 March 1999

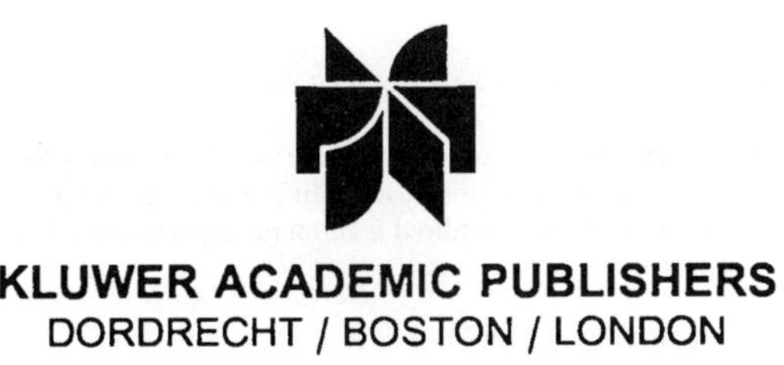

KLUWER ACADEMIC PUBLISHERS
DORDRECHT / BOSTON / LONDON

Library of Congress Cataloging in-Publication Data is available.

ISBN 0-7923-8755-4

Published by Kluwer Academic Publishers, BV
P.O. Box 17, 3300 AA Dordrecht, The Netherlands.

Sold and distributed in North, Central and South America
by Kluwer Academic Publishers, PO Box 358,
Accord Station, Hingham, MA 02018–0358, USA.

In all other countries, sold and distributed
by Kluwer Academic Publishers, Distribution Center,
P.O. Box 322, 3300 AH Dordrecht, The Netherlands

Printed on acid-free paper

Printed and bound in Great Britain by MPG Books.

Contents

SECTION III: CLINICAL TRIALS

SECTION IV: OTHER CHOLESTATIC CONDITIONS

SECTION V: ALCOHOLIC AND OTHER LIVER DISEASES

SECTION VI: BILE ACID THERAPY

List of Principal Authors

H.A. Ahmed
Department of Gastroenterology,
  Endocrinology and Metabolism
St George's Hospital Medical School
Cranmer Terrace
London SW17 0RE
UK

M.F. Bassendine
Center for Liver Research
4th Floor William Leech Building
The Medical School
Framlington Place
Newcastle-upon-Tyne NE2 4HH
UK

J.L. Boyer
Liver Center
Section of Digestive Diseases
Yale University School of Medicine
333 Cedar Street
New Haven CT 06520-8019
USA

M.C. Carey
Harvard Medical School
Thorn 1430–Gastroenterology
  Division
Brigham and Women's Hospital
75 Francis Street
Boston, MA 02115-6195
USA

C. Colombo
Department of Pediatrics,
University of Milan and Sassari
Via San Pietro 12
I-07100 Sassari
Italy

R.H. Dowling
Gastroenterology Laboratory
4th Floor, North Wing
St Thomas' Hospital
London SE1 7EH
UK

C.A. Einarsson
Department of Gastroenterology
Huddinge University Hospital
K63
SE-141 86 Huddinge
Sweden

H. Ghodse
Department of Psychiatry of Addictive
  Behaviour and Psychological
  Medicine
St George's Hospital Medical School
Cranmer Terrace
London SE17 0RE
UK

T. Gilat
Department of Gastroenterology
Tel-Aviv Sourasky Medical Center
6 Weizman St,
64239 Tel Aviv
Israel

P.C. Hayes
Department of Medicine (RIE)
The University of Edinburgh
Royal Infirmary
Lauriston Place
Edinburgh EH3 9YW
UK

LIST OF PRINCIPAL AUTHORS

J. Heathcote
Division of Gastroenterology
Toronto Western Hospital
University of Toronto West Wing
  4-828
399 Bathhurst Street
Toronto, ONT M5T 2S8
Canada

K.W. Heaton
Claverham House
Claverham
North Somerset
BS49 4QD
UK

A.F. Hofmann
Division of Gastroenterology
Department of Medicine (0813)
University of California, San
  Diego
La Jolla, CA 92093-0813
USA

R.P. Jazrawi
Department of Gastroenterology,
  Endocrinology and Metabolism
St George's Hospital Medical
  School
Cranmer Terrace
London SW17 0RE
UK

A.G. Johnson
Division of Surgical and Anaesthetic
  Sciences
Floor K
Royal Hallamshire Hospital
Sheffield S10 2JF
UK

A. Lanzini
Medicine 1
Spedali Civili
Piazzale degli Spedali Civili 1
25100 Brescia
Italy

U. Leuschner
Medical Clinic II
University Hospital
Theodor-Stern-Kai 7
D-60590 Frankfurt/Main
Germany

C.S. Lieber
Alcohol Research and Treatment
  Center
Liver Diseases and Nutrition Section
Bronx VA Medical Center
130 West Kingsbridge Road
Bronx
New York NY 10468-3992
USA

A.G. Lim
Department of Gastroenterology,
  Endocrinology and Metabolism
St George's Hospital Medical School
Cranmer Terrace
London SW17 0RE
UK

P. Milkiewicz
Liver Unit
Liver Research Labs
Queen Elizabeth Hospital
Edgbaston
Birmingham B15 2TH
UK

T.C. Northfield
Department of Gastroenterology,
  Endocrinology and Metabolism
St George's Hospital Medical School
Cranmer Terrace
London SW17 0RE
UK

T. Peters
Department of Clinical Biochemistry
King's College School of Medicine
Denmark Hill
Bessemer Road
London SE5 9PJ
UK

J.M.C. Stenner
Department of Gastroenterology,
  Endocrinology and Metabolism
St George's Hospital Medical School
Cranmer Terrace
London SW17 0RE
UK

J. Reichen
Department of Clinical Pharmacology
Murtenstrasse 35
CH 3010 Berne
Switzerland

E. Roda
Dipartimento di Medicina Interna e
    Gastroenterologia
Policlinico S. Orsola-Malpighi
Via Massarenti 9
40126 Bologna
Italy

G. Sauter
Department of Medicine II
Klinikum Grosshadern
81366 Munich
Germany

K.D.R. Setchell
Clinical Mass Spectrometry
NRB-R029
Children's Hospital Medical Center
3333 Burnet Avenue
Cincinnati, OH 45229-3039
USA

M. Stellini
c/o Professor Dowling
Gastroenterology Laboratory
Division of Medicine
4th Floor, North Wing
St Thomas' Hospital
London SE1 7EH
UK

A. Stiehl
Medizinische Universitatsklinik
Bergheimerstr. 58
D-69115 Heidelberg
Germany

R. Thompson
Department of Child Health
Guy's, King's and St Thomas' School
    of Medicine
Denmark Hill Campus
Bessemer Road
London SE5 9PJ
UK

H.J. Verkade
Department of Pediatrics
    Laboratory Center
CMC IV, Rm Y-2115
University Hospital Groningen
P.O. Box 30.001
NL-9700 RB Groningen
The Netherlands

A. Verma
Department of Gastroenterology,
    Endocrinology and Metabolism
St George's Hospital Medical School
Cranmer Terrace
London SW17 0RE
UK

R. Williams
Institute of Hepatology
University College London and
    University College London
    Hospitals
69-75 Chenies Mews
London WC1E 6HX
UK

P.L. Zentler-Munro
Department of Medicine
Raigmore Hospital
Old Perth Road
Inverness IV2 3UJ
UK

Introduction

This book contains the contributions of the speakers at the second Falk workshop on bile acids to be held in the UK. This second meeting, held at the Royal Institution of Great Britain on 29th and 30th March, 1999, commemorated the bicentenary of the Royal Institution, where the first scientific meeting was held in March 1799. The formal lectures were held in the same lecture hall as that used by Michael Faraday, the presiding genius of the Royal Institution in the 19th century, as well as by its fifteen Nobel Laureates in the 20th century.

The main interest in bile acid therapy in recent years has been in cholestatic liver disease. This workshop was convened not only to discuss this, but also to move on to examine the possible use of bile acids in alcoholic liver disease, and to move back to re-examine their role in biliary disease. With respect to cholestatic liver disease, discussion focused on physiology, pathophysiology and epidemiology; with respect to alcoholic liver disease, it focused on pathogenesis and clinical aspects, and on broader aspects of alcohol abuse and metabolism. Discussion of cholesterol gallstone disease focused on pathogenesis in relation to the liver, the bile, the gallbladder and the large intestine. In recent years, non-surgical therapy has been eclipsed by laparoscopic cholecystectomy, but the roles of bile acid therapy, lithotripsy and contact dissolution were reassessed by experts in the field.

Discussion then moved on to other conditions in which bile acids have a role, including colonic neoplasia, chronic pancreatitis and cystic fibrosis. In the final lecture, Alan Hofmann emphasised the continuing importance of bile acids and assessed their role in the next millennium. He incorporated a practical demonstration of the physical chemistry of lipids at the podium, with the assistance of Martin Carey, in keeping with the traditions of the Royal Institution's demonstrations in physics and chemistry over the last 200 years. The proceedings as a whole were in keeping with Dr. Falk's tradition of mixing good science with good social events, the delegates' dinner being held in the Cafe Royal nearby.

Tim Northfield

Section I
Cholestatic liver disease: physiology, pathogenesis and epidemiology

1
Cellular and molecular mechanisms of bile salt transport in health and disease

J.L. BOYER

Bile salts play an important role in the generation of bile secretion and in the pathophysiology of cholestasis. Much has been learned in recent years about the cellular and molecular transport mechanisms that are involved in these processes and their alterations in cholestatic liver injury[1]. Bile is formed by the generation of osmotic gradients within the lumen of the bile canaliculus and is composed of both bile salt-dependent and bile salt-independent components. Bile salt-dependent bile secretion is primarily dependent on the enterohepatic circulation of bile salts, which is maintained by a series of membrane transport proteins in the liver and ileum. In the liver, conjugated bile salts are efficiently removed from the portal circulation primarily by a high affinity ~ 50 kDa transport protein on the hepatic sinusoidal membrane, the sodium taurocholate co-transporting polypeptide (NTCP)[2]. The inwardly directed sodium gradient provides the driving force for this process. Unconjugated bile salts are taken up primarily by several multi-specific organic anion transporting polypeptides (OATP1 and 2), which also transport a variety of other organic solutes[2]. Bile salts then bind to a cytosolic binding protein, 3-hydroxysteroid-dehydrogenase[3], and rapidly diffuse to the canalicular membrane where they are excreted into bile by the bile salt export pump, BSEP, a member of the ATP binding cassette gene family[4]. The ileal bile salt transporter, ISBT, a sodium coupled co-transporting polypeptide on the brush border, then removes the majority of the bile salt pool from the intestinal lumen[5]. Bile salts probably enter the portal circulation from the ileum by way of an organic anion exchange protein (?OATP3 or 4) on the basolateral membrane whose molecular identity has not yet been firmly established. ISBT is also located on the luminal membrane of cholangiocytes where it could function to maintain a cholehepatic circulation for bile salts[6,7].

During cholestatic liver injury, bile salts accumulate in the liver and transcriptional and post-transcriptional alterations in some of the bile salt transporters occur. Studies based on several animal models of cholestasis in the rat show that the hepatic uptake of bile salts is reduced by down-regulation of both

Ntcp and Oatp[8–13]. In cholestasis induced by bacterial endotoxin (LPS), there is a loss of specific transcription factors (HNF-1 and footprint B) that regulate the expression of Ntcp at the level of gene transcription[11]. These responses to cholestatic liver injury can be interpreted as protecting the liver from further accumulations of potentially toxic bile salts. In contrast to the hepatic uptake mechanisms for bile salts, the canalicular bile salt excretory pump is only modestly down-regulated and appears to maintain its canalicular location and capacity to excrete bile salts during cholestasis, at least when produced by bile duct obstruction[14,15]. This is in contrast to mutations in the human BSEP gene, which are associated with marked reductions in bile salts in bile and result in progressive familial intrahepatic cholestasis, type 2 in infants[16]. Further details of the molecular regulation of hepatocellular transport systems in cholestasis can be found in a recent review[17].

REFERENCES

1. Trauner M, Meier PJ, Boyer JL. Molecular pathogenesis of cholestasis. N Engl J Med. 1998;339:1217–1227.
2. Meier PJ, Eckhardt U, Schroeder A, Hagenbuch B, Stieger B. Substrate specificity of sinusoidal bile acid and organic anion uptake systems in rat and human liver. Hepatology. 1997;26:1667–1677.
3. Stolz A, Takikawa H, Ookhtens M, Kaplowitz N. The role of cytoplasmic proteins in hepatic bile acid transport. Annu Rev Physiol. 1989;51:161–176.
4. Gerloff T, Stieger B, Hagenbuch B et al. The sister of P-glycoprotein represents the canalicular bile salt export pump of mammalian liver. J Biol Chem 1998;273:10046–10050.
5. Wong MH, Oelkers P, Dawson PA. Identification of a mutation in the ileal sodium-dependent bile acid transporter gene that abolishes transport activity. J Biol Chem. 1995;270:27228–27234.
6. Lazaridis KN, Pham L, Tietz P et al. Rat cholangiocytes absorb bile acids at their apical domain via the ileal sodium-dependent bile acid transporter. J Clin Invest. 1997;100:2714–2721.
7. Alpini G, Glaser SS, Rodgers R et al. Functional expression of the apical Na+-dependent bile acid transporter in large but not small rat cholangiocytes. Gastroenterology. 1997;113:1734–1740.
8. Gartung C, Ananthanarayanan M, Rahman MA et al. Down-regulation of expression and function of the rat liver Na+/bile acid cotransporter in extrahepatic cholestasis. Gastroenterology. 1996;110:199–209.
9. Moseley RH, Wang W, Takeda H et al. Effect of endotoxin on bile acid transport in rat liver: a potential model for sepsis-associated cholestasis. Am J Physiol. 1996;271:G137–G146.
10. Simon FR, Fortune J, Iwahashi M, Gartung C, Wolkoff A, Sutherland E. Ethinyl estradiol cholestasis involves alterations in expression of liver sinusoidal transporters. Am J Physiol. 1996;34:G1043–G1052.
11. Trauner M, Arrese M, Lee H, Boyer JL, Karpen S. Endotoxin downregulates rat hepatic ntcp gene expression via decreased activity of critical transcription factors. J Clin Invest. 1998;101:2092–2100.
12. Gartung C, Trauner M, Schlosser SF, Hagenbuch B, Meier PJ, Boyer JL. Sodium-independent uptake of bile acids is unaffected by down-regulation of an organic anion transporter (oatp) in rat liver during cholestasis produced by common bile duct ligation (CBDL). Hepatology. 1996;24:369A.
13. Dumont M, Jacquemin E, D'Hont C et al. Expression of the liver Na+-independent organic anion transporting polypeptide (oatp-1) in rats with bile duct ligation. J Hepatol. 1997;27:1051–1056.
14. Lee JM, Trauner M, Soroka C, Steiger B, Meier PJ, Boyer JL. The molecular expression of the bile salt excretory pump, sister of P-glycoprotein (SPGP), is selectively preserved in cholestatic liver injury. Hepatology. 1998;28(4):429A.

15. Vos TA, Guido J, Hooiveld EJ et al. Up-regulation of the multidrug resistance genes, Mrp1 and Mdr1b, and down-regulation of the organic anion transporter, Mrp2, and the bile salt transporter, Spgp, in endotoxemic rat liver. Hepatology. 1998;28:1637–1644.
16. Strautnieks SS, Bull L, Knisely AS et al. A gene encoding a liver-specific ABC transporter is mutated in progressive familial intrahepatic cholestasis. Nature Genet. 1998;20:233–238.
17. Trauner M, Meier PJ, Boyer JL. J Hepatol. 1999;31:165–178.

2
Effect of bile duct ligation and bile salts on the activity of 11β-hydroxysteroid dehydrogenase: another explanation for mineralocorticoid excess in biliary cirrhosis in the rat

J. REICHEN, B. FREY and F.J. FREY

INTRODUCTION

Advanced liver disease is characterized by mineralocorticoid excess, which leads to sodium retention and ascites[1] and which is traditionally attributed to the effects of vasodilation on the renin-angiotensin system[2]. However, mineralocorticoids are not the only steroid hormones potentially affected in chronic liver disease: some patients with alcoholic liver disease exhibit Cushingoid features which disappear after abstinence[3].

Inhibition of 11β-hydroxysteroid dehydrogenase might also contribute to both mineralo- and glucocorticoid excess. This enzyme reduces endogenous and exogenous 11β-hydroxy to the inactive 11-keto steroids and thereby protects the mineralocorticoid receptor from mineralocorticoid excess. Two isoforms have been cloned[4,5]. The tissue distribution and properties of the two isoenzymes are reported in Table 1.

Table 1. Isoenzymes of 11β-hydroxysteroid dehydrogenase

	Type 1	Type 2
Localization	liver	distal renal tubule
	proximal renal tubule	colon
co-factor	NADP	NAD
protection from excess	glucocorticoid	mineralocorticoid

We therefore investigated activity, protein mass, and mRNA in liver and kidney of bile duct ligated rats.

METHODS

The methods are reported full in our original publication[6]. In brief, the common bile duct of male Sprague–Dawley rats was ligated under pentobarbital anaesthesia. Sham-operated animals served as controls. The animals were studied 4 weeks after surgery, when cirrhosis is fully established[7].

Enzyme activity in liver and kidney homogenate was determined according to Lakshmi and Monder[8]. Protein mass was determined by Western blotting using polyclonal antibodies kindly provided by C. Monder New York (isoenzyme 1) and Z. Krozowski, Melbourne (isoenzyme 2). Total RNA was isolated by the guanidium thiocyanate method. After reverse transcription the RNAs for the two 11β-hydroxy steroid dehydrogenases, and for GAPDH as an internal standard[9], were amplified by the polymerase chain reaction.

The effect of bile and individual bile salts was tested in vitro in Cos-1 cells transfected with the cDNAs for either of the two isoenzymes.

RESULTS AND DISCUSSION

At 4 weeks, all bile duct ligated animals had portal hypertension and a nodular liver (Table 2).

The activity of BHSDH-1 was much higher in liver than in kidney (Figure 1). Oxidase activity (assessed using corticosterone as substrate) was significantly reduced after bile duct ligation; in contrast reductase activity (assessed using dehydrocorticosterone as substrate) was unaffected (Figure 1). This finding could explain the elevation of endogenous gluococorticoids seen in cholestatic rats[10], and may contribute to the increased susceptibility to infection in obstructive jaundice[11,12].

As expected, BHSDH-2 activity was not detectable in liver but was reduced by 27% ($p < 0.01$) in renal tissue from cirrhotic rats (Figure 1). This permits glucocorticoids to act as mineralocorticoids at the aldosterone receptor. This observation potentially reconciles the conflicting data about the onset of hyperaldosteronism and sodium retention in cirrhotic liver disease[13–16].

Table 2. Characteristics of control (CTR; $n = 5$) and cirrhotic rats (BDL; $n = 7$).

	CTR	BDL
Portal pressure (cm H_2O)	12.4 ± 0.7	$20.2 \pm 2.1^*$
Alkaline phosphatase (IU/l)	155 ± 41	$605 \pm 288^*$
Serum bilirubin (μmol/l)	2 ± 0	$130 \pm 26^*$
Serum bile acids (μmol/l)	3 ± 2	$91.5 \pm 51^*$

Results are given as mean $\pm$ SD. $^*p < 0.05$ (Student's t-test).

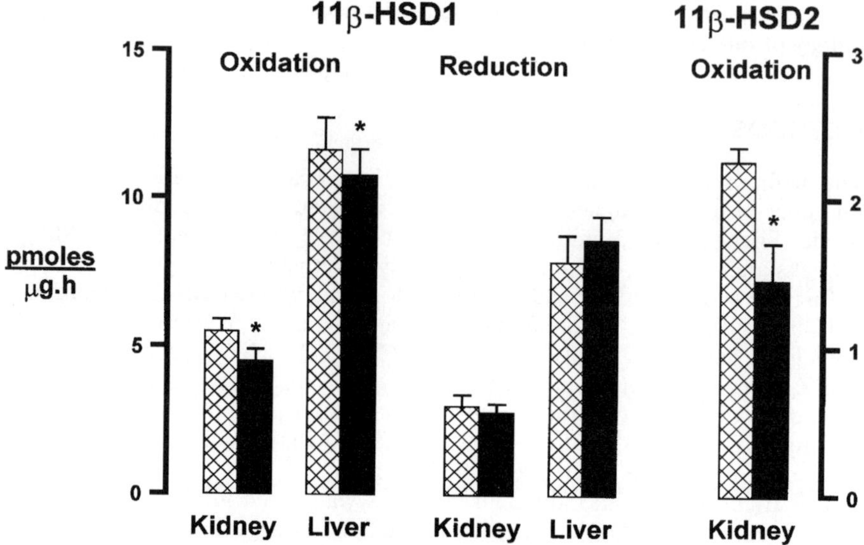

Figure 1. Activity of the 11β-hydroxysteroid dehydrogenase in liver and kidney of control (⊠) and cirrhotic (■) rats. Mean ± 1 sd are given. Significant differences (Student's *t*-test) are indicated by an asterisk. Redrawn from ref. 6 with permission from the publisher.

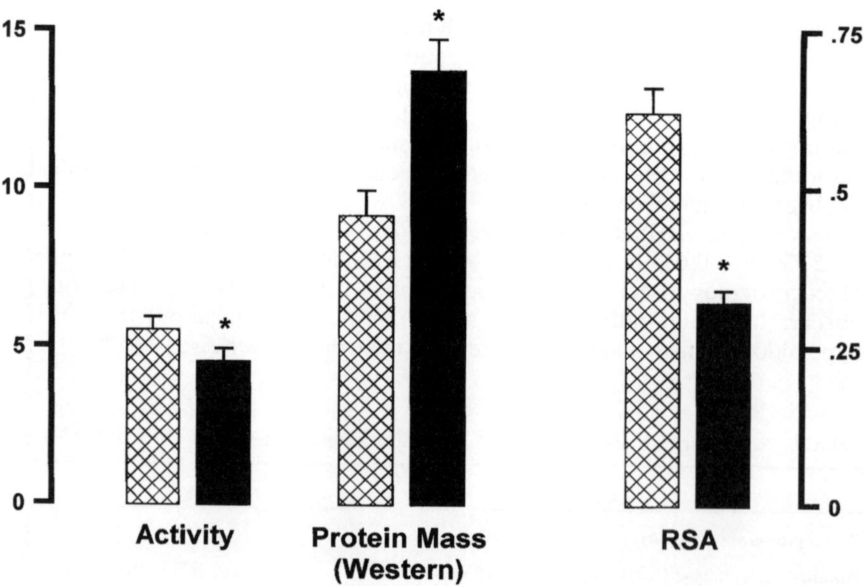

Figure 2. Activity, protein mass and ratio thereof (specific activity) of 11β-hydroxysteroid dehydrogenase type 1 in renal tissue of control (⊠) and cirrhotic (■) rats. Mean ± 1 sd are given. All three parameters were significantly lower in tissue from bile duct ligated animals suggesting posttranslational modification and/or the presence of an endogenous inhibitor.

The protein mass of BHSDH-1 was reduced by 58% in liver but, paradoxically, increased by 50% in renal tissue. Its relative specific activity, calculated from activity and protein mass, was markedly decreased in renal tissue (Figure 2). BHSDH-2 protein mass, in contrast, remained constant; thus, the relative specific activity for type 2 was also lower in renal tissue (not shown). BHSDH-2 protein was not detectable in liver.

RNA for BHSDH-1 was markedly decreased in liver but not kidney (Figure 3). The expression of the housekeeping gene GAPDH, which is known to be unaffected by bile duct ligation[9], remained constant, and the data shown in Figure 3 are therefore normalized for this gene. In contrast to type 1, BHSDH-2 RNA was markedly decreased in renal tissue from bile duct ligated rats (Figure 3). Thus, the decrease in BHSDH-2 activity, but not BHSDH-1 activity, in renal tissue could be due to decreased translation.

The reduced activity of BHSDH-1 and BHSDH-2 in renal tissue is compatible with a post-translational modification and/or the presence of endogenous inhibitors. This is supported by the normal mRNA levels of BHSDH-1, but for BHSDH-2 down-regulation at the translational level has been postulated. A post-translational modification could be related to cytokines such as tumour necrosis factor α (TNF-α) since this cytokine has been shown to induce a similar shift in oxidative versus reductive activity in renal mesangial cells[17]. This hypothesis is very attractive since endotoxin, a potent inducer of TNF-α, is thought to play a major role in the changes seen in obstructive jaundice[18] and liver cirrhosis[19,20].

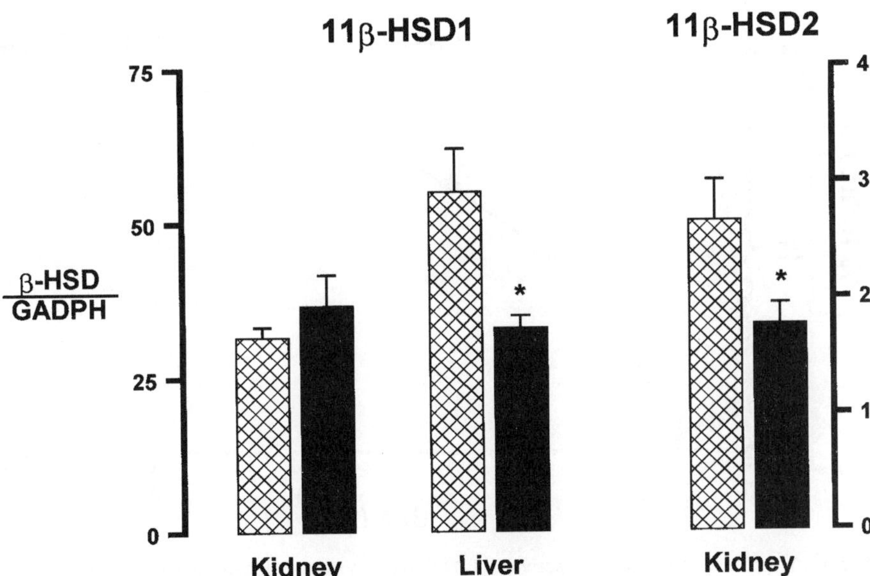

Figure 3. RNA for 11β-hydroxysteroid dehydrogenase in liver and kidney of control (⊠) and cirrhotic (■) rats. Mean ± 1 sd are given. Significant differences (Student's *t*-test) are indicated by an asterisk. Redrawn from ref. 6 with permission from the publisher.

We were interested, however, to further explore the hypothesis that endogenous inhibitors could contribute to the reduced activity of renal BHSDHs. We therefore incubated COS-1 cells transfected with either of the two isoenzymes. A dose-dependent inhibition was found for BHSDH-1 (Figure 4) which was maximal at 1% (v/v) of bile (about 30 μM/l bile salt concentration). For BHSDH-2, in contrast, activation occurred at low bile concentrations, and inhibition only at higher concentrations: maximal inhibition was achieved only at 5% (about 150 μM/l).

We then investigated the influence of different bile salts. Taurocholate and chenodeoxycholate inhibited both isoenzymes in a dose-dependent fashion between 1 and 500 μM/l, the IC_{50} being 8 and 23 μM for taurocholate and chenodeoxycholate, respectively. These comparatively low IC_{50}s, particularly for taurocholate (which is less hydrophobic and toxic), argues against this being a toxic effect. To further explore this, several other bile salts were studied at concentrations of 50 and 500 μM/l. The results for 50 μM/l (Figure 5) again show no relationship between hydrophobicity and inhibitory capacity. This contrasts clearly with the toxic effects of bile salts in many other systems[21–23].

Thus, bile salts inhibit both isoenzymes of BHSDH at almost physiological concentrations and certainly at concentrations seen in vivo in the present experiments. This does not preclude the possibility that other cholephiles contribute to the inhibition of BHSDHs.

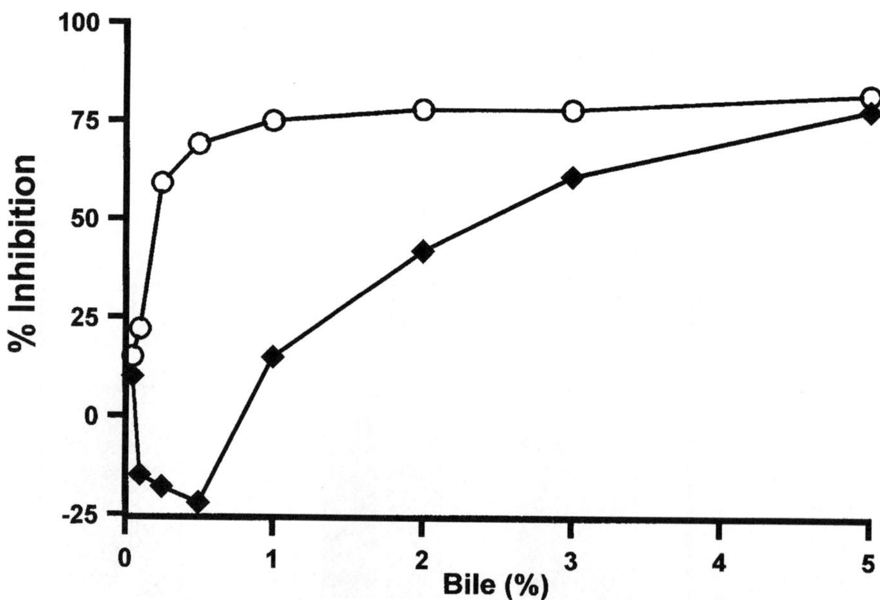

Figure 4. Effect of bile on the activity of 11β-hydroxysteroid dehydrogenase in COS-1 cells transfected with the cDNA for either isoenzyme. Type 1 (○) was inhibited in a dose-dependent fashion, with maximum inhibition being achieved at 1% (v/v). In contrast, the effect of bile on type 2 (◆) was biphasic, activation at lower concentrations being followed by a dose-dependent inhibition starting at 1% (v/v). Redrawn from ref. 6 with permission from the publisher.

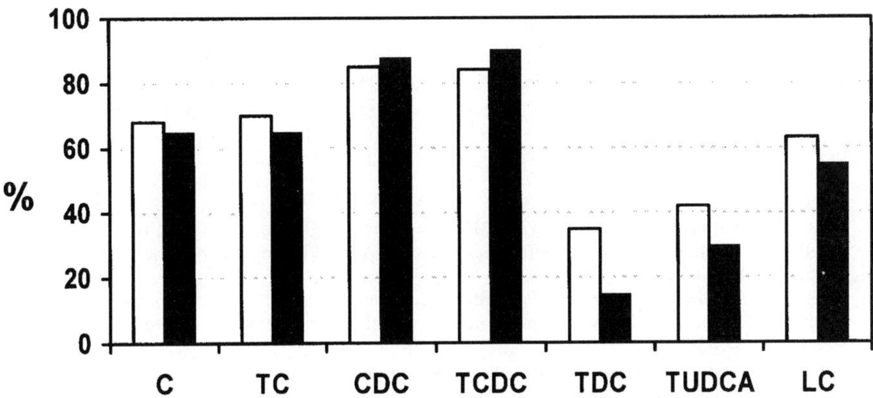

Figure 5. Inhibition of type 1 (□) and type 2 (■) 11β-hydroxysteroid dehydrogenase by different bile salts: cholate (C), taurocholate (TC), chenodeoxycholate (CDC) and its taurine conjugate (TCDC), taurodeoxycholate (TDC), tauroursodeoxycholate (TUDCA) and lithocholate (LC). There was no discernible relation between inhibitory potency and hydrophobicity. Redrawn from (6) with permission from the publisher.

CONCLUSIONS

Inhibition of 11β-hydroxysteroid dehydrogenase could contribute to sodium retention in portal hypertension by permitting glucocorticoids access to the mineralocorticoid receptor, thereby allowing them to act as mineralocorticoids. This could also explain the Cushingoid features seen in some patients with chronic liver disease, and the increased susceptibility of patients with obstructive jaundice and cirrhosis to infection. Further studies in other animal models are needed to permit generalization of our findings.

Acknowledgements

Supported by a grant (# 32.35349) from the Swiss National Foundation for Scientific Research to JR.

REFERENCES

1. Bosch J, Arroyo V, Betriu A et al. Hepatic hemodynamics and the renin-angiotensin-aldosterone system in cirrhosis. Gastroenterology. 1980;78:92–99.
2. Arroyo V, Bernardi M, Epstein M, Henriksen JH, Schrier RW, Rodés J. Pathophysiology of ascites and functional renal failure in cirrhosis. J Hepatol. 1988;6:239–257.
3. Rees LH, Besser GM, Jeffcoate WJ, Goldie DJ, Marks V. Alcohol-induced pseudo-Cushing's syndrome. Lancet. 1997;1:726–728.
4. Agarwal AK, Monder C, Eckstein B, White PC. Cloning and expression of rat cDNA encoding corticosteroid 11β-hydroxysteroid dehydrogenase. J Biol Chem. 1989;264:18939–18943.
5. Albitson AL, Obeyesekere VR, Smith RE, Krozowski Z. Cloning and tissue distribution of the human 11β-hydroxysteroid dehydrogenase type 2 enyme. Mol Cell Endocrinol. 1994;105:R11–R17.
6. Escher G, Nawrocki A, Staub T et al. Down-regulation of hepatic and renal 11β-hydroxysteroid dehydrogenase in rats with liver cirrhosis. Gastroenterology. 1998;114:175–184.

7. Gross JB, Reichen J, Zeltner T, Zimmermann A. The evolution of changes in quantitative liver function tests in a rat model of cirrhosis: Correlation with morphometric measurement of hepatocyte mass. Hepatology. 1987;7:457–463.
8. Lakhsmi V, Monder C. Evidence for independent 11-oxidase and 11-reductase activity of 11β-hydroxysteroid dehydrogenase: Enzyme latency, phase transitions, and lipid requirement. Endocrinology. 1985;116:552–560.
9. Elsing C, Reichen J, Marti U, Renner EL. Hepatocellular Na+/H+ exchange is activated at transcriptional and posttranscriptional level in rat biliary cirrhosis. Gastroenterology. 1994;107:468–478.
10. Tjandra K, Kubes P, Rioux K, Swain MG. Endogenous glucocorticoids inhibit neutrophil recruitment to inflammatory sites in cholestatic rats. Am J Physiol Gastrointest Liver Physiol. 1996;270:G821–G825.
11. Ding JW, Andersson R, Soltesz V, Willen R, Bengmark S. Obstructive jaundice impairs reticuloendothelial function and promotes bacterial translocation in the rat. J Surg Res. 1994;57:238–245.
12. Leung JWL, Ling TKW, Chan RCY et al. Antibiotics, biliary sepsis and bile duct stones. Gastrointest Endosc. 1994;40:716–721.
13. Jimenez W, Martinez Pardo A, Arroyo V et al. Temporal relationship between hyper-aldosteronism – sodium retention and ascites formation in rats with experimental cirrhosis. Hepatology. 1985;5:245–250.
14. Wood LJ, Massie D, McLean AJ, Dudley FJ. Renal sodium retention in cirrhosis: tubular site and relation to hepatic dysfunction. Hepatology. 1988;8:831–836.
15. Wensing G, Sabra R, Branch RA. The onset of sodium retention in experimental cirrhosis in rats is related to a critical threshold of liver function. Hepatology. 1990;11:779–786.
16. Wong F, Liu P, Allidina Y, Blendis L. Pattern of sodium handling and its consequences in patients with preascitic cirrhosis. Gastroenterology. 1995;108:1820–1827.
17. Escher G, Galli I. Vishwanath BS, Frey BM, Frey FJ. Tumor necrosis factor a and interleukin 1β enhance the cortisone/cortisol shuttle. J Exp Med. 1997;186:189–198.
18. Clements WD, Erwin P, McCaigue MD, Halliday I, Barclay GR, Rowlands BJ. Conclusive evidence of endotoxaemia in biliary obstruction. Gut. 1998;42:293–299.
19. Guarner C, Soriano G, Tomas A et al. Increased serum nitrite and nitrate levels in patients with cirrhosis – relationship to endotoxemia. Hepatology. 1993;18:1139–1143.
20. Le Moine O, Soupison T, Sogni P et al. Plasma endotoxin and tumor necrosis factor-a in the hyperkinetic state of cirrhosis. J Hepatol. 1995;23:391–395.
21. Heuman DM, Pandak WM, Hylemon PB, Vlahcevic ZR. Conjugates of ursodeoxycholate protect against cytotoxicity of more hydrophobic bile salts: in vitro studies in rat hepatocytes and human erythrocytes. Hepatology. 1991;14:920–926.
22. Krähenbühl S, Talos C, Fischer S, Reichen J. Toxicity of bile acids on the electron transport chain of isolated rat liver mitochondria. Hepatology. 1994;19:471–479.
23. Salvioli G, Gaetti E, Panini R, Lugli R, Pradelli JM. Different resistance of mammalian red blood cells to hemolysis by bile salts. Lipids. 1993;28:999–1003.

3
Immunological aspects of cholestatic liver disease

M.F. BASSENDINE and D.E.J. JONES

Primary biliary cirrhosis (PBC) can be considered as a model autoimmune cholestatic liver disease in which breakdown of tolerance to non-organ specific mitochondrial (M2) antigens is accompanied by focal immune-mediated damage to biliary epithelial cells (BEC) lining the small intrahepatic bile ducts. This results in loss of bile ducts, chronic cholestasis, scarring (or fibrosis), the

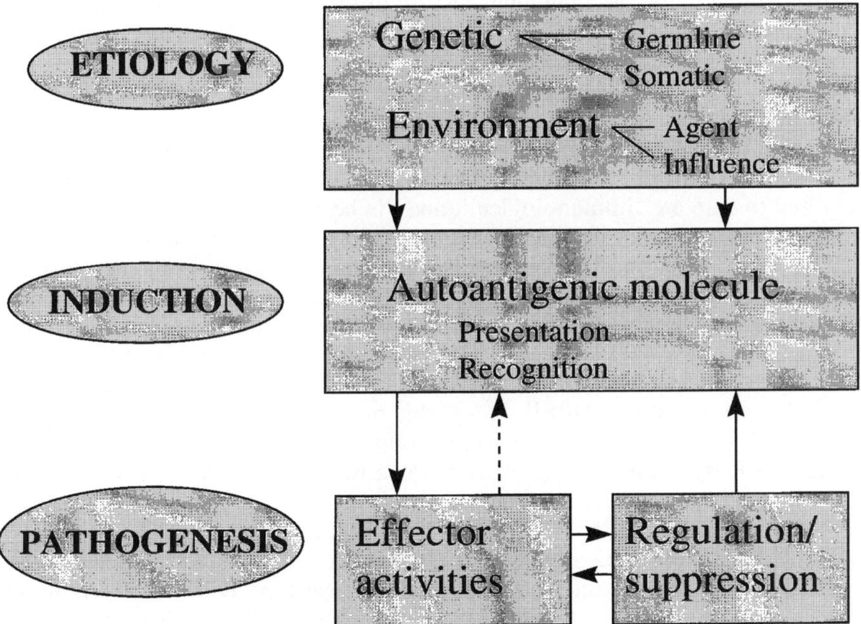

Figure 1. The components of autoimmunity can be divided into aetiological factors, leading to induction of the abnormal immune response and pathogenesis which involves both effector and immunoregulatory mechanisms.

development of cirrhosis and ultimately liver failure and death or liver transplantation. The loss of tolerance to M2 antigens is an early event in the progression of this disease: antimitochondrial antibodies are detectable in serum before liver function tests become abnormal and long before the onset of symptoms[1,2]. The maintenance of tolerance to self requires very intricate and sequentially gated mechanisms which are far from being clearly understood. This review discusses what is known of immune abnormalities in PBC from the perspective of the components of autoimmunity in general (Figure 1).

AETIOLOGY OF PBC

Autoimmune diseases such as PBC appear to develop in genetically susceptible individuals, with the expression of disease being modified by permissive and protective environments.

Immunogenetic influences

PBC is associated with a variety of other autoimmune diseases, and also occurs in familial clusters, suggesting that genetic factors play a significant role in determining susceptibility to the disease[3,4]. The relative risk (λ_s) in siblings has been estimated to lie between 10 and 100[5,6], as in other autoimmune diseases where it is thought that genetic influences may contribute up to 50% of the total risk. A single report has suggested discordant disease in monozygotic twins[7], confirming that increased individual susceptibility and environmental factors are both necessary for the development of PBC[8]. Familial clustering in all auto-immune diseases has provided the impetus for the search for putative susceptibility loci. The searches for linkage through the genome in other autoimmune disorders such as type 1 (insulin dependent) diabetes mellitus[9] has shown that these diseases are polygenic, so that no single gene is either necessary or sufficient for disease development. Most candidates for susceptibility loci identified to date are 'immunological', and the best studied lie within the major histocompatibility complex (MHC) on the short arm of chromosome 6. The MHC is highly polymorphic: it comprises three distinct groups of genes, termed human leucocyte antigens (HLA) class I, class II and class III[10] which encode various products involved in the interactions of cells with antigen-specific receptors on the surface of T cells, and related to the immune response to foreign antigen presentation. PBC has been consistently reported to be associated with the HLA class II antigen DR8[11, 12], and this has been confirmed by genotyping studies in both Caucasian and Japanese populations[13–15]. The relative risk of developing PBC if one carries HLA DR8 is between 2 and 7[16] but, as noted above, this antigen is neither necessary nor sufficient for the development of PBC. Indeed, in Caucasian populations DR8 accounts for 11–36% of patients, whereas in Japanese patient groups the prevalence of DR8 varies between 38 and 79%. It has been suggested that another genotype DPB1*0501 is more strongly associated with PBC than DR8 in Japanese patients[17], but this has not been confirmed in Caucasian patients[18]. Conversely it has been reported that resistance to PBC is associated with DQA1*0102[19]. Some researchers have sought associations between the HLA class III region and PBC, in the light of complement abnormalities in PBC[20]. The complement allotype C4B2, studied in isolation, was found in 15 of 33 patients (45%) compared with 53 of 307 (17%) controls[21], but a more recent study has suggested that HLA-DR8 and C4B2 are in linkage disequilibrium and that C4B2 is not an independent susceptibility locus. Indeed, a genetic marker located midway between HLA-DR8 and C4B2 termed G91 appears to be the telomeric limit for the gene associated with HLA-DR8 that encodes susceptibility to PBC[22]. One small study has reported an association between PBC and the complement allotype C4AQ0[12], but this is known to be in linkage disequilibrium with HLA-DR3 and the association may be due to the presence of HLA-DR3 on the haplotype[23] rather than C4AQ0.

The clustering of autoimmune diseases within the same individual or family suggests that the same genes may be involved in different diseases. This is supported by the recent demonstration that 65% of the non-MHC loci for susceptibility to autoimmunity identified to date map non-randomly into 18 distinct clusters[24]. One such locus is the cytotoxic T lymphocyte-associated antigen-4 (CTLA-4) gene (located on chromosome 2q 33 and identified as IDDM 12 by genome scanning methods), which is associated with susceptibility not only to insulin-dependent diabetes mellitus[25,26] but also to autoimmune thyroid disease[27,28]. CTLA-4 is a T cell surface molecule which interacts, in competition with the costimulatory molecule CD28, with the ligands B7-1 and B7-2 on antigen presenting cells to influence the induction, maintenance and, particularly, termination of peripheral T cell responses[29,30]. The net interaction of CD28 and CTLA-4 with their ligands may influence the nature of the resulting T cell responses by determining the extent and kinetics of T cell activation. We have recently studied the CTLA-4 exon 1 polymorphism (A/G encoding for threonine or alanine respectively) in PBC and reported that it is the first non-MHC gene to be identified as a susceptibility locus for PBC[31]. Our data support the hypothesis that clinically distinct autoimmune diseases may be controlled by a common set of susceptibility genes, which might bias the development of the immune repertoire towards autoimmune reactivity.

Environmental influences

Although little is known of the role of the environment in the aetiology of PBC, an early epidemiological study in the North of England generated great interest. Triger reported that the prevalence of PBC in Sheffield within an area supplied with water from one reservoir was 10 times that in the area supplied by the other four city reservoirs, suggesting a link between PBC and water supply[32]. No other group has yet been able to confirm a similar link. Studies suggesting a role for an infectious agent in the induction of PBC also remain unconfirmed. Such infectious agents are usually considered to operate by molecular mimicry, whereby close homology between a constituent protein of the infectious agent and a host protein results in the protective response to the organism 'cross-reacting' with self. As it is now recognized that the immunodominant mitochondrial autoantigens in PBC are not only non-organ specific but also non-species specific and ubiquitous, the molecular mimicry hypothesis is gaining favour. Sera from patients with tuberculosis recognize the major M2a autoantigen[33], suggesting that atypical mycobacteria may act as a trigger for the breakdown of self-tolerance in PBC[34]. Data from other studies[35,36] however, do not support a role for mycobacterial antigens in the pathogenesis of PBC. In view of the ubiquitous nature of the M2 antigens (see below) it could be hypothesized that challenge of the immune system of a genetically predisposed individual with these antigens from a variety of different sources could lead to the production of AMA and trigger the initiating event in the sequentially gated mechanisms involved in loss of self-tolerance.

INDUCTION OF PBC

The essential components for the induction of an autoimmune response are the autoantigen, the mechanisms involved in the presentation of the autoantigenic epitope(s) to the immune system, and the recognition of the epitope in such a way that tolerance is broken down.

Mitochondrial autoantigens and autoantibodies

The last decade has seen an explosion of knowledge in this area following the initial reports that AMA in PBC sera react predominantly with two components of pyruvate dehydrogenase complex (PDC) – the E2 component (also termed dihydrolipoamide acetyltransferase) and E3 binding protein (E3BP, previously termed protein X)[37,38]. In order to understand how molecular mimicry might operate it is necessary to summarize briefly what is known of the biochemical nature of these autoantigens[39,40].

PDC-E2 has a highly segmented structure that has been conserved in evolution: it comprises, from the N terminus, one to three lipoyl domains, a peripheral subunit-binding domain and an inner acyltransferase catalytic domain[41], which binds to other copies of E2 to form the symmetrical core of the multienzyme complex. E3BP also has a multidomain substructure, consisting of an amino-terminal lipoyl domain, followed by an E3-binding domain and then a carboxyl-terminal E2-binding domain[42] (Figure 2).

All experimental data indicate that the immunodominant B-cell epitopes in PBC are located within the lipoyl domains[43,44]. The three-dimensional structure of the inner lipoyl domain from human PDC-E2 has now been determined by means of nuclear magnetic resonance spectroscopy[45]: it resembles the lipoyl

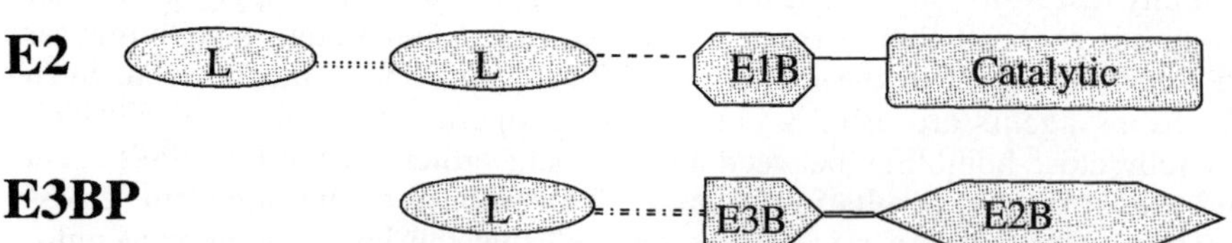

Figure 2. Diagrammatic representation of the structural domains of the E2 components of the 2-oxo acid dehydrogenase complexes and the E3 binding protein (E3BP, previously termed protein X) component of pyruvate dehydrogenase complex. L indicates the lipoyl domain to which the essential co-factor, lipoic acid, is covalently attached and B the subunit binding domain(s).

domains of bacterial PDC-E2s[46–48] comprising two antiparallel β sheets, each of which contains three major strands and one minor strand. The lipoylation site (lysine residue) is physically exposed at the tip of a tight turn in one of the β-sheets, and the N and C-terminal residues are close together at the other end of the molecule. AMA in PBC patients' sera recognize this physically exposed lipoylation site and other distinctive surface conformational features at the tip of the β-turn in the lipoyl domain; in the assembled multienzyme complex these extend outwards from the inner core and interdigitate between the E1 and E3 components on the surface of the complex. It is notable that in the β strand residues 41–48, which precede the highly conserved DKA triplet of the lipoyl β turn, six of the eight residues are completely conserved between human PDC-E2 and E3BP[49] but differ from the corresponding sequences of *E. coli* PDC-E2. This suggests that the immunodominant B-cell epitope in PBC comprises the 41–48 β strand and the following β turn with the attached lipoyl moiety (residues 49–53). The observation that monoclonal antibodies derived from fusions of circulating B lymphocytes from patients with PBC show significantly stronger binding to lipoyl-containing domains than their unlipolyated counterparts strengthens this conclusion[50].

A striking property of AMA in PBC sera is their capacity to rapidly inactivate the catalytic function of PDC in vitro[38]. This assay has been used to demonstrate autoantibodies in PBC sera that inhibit PDC function but do not show reactivity in an immunoblot with recombinant human PDC-E2[51]. These non-blotting inhibitory AMA are presumed to react with exclusively conformational determinant(s) perhaps presented by the tertiary structure of the entire multienzyme complex. Interestingly AMA in PBC sera have also been shown to inhibit the mammalian PDC strongly (99%), yeast PDC only moderately (70%), and *E. coli* PDC weakly (26%)[52]. At first sight these results do not appear to support the concept of molecular mimicry/cross-reactivity as an explanation for the origin of mitochondrial autoantibodies, but they do not engage the question of T cell recognition of autoantigen. T cells respond to nonapeptide sequences but may require only one or two critical residues appropriately aligned in the groove of MHC molecules[53], so that molecular mimicry is more likely to operate at the T cell rather than B cell level.

T cell responses to autoantigen

Several studies have examined the T cell response to mitochondrial autoantigens[54]. We have shown that peripheral blood T cells from PBC patients respond to biochemically purified PDC-E2 and E3BP[55,56] suggesting a possible role in the disease process. Attempts to localize the T cell autoepitopes within PDC-E2 have, however, generated contradictory results. One T cell cloning study has identified a single dominant epitope contained within the dominant B cell epitope represented by amino acids 40–53 and spanning the lipoyl binding lysine residue within the lipoyl domain[57]. This study also demonstrated that these T cell clones cross-reacted with the corresponding peptide from *E. coli*, raising the possibility that molecular mimicry may be involved in the induction of PBC at a T cell level. Our experiments have shown that the lipoylation state of this 14-residue peptide does not affect the T cell response, and also suggested that it is not a universal immunodominant T cell epitope in PBC patients: there may be T cell autoepitopes within PDC-E2/E3BP which lie outside this peptide in some patients[58].

Autoantigen presentation and recognition

Evidence from immunohistochemical studies and fluorescence-activated cell sorter analysis of mononuclear cells isolated from PBC liver suggests that the mononuclear cell infiltrate in the portal tracts consists predominantly of activated CD4$^+$ and CD8$^+$ T lymphocytes and that Th1 cells are the more prominent T cell subset[59,60]. Damage to biliary epithelial cells (BEC), is moreover accompanied by up-regulation of cell-surface markers, such as class II MHC and the adhesion molecule ICAM-1[61] which are typically induced by T cell cytokines, a finding that suggests local T cell activation. It has been suggested, therefore, that BEC may be capable of presenting autoantigen to CD4$^+$ lymphocytes infiltrating the liver, and of initiating an intrahepatic immune response. We have shown this is unlikely to occur via the classic T cell co-stimulatory molecules B7-1 or B7-2 as human intrahepatic BEC do not express these CD28 ligands at either mRNA or protein level and are unable to activate T cells to produce IL-2 and a lympho-proliferative response in vitro[62]. CD40, however, can act as an accessory molecule implicated in T cell stimulation in a B7/CD28 independent manner. CD40 is a 50 kDa glycoprotein of the tumour necrosis factor/nerve growth receptor superfamily and its ligand is expressed on activated CD4$^+$ T cells. BEC have recently been shown to express CD40 constitutively and this expression was up-regulated by the pro-inflammatory cytokine interferon γ, suggesting that the susceptibility of BEC to T cell recognition may be increased during an inflammatory response. CD40/CD40L interaction has been shown to be involved in the production of IL-12, a key cytokine for the development of Th1 cytotoxic responses. These data suggest that BEC may participate in the recruitment of inflammatory cells by a B7 independent pathway.

Several studies have shown that the PBC autoantigen(s) PDC-E2 and/or E3BP are aberrantly expressed on the surface of biliary epithelium[63–66] in PBC livers, and it is suggested that this abnormality relates to the pathogenesis of bile duct lesions. It remains unclear whether AMA are involved in the pathogenesis of bile duct damage, but the presence of a target antigen on the membrane of BEC may render the cells susceptible to antibody mediated cytotoxicity. If the initial T cell response in PBC is to foreign PDC-E2 and/or PDC-E3BP, and T cells are recruited that react with shared autologous motifs[67], then cytotoxic T cell responses would be aimed at the BEC with membrane expression of the autoantigen.

PATHOGENESIS OF PBC

The processes that initiate and regulate the slow pathogenesis of PBC are poorly understood. The inflammatory cell-mediated immune processes may be principally mediated by the CD4$^+$ helper T-cells of the Th1 regulatory subset. A better understanding of the mechanisms involved in chronic non-suppurative destructive cholangitis (NSDC) may lead to more effective medical therapies for PBC, and this has provided the impetus for the search for a reproducible animal model. A number of models of NSDC have been reported in several different laboratory animal species[68]. We have recently identified a strain of mouse (SJL) which develops both AMA and bile duct damage similar to the early stages of PBC when sensitized with purified mitochondrial antigen and complete Freund's adjuvant by the intraperitoneal route[69]. The susceptibility of this strain may result in part from a tendency of SJL mice to preferentially mount CD4$^+$ T cell responses of the Th1 subset. This in turn may be due to a defect in inducible interleukin-4 production, which is involved in regulating pathogenic Th1 responses[70,71]. This experimental model of NSDC, which we have termed experimental autoimmune cholangitis, should be of value in unravelling the complex immunopathogenesis of NSDC and in the development of novel, immune-based therapeutic modalities.

REFERENCES

1. Mitchison HC, Bassendine MF, Hendrick AM et al. Positive antimitochondrial antibody but normal liver function tests: is this primary biliary cirrhosis? Hepatology. 1986;6:1279–1284.
2. Metcalf JV, Mitchison HC, Palmer JM, Jones DEJ, Bassendine MF, James OFW. Natural history of early primary biliary cirrhosis. Lancet. 1996;348:1399–1402.
3. Bach N, Schaffner F. Familial primary biliary cirrhosis. J Hepatol. 1994;20:698–701.
4. Brind AM, Bray GP, Portmann BC, Williams R. Prevalence and pattern of familial disease in primary biliary cirrhosis. Gut. 1995;36:615–617.
5. Jones DEJ, Watt FE, Metcalf JV, Bassendine MF, James OFW. Familial primary biliary cirrhosis reassessed: a geographically-based population study. J Hepatol. 1999;30:402–407.
6. Vyse TJ, Todd JA. Genetic analysis of autoimmune disease. Cell. 1996;85:311–318.
7. Kaplan MM, Rabson AR, Lee YM, Williams DL, Montaperto PA. Discordant occurrence of primary biliary cirrhosis in monozygotic twins. New Engl J Med. 1994;331:952.
8. Douglas JG, Finlayson NDC. Are increased individual susceptibility and environmental factors both necessary for the development of primary biliary cirrhosis? Br Med J. 1970;2:419–420.
9. Todd JA. Genetic analysis of type 1 diabetes using whole genome approaches. Proc Natl Acad Sci USA. 1995;92:8560–8565.
10. Bodmer JG, Marsh SG, Albert ED et al. Nomenclature for factors of the HLA system. Human Immunol. 1997;53:98–128.
11. Gores GJ, Moore SB, Fisher LD, Powell FC, Dickson ER. Primary biliary cirrhosis: associations with class II major histocompatibility antigens. Hepatology. 1987;7:889–892.
12. Manns MP, Bremm A, Scheider PM et al. HLA-DRw8 and complement C4 deficiency as risk factors in primary biliary cirrhosis. Gastroenterology. 1991;101:1367–1373.
13. Underhill J, Donaldson P, Bray G, Doherty D, Portmann B, Williams R. Susceptibility to primary biliary cirrhosis is associated with the HLA-DR8-DQB1*0402 haplotype. Hepatology. 1992;16:1404–1408.
14. Gregory WL, Mehal W, Dunn AN et al. Primary biliary cirrhosis: contribution of HLA class II allele DR8. Q J Med. 1993;86:393–399.
15. Onishi S, Sakamaki T, Maeda T et al. DNA typing of HLA class II genes; DRB1*0803 increases the susceptibility of Japanese to primary biliary cirrhosis. J Hepatol. 1994;21:1053–1060.
16. Agarwal K, Jones DEJ, Bassendine MF. Genetic susceptibility to primary biliary cirrhosis. Eur J Gastroenterol Hepatol. 1999; in press.
17. Seki T, Kiyosawa K, Ota M et al. Association of primary biliary cirrhosis with human leucocyte antigen DPB1*0501 in Japanese patients. Hepatology. 1993;18:73–78.
18. Underhill JA, Donaldson PT, Doherty DG, Manabe K, Williams R. HLA DPB polymorphism in primary sclerosing cholangitis and primary biliary cirrhosis. Hepatology. 1995;21:959–962.
19. Begovich AB, Klitz W, Moonsamy PV, Van de Water J, Peltz G, Gershwin ME. Genes within HLA class II region confer both predisposition and resistance to primary biliary cirrhosis. Tissue Antigens. 1994;43:71–77.

20. Potter BJ, Elias E, Jones EA. Hypercatabolism of the third component of complement in patients with primary biliary cirrhosis. J Lab Clin Med. 1976;88:427–439.
21. Briggs DC, Donaldson PT, Hayes P, Welsh KI, Williams R, Neuberger JM. A major histocompatibility complex class III allotype (C4B2) associated with primary biliary cirrhosis (PBC). Tissue Antigens. 1987;29:141–145.
22. Mehal WZ, Gregory WL, Lo Y-MD et al. Defining the immunogenetic susceptibility to primary biliary cirrhosis. Hepatology. 1994;20:1213–1219.
23. Ercilla G, Pares A, Arriaga F et al. Primary biliary cirrhosis associated with HLA-DRw3. Tissue Antigens. 1979;14:449–452.
24. Becker KG, Simon RM, Bailey-Wilson JE et al. Clustering of non-major histocompatibility complex susceptibility loci in human autoimmune diseases. Proc Natl Acad Sci USA. 1998;95:9979–9984.
25. Marron MP, Raffel LJ, Garchon HJ et al. Insulin-dependent diabetes mellitus (IDDM) is associated with CTLA-4 polymorphisms in multiple ethnic groups. Human Mol Genet. 1997;6:1275–1282.
26. Donner H, Rau H, Walfish PG et al. CTLA-4 alanine-17 confers genetic susceptibility to Graves' disease and to Type 1 diabetes mellitus. J Clin Endocrinol Metab. 1997;82:143–146.
27. Nistico L, Buzzeti R, Pritchard LE et al. The CTLA-4 region of chromosome 2q33 is linked to, and associated with, type 1 diabetes. Human Mol Genet. 1996;5:1075–1080.
28. Kotsa K, Watson PF, Weetman AP. A CTLA-4 gene polymorphism is associated with both Graves disease and autoimmune hypothyroidism. Clin Endocrinol. 1997;46:551–554.
29. Thompson CB, Allison JP. The emerging role of CTLA-4 as an immune attenuator. Immunity. 1997;7:445–450.
30. Bluestone JA. Is CTLA-4 a master switch for peripheral T cell tolerance? J Immunol. 1997;158:1989–1993.
31. Agarwal K, Grove J, Pearce S, Daly A, Jones DEJ, Bassendine MF. CTLA-4 gene polymorphism associated with primary biliary cirrhosis. Hepatology. 1998;28:404A.
32. Triger DR. Primary biliary cirrhosis: an epidemiological study. Br Med J. 1980;281:772–775.
33. Klein R, Wiebel M, Engelhart S, Berg PA. Sera from patients with tuberculosis recognize the M2a-epitope (E2-subunit of pyruvate dehydrogenase) specific for primary biliary cirrhosis. Clin Exp Immunol. 1993;92:308–316.
34. Vilagut L, Vila J, Vinas O et al. Cross-reactivity of anti-*Mycobacterium gordonae* antibodies with the major mitochondrial autoantigens in primary biliary cirrhosis. J Hepatol. 1994;21:673–677.
35. O'Donohue J, McFarlane B, Bomford A, Yates M, Williams R. Antibodies to atypical mycobacteria in primary biliary cirrhosis. J Hepatol. 1994;21:887–889.
36. Jones DEJ, Palmer JM, Leon MP, Yeaman SJ, Bassendine MF, Diamond AG. T cell responses to Tuberculin-purified protein derivative in primary biliary cirrhosis: evidence for defective T-cell function. Gut. 1997;40:277–283.
37. Yeaman SJ, Fussey SP, Danner DJ, James OFW, Bassendine MF. Primary biliary cirrhosis: identification of two major M2 mitochondrial autoantigens. Lancet. 1998;i:1067–1070.
38. Van de Water J, Fregeau D, Davis P et al. Autoantibodies of primary biliary cirrhosis recognize dihydrolipoamide acetyltransferase and inhibit enzyme function. J Immunol. 1988;141:2321–2324.
39. Bassendine MF, Jones OFW, Yeaman SJ. Biochemistry and autoimmune response to the 2-oxoacid dehydrogenase complexes in primary biliary cirrhosis. Semin Liver Dis. 1997;17:49–60.
40. Bassendine MF, Jones DEJ. Antimitochondrial and other autoantibodies in primary biliary cirrhosis. In: Krawitt E, Wiesner H R, Nishioka M, eds. Autoimmune Liver Diseases, 2nd edn. Amsterdam: Elsevier Science, 1998:287–304.
41. Perham RN. Domains, motifs and linkers in 2-oxo acid dehydrogenase multienzyme complexes: a paradigm in the design of a multifunctional protein. Biochemistry. 1991;30:8501–8512.
42. Maeng CY, Yazdi MA, Reed LJ. Stoichiometry of binding of mature and truncated forms of the dihydrolipoamide dehydrogenase-binding protein to the dihydrolipoamide acetyltransferase core of the pyruvate dehydrogenase complex from *Saccharomyces cerevisiae*. Biochemistry. 1996;35:5879–5882.

43. Tuaillon N, Andre C, Briand JP, Penner E, Muller S. A lipoyl synthetic octapeptide of dihydrolipoamide acetyltransferase specifically recognized by anti-M2 autoantibodies in primary biliary cirrhosis. J Immunol. 1992;148:445–450.
44. Quinn J, Diamond AG, Palmer JM, Bassendine MF, James OFW, Yeaman SJ. Lipoylated and unlipoylated domains of human PDC-E2 as autoantigens in primary biliary cirrhosis: significance of lipoate attachment. Hepatology. 1993;18:1384–1391.
45. Howard MJ, Fuller C, Broadhurst W et al. Three-dimensional structure of the major autoantigen in primary biliary cirrhosis. Gastroenterology. 1998;115:1–9.
46. Green JD, Laue ED, Perham RN, Ali ST, Guest JR. Three-dimensional structure of a lipoyl domain from the dihydrolipoyl acetyltransferase component of the pyruvate dehydrogenase multienzyme complex of *Escherichia coli*. J Mol Biol. 1995;248:328–343.
47. Dardel F, Davis AL, Laue ED, Perham RN. Three-dimensional structure of the lipoyl domain from *Bacillus stearothermophilus* pyruvate dehydrogenase complex. J Mol Biol. 1993;229:1037–1048.
48. Berg A, Vervoort J, de Kok A. Three-dimensional structure in solution of the N-terminal lipoyl domain of the pyruvate dehydrogenase complex from *Azotobacter vinelandii*. Eur J Biochem. 1997;244:352–360.
49. Harris RA, Bowker-Kinley MM, Wu P, Jeng J, Popov KM. Dihydrolipoamide dehydrogenase-binding protein of the human pyruvate dehydrogenase complex. J Biol Chem. 1997;272: 19746–19751.
50. Thomson RK, Davis Z, Palmer JM et al. Immunogenetic analysis of a panel of monoclonal IgG and IgM anti-pyruvate dehydrogenase complex antibodies derived from patients with primary biliary cirrhosis. J Hepatol. 1998;28:582–594.
51. Rowley MJ, McNeilage JL, Armstrong JM, Mackay IR. Inhibitory autoantibody to a conformational epitope of the pyruvate dehydrogenase complex, the major autoantigen in primary biliary cirrhosis. Clin Immunol Immunopathol. 1991;60:356–370.
52. Teoh KL, Mackay IR, Rowley MJ, Fussey SP. Enzyme inhibitory autoantibodies to pyruvate dehydrogenase complex in primary biliary cirrhosis differ for mammalian, yeast and bacterial enzymes: implications for molecular mimicry. Hepatology. 1994;19:1029–1033.
53. Ohno S. How cytotoxic T cells manage to discriminate nonself from self at the nonapeptide level. Proc Natl Acad Sci USA. 1992;89:4643–4647.
54. Van de Water J, Ansari A, Prindiville T et al. Heterogeneity of autoreactive T cell clones specific for the E2 component of the pyruvate dehydrogenase complex in primary biliary cirrhosis. J Exp Med. 1995;181:723–733.
55. Jones DEJ, Palmer JM, Yeaman SJ, James OFW, Bassendine MF, Diamond AG. T cell responses to components of pyruvate dehydrogenase complex in primary biliary cirrhosis. Hepatology. 1995;21:995–1002.
56. Jones DEJ, Palmer JM, Yeaman SJ, Bassendine MF, Diamond AG. T cell responses to native human proteins in primary biliary cirrhosis. Clin Exp Immunol. 1997;107:562–568.
57. Shimoda S, Nakamura M, Ishibishi H, Hayashida K, Niho Y. HLA DRB4 0101 restricted immunodominant T cell autoepitope of pyruvate dehydrogenase complex in primary biliary cirrhosis: evidence of molecular mimicry in human autoimmune disease. J Exp Med. 1995;181:1835–1845.
58. Palmer JM, Diamond A, Yeaman SJ, Bassendine MF, Jones DEJ. T cell responses to the putative dominant autoepitope in primary biliary cirrhosis. Clin Exp Immonol. 1999;115:in press.
59. Shindo M, Mullin GE, Braun-Elwert L, Bergasa NV, Jones EA, James SP. Cytokine mRNA expression in the liver of patients with primary biliary cirrhosis (PBC) and chronic hepatits B (CHB). Clin Exp Immunol. 1996;105:254–259.
60. Harada K, Van de Water J, Leung PS et al. In situ nucleic acid hybridization of cytokines in primary biliary cirrhosis: predominance of the Th1 subset. Hepatology. 1997;25: 791–796.
61. Yasoshima M, Nakanuma Y, Van de Water J, Gershwin ME. Immunohistochemical analysis of adhesion molecules in the micro-environment of portal tracts in relation to aberrant expression of PDC-E2 and HLA-DR on the bile ducts in primary biliary cirrhosis. J Pathol. 1995;175:319–325.
62. Leon MP, Bassendine MF, Wilson JL, Ali S, Thick M, Kirby JA. Immunogenicity of biliary epithelium: Investigation of antigen presentation to CD4+ T cells. Hepatology. 1996;24:562–567.

63. Joplin R, Gordon Lindsay J, Johnson GD, Strain A, Neuberger J. Membrane dihydrolipoamide acetyltransferase (E2) on human biliary epithelial cells in primary biliary cirrhosis. Lancet. 1992;339:93–94.
64. Van de Water J, Turchany J, Leung PS et al. Molecular mimicry in primary biliary cirrhosis. Evidence for biliary epithelial expression of a molecule cross-reactive with pyruvate dehydrogenase complex-E2. J Clin Invest. 1993;91:2653–2664.
65. Joplin RE, Johnson GD, Matthews JB et al. Distribution of pyruvate dehydrogenase dihydrolipoamide acetyltransferase (PDC-E2) and another mitochondrial marker in salivary gland and biliary epithelium from patients with primary biliary cirrhosis. Hepatology. 1994;19:1375–1380.
66. Joplin R, Wallace LL, Lindsay JG, Yeaman SJ, Palmer JM, Neuberger JM. Pyruvate dehydrogenase-X (PDH-X) is associated with the biliary epithelial cell (BEC) plasma membrane in primary biliary cirrhosis (PBC). Hepatology. 1996;24:165A.
67. Mamula MJ, Lin RH, Janeway CA, Hardin JA. Breaking T cell tolerance with foreign and self co-immunogens: a study of autoimmune T and B cell epitopes of cytochrome c. J Immunol. 1992;149:789–795.
68. Howell CD, Li J, Chen W. Animal models of primary biliary cirrhosis. In: Keith D. Lindor EJH, Poupon R, eds. Primary Biliary Cirrhosis: From Pathogenesis to Clinical Treatment. Dordrecht, The Netherlands: Kluwer Academic Publishers PV, 1998:53–63.
69. Bassendine MF, Palmer JM, DeCruz D et al. Approaches to a murine model of AMA positive non-suppurative destructive cholangitis. J Hepatol. 1998;28:124.
70. Yoshimoto T, Bendelac A, Hu-Li J, Paul WE. Defective IgE production by SJL mice is linked to the absence of CD4+, NK1.1+ T cells that promptly produce interleukin 4. Proc Natl Acad Sci USA. 1995;92:11931–11934.
71. Beutner U, Launois P, Ohteki T, Louis JA, MacDonald HR. Natural killer-like T cells develop in SJL mice despite genetically distinct defects in NK1.1 expression and in inducible interleukin-4 production. Eur J Immunol. 1997;27:928–934.

Section II
Bile acid therapy

4
The optimum dose of ursodeoxycholic acid in primary biliary cirrhosis

A. VERMA, R.P. JAZRAWI, H.A. AHMED and T.C. NORTHFIELD

INTRODUCTION

In 1985 Leuschner reported that serum transaminase levels improved in patients with chronic hepatitis who were undergoing gallstone dissolution therapy with UDCA[1]. This led to several studies of UDCA therapy in PBC, with the first report appearing in 1986[2]. UDCA is now established as the treatment of choice in PBC as it is safe and well tolerated[3], improves liver enzymes[4-11], improves immunological markers[12-16], improves histology in some studies[7,10], may retard the onset of complications[17], improves survival[18,19] and, in a recent cost analysis, results in a saving of $1372 per patient per year compared with placebo[20].

Eight randomized control trials of the use of UDCA in PBC have been published (Table 1). One of these studies used 7.7 mg/kg/day[11], one 8.7 mg/kg/day[5], two 10 mg/kg/day[4,6], one 10–12 mg/kg/day[10] and three 13–15 mg/kg/day[9,21,22]. These doses largely reflect the doses of UDCA used in gallstone dissolution[23]. At the lowest dose the cost of treatment per patient per year is £422 (based on a 65 kg patient using Ursofalk®), with the highest dose costing twice as much.

Table 1. The dose of UDCA used in randomized control studies

Study	Dose (mg/kg)
Eriksson et al. 1997[11]	7.7
Battezzati et al. 1993[5]	8.7
Leuschner et al. 1989[4]	10
Turner et al. 1994[6]	10
Combes et al. 1995[10]	10–12
Heathcote et al. 1994[9]	14
Poupon et al. 1991[21]	13–15
Lindor et al. 1994[22]	13–15

Given the prevalence of PBC in the UK of up to 14 800 (based on the prevalence of 328/million of the adult population[24] and the census[25]), the dose used has considerable cost implications.

DOSE–RESPONSE STUDIES IN PRIMARY BILIARY CIRRHOSIS

Podda et al. studied 30 patients with PBC, giving them 250/500/750 mg in random order and measuring the levels of liver enzymes in blood and bile acids in bile[26]. They found significant reduction in the liver enzymes and bilirubin with all doses of UDCA, the magnitude of the response being roughly proportional to the degree of enrichment of the biliary bile acids with UDCA. The 500 and 750 mg doses were superior to 250 mg, but statistically there was no difference between the 500 and 750 mg. The authors therefore concluded that the optimum dose was 500 mg (equivalent to 8 mg/kg/day). However, in this study there was a large variation in the severity of the disease between patients: some were asymptomatic and anicteric while others were symptomatic and icteric (the histological stage of the patients was not defined). There was no washout period between the doses, and there may therefore have been a carry-over effect from the previous dose. There was a trend for liver enzymes to improve most with the highest dose. We felt that there was scope for trying higher doses. The use of higher doses of UDCA has also been suggested by Jorgensen et al. who showed that patients with the highest enrichment of their bile acids with UDCA were more likely to achieve biochemical normalization[27].

We studied 24 early (stage I and II) PBC patients to determine the optimum dose of UDCA, using alkaline phosphatase (ALP), alanine transaminase (ALT) and gamma glutamyl transferase (γGT) as markers of efficacy[28]. The patients were given 0, 300, 600, 900 and 1200 mg of UDCA for 8 weeks each, with 4 week washout periods between doses. In this study, only patients with histologically confirmed early stage PBC were recruited, in order to reduce the confounding effect of disease stage. Eight weeks of treatment was considered sufficient to record the effects of a particular dose: liver function tests do continue to improve with longer treatment, but the maximal effect has usually taken place by 8 weeks[21]. Furthermore, the enrichment of the bile acid pool by UDCA rises sharply initially and reaches a plateau within 3 months[29]. In order to remove the effect of the previous dose of UDCA, and as the half life of UDCA is approximately 3.5–7 days[29], there was a washout period of 4 weeks between doses (equivalent to 4–8 half life intervals). This was confirmed in the present study by the fact that the liver function tests returned to similar baseline values after each washout period.

We analysed our results using the absolute changes in liver enzyme levels (Figure 1). A clear dose–response effect was demonstrated in this study for all the variables except albumin and conjugated bilirubin. On placebo, liver function tests deteriorated. All the doses of UDCA were superior to placebo. Our results clearly show that both 900 and 1200 mg of UDCA per day are superior to the lower doses. The optimum dose of UDCA therefore appeared to be either 900 or 1200 mg UDCA daily, without a significant difference between the two doses. With respect to symptoms, our results showed that pruritus increased with dose, but only the 1200 mg dose increased pruritus significantly compared with

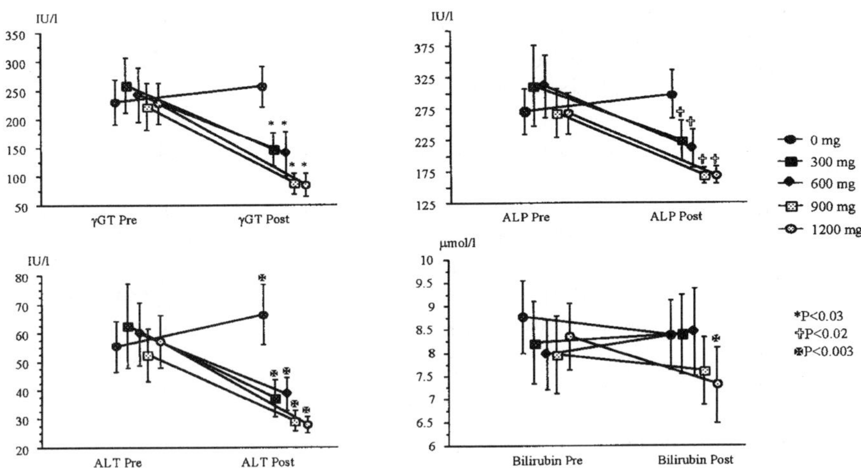

Figure 1. Changes in the liver tests on UDCA therapy.

Table 2. Mean (SEM) scores for the change in symptoms of the patients at the end of the dose compared to the beginning of the dose

	Placebo	300 mg	600 mg	900 mg	1200 mg
Lethargy	−0.44 (0.13)	0.00 (0.11)*	0.22 (0.14)*	0.13 (0.13)*	0.17 (0.12)*
Pruritus	−0.16 (0.19)	−0.13 (0.17)	0.17 (0.15)	0.17 (0.15)	0.35 (0.22)*
Diarrhoea	−0.08 (0.06)	0.00 (0.06)	−0.04 (0.10)	0.04 (0.08)	0.04 (0.08)

*$p < 0.05$ compared with placebo.

placebo (Table 2). We therefore conclude that the most efficacious dose of UDCA in PBC patients is 900 mg/day (equivalent to 12–15 mg/kg/day) as it produces the greatest reduction in LFTs without increasing symptoms.

SURVIVAL AND DOSE

The only hard end point for UDCA therapy in PBC is the effect on survival and/or time to transplantation. Although UDCA does improve survival/time to transplantation[18,19], no study has compared the efficacy of different doses in this respect. However, there are two studies which may begin to shed some light on this issue[11,19].

Poupon *et al.* reported the combined analysis from three randomised control trials of UDCA in PBC, from France, Canada and America[19]. In the French and Canadian studies, all patients were randomised to UDCA (13–15 mg/kg/day and 14 mg/kg/day respectively) or placebo. After two years, all patients on placebo were put on UDCA, whilst those already on UDCA continued with it. In the American study, all patients continued on UDCA (13–15 mg/kg/day) for four years. In total 553 patients were studied.

Ericksson *et al.* conducted the Swedish Multicentre trial of UDCA in PBC[11]. In this patients were randomised to UDCA (7.7 mg/kg/day) or placebo. At the end of two years, patients on placebo were offered UDCA (with 65% taking up this offer), whilst those already on UDCA continued with it (80%) for a further two years.

At 4 years both these studies analysed their data according to which group patients were originally allocated at the beginning of the trial, UDCA or placebo. The results on survival free of transplantation are very different. In the combined analysis study, there was a clear survival advantage for those allocated to UDCA compared with placebo ($p < 0.001$; relative risk 1.9; 95% confidence interval, 1.3–2.8). However, in the Swedish trial there was no difference between the two groups for survival without transplantation.

There are problems in comparing two studies in this manner. The patient mix was different, with 24% of patients in the combined analysis study being stage 4 compared with 9% in the Swedish trial. The numbers were different, with 553 in the combined analysis study and 116 in the Swedish trial, which affects the power of the studies to detect a difference. The only way to show that the difference in the results on survival was due to the different doses used in the two trials would be to analyse the raw data of the two trials together, controlling for other confounders (stage, bilirubin). Despite these limitations, one glaring difference between these studies is that the study that showed the survival advantage for UDCA[19], used the higher dose of 13–15 mg/kg/day.

CONCLUSION

The optimum dose of UDCA in PBC is 12–15 mg/kg/day. This conclusion is based on the effect on liver tests and symptoms in the second dose–response study, and the survival advantage shown in the combined analysis study compared with the Swedish trial.

Acknowledgement

The dose response study conducted by the authors was sponsored by CP Pharmaceuticals Limited, Wrexham, UK.

REFERENCES

1. Leuschner U, Leuschner M, Sieratzki J, Kurtz W, Hubner K. Gallstone dissolution with ursodeoxycholic acid in patients with chronic active hepatitis and two years follow-up. A pilot study. Dig Dis Sci. 1985;30:642–649.
2. Fisher MM, Paradine ME. Influence of ursodeoxycholic acid (UDCA) on biochemical parameters in cholestatic liver disease. Gastroenterology. 1986;90:1725.
3. Kaplan MM. Primary biliary cirrhosis. N Engl J Med. 1996;335:1570–1580.
4. Leuschner U, Fischer H, Kurtz W et al. Ursodeoxycholic acid in primary biliary cirrhosis: results of a controlled double-blind trial. Gastroenterology. 1989;97:1268–1274.
5. Battezzati PM, Podda M, Bianchi FB et al. Ursodeoxycholic acid for symptomatic primary biliary cirrhosis. Preliminary analysis of a double-blind multicenter trial. Italian Multicenter Group for the Study of UDCA in PBC. J Hepatol. 1993;17:332–338.
6. Turner IB, Myszor M, Mitchison HC, Bennett MK, Burt AD, James OF. A two year controlled trial examining the effectiveness of ursodeoxycholic acid in primary biliary cirrhosis. J Gastroenterol Hepatol. 1994;9:162–168.

7. Poupon RE. Poupon R, Balkau B. Ursodiol for the long-term treatment of primary biliary cirrhosis. The UDCA-PBC Study Group. N Engl J Med. 1994;330:1342–1347.

8. Floreani A, Zappala F, Mazzetto M, Naccarato R, Plebani M, Chiaramonte M. Different response to ursodeoxycholic acid (UDCA) in primary biliary cirrhosis according to severity of disease. Dig Dis Sci. 1994;39:9–14.

9. Heathcote EJ, Cauch-Dudek K, Walker V et al. The Canadian multicenter double-blind randomized controlled trial of ursodeoxycholic acid in primary biliary cirrhosis. Hepatology. 1994;19:1149–1156.

10. Combes B. Carithers RL, Maddrey WC et al. A randomized, double-blind, placebo-controlled trial of ursodeoxycholic acid in primary biliary cirrhosis. Hepatology. 1995;22:759–766.

11. Eriksson LS, Olsson R, Glauman H et al. Ursodeoxycholic acid treatment in patients with primary biliary cirrhosis. A Swedish multicentre, double-blind, randomized controlled study. Scand J Gastroenterol. 1997;32:179–186.

12. Lim AG, Wolfhagen HJ, Verma A et al. Soluble intercellular adhesion molecule-1 in primary biliary cirrhosis: effect of ursodeoxycholic acid and immunosuppressive therapy. Eur J Gastroenterol Hepatol. 1997;9:155–161.

13. Ide T, Sata M, Nakano H, Suzuki H, Tanikawa K. Increased serum IgM class anti-lipid A antibody and therapeutic effect of ursodeoxycholic acid in primary biliary cirrhosis. Hepato-Gastroenterology. 1997;44:1569–1573.

14. Kisand KE, Kisand KV, Karvonen AL, Vuoristo M, Mattila J, Makinen JUR. Antibodies to pyruvate dehydrogenase in primary biliary cirrhosis: correlation with histology. APMIS. 1998;106:884–892.

15. Yoshikawa M, Matsui Y, Kawamoto H et al. Intragastric administration of ursodeoxycholic acid suppresses immunoglobulin secretion by lymphocytes from liver, but not from peripheral blood, spleen or Peyer's patches in mice. Int J Immunopharmacol. 1998;20:29–38.

16. Sasatomi K, Noguchi K, Sakisaka S, Sata M, Tanikawa K. Abnormal accumulation of endotoxin in biliary epithelial cells in primary biliary cirrhosis and primary sclerosing cholangitis. J Hepatol. 1998;29:409–416.

17. Lindor KD, Jorgensen RA, Therneau TM, Malinchoc M, Dickson ER. Ursodeoxycholic acid delays the onset of esophageal varices in primary biliary cirrhosis. Mayo Clin Proc. 1997;72:1137–1140.

18. Lindor KD, Therneau TM, Jorgensen RA, Malinchoc M, Dickson ER. Effects of ursodeoxycholic acid on survival in patients with primary biliary cirrhosis. Gastroenterology. 1996;110:1515–1518.

19. Poupon RE, Lindor KD, Cauch-Dudek K, Dickson ER, Poupon R, Heathcote EJ. Combined analysis of randomized controlled trials of ursodeoxycholic acid in primary biliary cirrhosis. Gastroenterology. 1997;113:884–890.

20. Pasha T, Heathcote EJ, Gabriel S et al. Cost-effectiveness of ursodeoxycholic acid therapy in primary biliary cirrhosis. Hepatology. 1999;29:21–26.

21. Poupon RE, Balkau B, Eschwege E, Poupon R. A multicenter, controlled trial of ursodiol for the treatment of primary biliary cirrhosis. UDCA-PBC Study Group. N Engl J Med. 1991;324:1548–1554.

22. Lindor KD, Dickson ER, Baldus WP et al. Ursodeoxycholic acid in the treatment of primary biliary cirrhosis. Gastroenterology. 1994;106:1284–1290.

23. Lanzini A, Northfield TC. Review article: bile acid therapy. Aliment Pharmacol Ther. 1990;4:1–24.

24. Metcalf J, Bhopal R, Howell J, Myszor M, James OFW. PBC: Increased incidence and prevalence together with geographical variation in one UK region. Gut. 1998;42(Supplement 1):A31.

25. Wisniewski D, editor. Annual Abstract of Statistics. London: HMSO; 1997. 10pp.

26. Podda M, Ghezzi C, Battezzati PM et al. Effect of different doses of ursodeoxycholic acid in chronic liver disease. Dig Dis Sci. 1989;34:59S–65S.

27. Jorgensen RA, Dickson ER, Hofmann AF, Rossi SS, Lindor KD. Characterization of patients with a complete biochemical response to ursodeoxycholic acid. Gut. 1995;36:935–938.

28. Verma A, Jazrawi RP, Ahmed HA et al. Optimum dose of ursodeoxycholic acid in primary biliary cirrhosis. Eur J Gastroenterol Hepatol. 1999;11:1069–76.

29. Ward A, Brogden RN, Heel RC, Speight TM, Avery GS. Ursodeoxycholic acid: a review of its pharmacological properties and therapeutic efficacy. Drugs. 1984;27:95–131.

5
Ursodeoxycholic acid – an immunomodulator in primary biliary cirrhosis?

A.G. LIM, R.P. JAZRAWI, H.A. AHMED and T.C. NORTHFIELD

Immune mechanisms are thought to play a key role in both the initiation and maintenance of bile duct damage in primary biliary cirrhosis (PBC). A raised immunoglobulin M (IgM) level is commonly observed. As in many autoimmune conditions, there is a disease-specific antibody – in this case, the anti-mitochondrial, and more specifically the M2, antibody. Histologically, the intra-hepatic bile ducts are infiltrated by T lymphocytes, B lymphocytes and plasma cells. Levels of cytokines, activation markers and adhesion molecules are all elevated. Whilst the pathogenesis of PBC remains obscure, immune-mediated damage directed towards the biliary epithelial cells is believed to be central.

Curiously, direct immunosuppressive treatment with azathioprine, corticosteroids, chlorambucil, cyclosporine or methotrexate has not been found to alter the natural progression of PBC significantly[1]. However, ursodeoxycholic acid (UDCA), a bile acid allegedly without known immune actions, improves clinical outcome in PBC. Its efficacy is probably related to its biochemical properties and actions. UDCA is less hydrophobic than endogenous bile acids, and is less damaging to cellular and subcellular structures, possibly through its membrane stabilizing actions. It also stimulates biliary secretion and, with it, the excretion of endogenous damaging hydrophobic bile acids[2]. Whether some of the beneficial effects of UDCA in PBC result from a reduction of immunological damage remains to be proven. Several groups have examined the effect of UDCA on a variety of markers of immune activity.

SERUM IgM

This is frequently elevated in PBC patients. A significant reduction in IgM levels following UDCA treatment has been reported in several studies[3-5]. Falls in serum immunoglobulin G (IgG) and immunoglobulin A (IgA) levels have been noted in some studies but not others[3,6,7]. The ability of UDCA to affect immunoglobulin production has also been reproduced in vitro. Micromolar concentrations of UDCA inhibited IgM, IgG and IgA production by peripheral blood mononuclear cells artificially stimulated with *Staphylococcus* Cowan I[8]. The bile acid concentrations used in these experiments are not directly cytotoxic and are similar to those achievable in vivo during UDCA therapy. A simplistic possibility is that UDCA directly inhibits mononuclear immunoglobulin production in treated patients. This effect on serum IgM is relatively non-specific but suggests an effect on humoral immunity.

ANTI-MITOCHONDRIAL ANTIBODIES

Anti-mitochondrial antibodies (AMA) can be demonstrated in more than 90% of PBC patients and are used as a common diagnostic tool. The major antigens to these antibodies have been identified as the sub-units of the 2-oxo-acid dehydrogenase family of inner mitochondrial membrane enzyme, but the exact role of these antibodies in pathogenesis of PBC is still uncertain[10]. The effect of UDCA on AMA titres in PBC has been examined but with differing results. Poupon et al. randomized 146 patients to either UDCA or placebo[3]. A significant reduction in AMA titres was observed at 2 years in the UDCA treated patients, but not the placebo group. Oka et al. randomized 45 PBC patients to either UDCA or placebo for 6 months[9]. By contrast, they found no significant change in AMA levels in either group.

HISTOLOGY

The effects of UDCA on the histological inflammatory pattern of immune activity is controversial. Improvements in histology have been reported by some, and disputed by others[3,5,6]. Batts et al. examined the effects of 2 years' treatment with UDCA on liver histology in PBC[11]. When the biopsies of 61 patients (32 receiving UDCA and 29 receiving placebo) were compared by a single blinded pathologist, no significant difference in the degree of inflammation between the two groups could be identified.

ADHESION MOLECULES

In PBC, there is a chronic inflammatory infiltrate, mainly of T lymphocytes, associated with damaged intrahepatic bile ducts. The establishment of this chronic inflammation in the liver depends on the recruitment of T lymphocytes from the circulation. This is sequentially orchestrated, and at a molecular level is dependent on the interactions between specific glycoproteins (adhesion molecules) and their respective ligands. There is initially a transient, reversible binding which causes the lymphocytes to roll on the vessel wall; strong adhesion then develops, followed by the lymphocytes migrating through intercellular endothelial junctions and into tissue. One of these adhesion molecules is intercellular adhesion molecule-1 (ICAM-1). It is a member of the immunoglobulin supergene family of adhesion molecules, and binds to the leucocyte integrin adhesion receptors, LFA-1 and

MAC-1. In health, there is minimal membrane expression of ICAM-1 in the liver. In PBC, up-regulation of ICAM-1 expression has been demonstrated on interlobular bile ducts, proliferating bile ductules, hepatocytes and infiltrating leucocytes.

sICAM-1 is the soluble form of this molecule. It is identical to ICAM-1, except for the lack of a transmembrane component. Significant elevations of sICAM-1 have been reported in a variety of inflammatory and autoimmune diseases. We have shown a marked elevation of sICAM-1 in PBC. Levels of sICAM-1 correlate with biochemical liver function tests, histological stage and disease severity in PBC[12]. We examined the effect of UDCA treatment for 12 months in 24 PBC patients[13]. A significant fall of 20% (median) in sICAM-1 levels was observed. It is possible that this fall in sICAM-1 reflects a fall in adhesion molecule production and, with it, the degree of lymphocyte recruitment. However, the possibility that this fall in sICAM-1 merely reflects improved hepatobiliary function and reduced cholestasis cannot be discounted. We have previously shown a correlation between sICAM-1 levels and biliary excretion rate examined by hepato-scintigraphy.

We also examined the effect of UDCA on other adhesion molecules, including soluble VCAM-1 and soluble E-selectin[14]. Elevations in these adhesion molecules in PBC are much less marked and the effects of therapy less clear.

T LYMPHOCYTE ACTIVATION MARKERS

When T lymphocytes arrive at their target of intrahepatic bile ducts, they are activated by exposure to the antigen. One of the important interactions is between T lymphocytes and fragments of proteins (antigens) embedded in the groove of major histocompatibility complex proteins present in hepatocytes and biliary epithelial cells. T lymphocyte activation then takes place in the presence of co-stimulatory signals. Interleukin-2 receptor (IL-2R) expression on T lymphocytes is a marker of activation. In PBC, as in other chronic liver diseases such as alcoholic liver disease and primary sclerosing cholangitis, there is an increase in the percentage of activated T lymphocytes in the circulation. We did not find any alteration in these levels in PBC patients treated with UDCA for 6 months[13].

Circulating levels of the soluble form of IL-2 receptor are also elevated in PBC. Treatment with UDCA did not significantly alter these levels. Our findings suggest that UDCA has little effect on T cell activation in PBC, but are at variance with the findings of Kurktschiev et al.[15] They examined the effect of UDCA therapy on membrane dipeptidyl IV (CD 26), a different marker of T lymphocyte activation, in PBC patients[8]. They demonstrated a reduction in the levels of activated peripheral blood lymphocytes, with normalization of dipeptidyl peptidase IV expression following UDCA therapy. The difference in the degree of activation, as measured by different markers of T lymphocyte activation, is difficult to explain.

CLASS I AND II MAJOR HISTOCOMPATIBILITY COMPLEX MOLECULES

In PBC, there is aberrant expression of human leucocyte antigen (HLA) class 1 molecules on hepatocytes, and aberrant expression of HLA class II molecules on biliary epithelial cells. Calmus et al. compared the hepatic HLA presentation in patients treated with UDCA for one year with those not on treatment[16]. UDCA reduced the aberrant expression of hepatocyte HLA class I expression, but not aberrant expression of HLA class II on biliary epithelial cells. Similar results were found when hepatic presentation of these molecules was compared before and after UDCA treatment[17]. The interpretation of data from these studies, which are based on liver biopsies, must allow for sampling error, particularly in the case of bile duct lesions which are focal and segmental.

HLA class I expression is an important part of the targeting of cell mediated immune damage to hepatocytes. It has been suggested that these findings indicate a reduction in HLA class I mediated immune injury in PBC. However, aberrant HLA class I expression is not specific to PBC; but also occurs in other hepatobiliary diseases, including autoimmune hepatitis, alcoholic liver disease and biliary tract obstruction. Furthermore, the ability of cholestasis to induce the expression of HLA class I molecules on hepatocytes has been demonstrated both experimentally in bile duct ligated rates and in patients with extrahepatic cholestasis[18]. These findings suggest that aberrant expression of HLA class I is most likely an epiphenomenon, and that the improvement on UDCA may simply reflect a reduction in cholestasis.

CYTOKINES

Bile acids such as cholic acid, deoxycholic acid and chenodeoxycholic acid can all inhibit lymphocyte function[19]. UDCA has been shown to reduce lymphocyte proliferation, which may be cytokine mediated[20]. The effect of UDCA on cytokine levels has been examined both in vitro and in vivo. The effect of UDCA on cytokine production in vitro has been evaluated by Yoshikawa et al.[8]. In their experiments, it is important to note that micromolar concentrations of UDCA were used and the viability of the cells was not affected. The levels in these experiments could be achieved in vivo in PBC patients receiving UDCA, where peripheral plasma concentrations are approximately 0.01–0.1 mmol/l. The bile acid concentration in portal venous plasma is even higher. They found that UDCA suppressed interleukin-2 and interleukin-4 and interferon-γ production by stimulated peripheral blood mononuclear cells, but did not affect interluekin-1 or interluekin-6 production. The suppression of interferon-γ is interesting as it is an important factor in the induction of aberrant major histocompatibility complex expression in inflammation. The lack of effect on interleukin-1, interleukin-6 and tumour necrosis factor production, was also reported by Calmus et al.[21]. The inhibition of interleukin-2 production was also found by Lacaille et al.[22].

The cytokine profile in PBC patients before and during treatment with UDCA has been examined. There are higher cytokine levels in patients with advanced disease. Serum levels of tumour necrosis factor, interleukin-8 and interleukin-12 fell significantly with treatment. Although the authors concluded that this reduction may reflect a mechanism of action of UDCA, this remains unsubstantiated[23].

CONCLUSION

UDCA was originally used for gallstone dissolution. There is no evidence of any immunomodulatory effect when used in this context. However, subsequent observations in PBC patients and in vitro experiments suggest that it has a down-regulating effect on several markers of immune activity. As the pathogenesis of PBC remains obscure and the exact immune mechanisms remain to be unravelled, the interpretation of these observations is difficult. Furthermore, improvements in cholestasis can result in 'improvements' in some measurements of immune activity. Whether UDCA actually has a meaningful action on the hitherto unclear immune mechanisms, thought to be of central importance in PBC, is still not known.

REFERENCES

1. Beuers U. Primary biliary cirrhosis: treatments other than ursodeoxycholic acid. In: Neuberger J, ed., Primary biliary cirrhosis. Eastbourne: Dunnsprint Ltd, 1999:115–118.
2. Lim A, Jazrawi R, Northfield T. The ursodeoxycholic acid story in primary biliary cirrhosis. Gut. 1995;37:301–305.
3. Poupon RE, Balkau B, Eschwege E et al. A multicentre controlled trial of ursodiol for the treatment of primary biliary cirrhosis. N Engl J Med. 1991;324:1548–1554.
4. Battezzati PM, Podda M, Bianchi R et al. Ursodeoxycholic acid for symptomatic primary biliary cirrhosis. J Hepatol. 1993;17:332–338.
5. Combes B, Carithers RL, Maddrey WC et al. A randomized, double blind placebo-controlled trial of ursodeoxycholic acid in primary biliary cirrhosis. Hepatology. 1995;22:759–766.
6. Heathcote JE, Cauch-Dudek K, Walker V et al. The Canadian multicentre double blind trial of ursodeoxycholic acid in primary biliary cirrhosis. Hepatology. 1994;19:1149–1156.
7. Eriksson LS, Olsson R, Glauman H et al. Ursodeoxycholic acid treatment in patients with primary biliary cirrhosis. Scand J Gastroenterol. 1997;32:179–186.
8. Yoshikawa M, Tsujii T, Matsumara K et al. Immunomodulatory effects of ursodeoxycholic acid on human responses. Hepatology. 1992;16:358–364.
9. Oka H, Toda G, Ikeda Y et al. A multi-centre double blind controlled trial of ursodeoxycholic acid for primary biliary cirrhosis. Gastroenterol Jpn. 1990;25:774–780.
10. Bassendine M, Fusey S, Mutimer D et al. Identification and characterization of four M2 mitochondrial autoantigens in primary biliary cirrhosis. Semin Liv Dis. 1989;9:124–131.
11. Batts KP, Jorgensen RA, Dickson ER, Lindor KD. Effects of ursodeoxycholic acid on hepatic inflammation and histological stage in patients with primary biliary cirrhosis. Am J Gastroenterol. 1996;91:2314–2317.
12. Lim AG, Jazrawi RP, Ahmed HA et al. Soluble intercellular adhesion molecule-1 in primary biliary cirrhosis: relationship with disease stage, immune activity and cholestasis. Hepatology. 1994;20:882–888.
13. Lim AG, Wolfhagen FHJ, Verma A et al. Soluble intercellular adhesion molecule-1 in primary biliary cirrhosis: effect of ursodeoxycholic acid and immunosuppressive therapy. Eur J Gastroenterol Hepatol. 1997;9:155–161.
14. Lim AG, Jazrawi RP, Levy JH et al. Soluble E-selectin and vascular cell adhesion molecule-1 (VCAM-1) in primary biliary cirrhosis. J Hepatol. 1995;22:416–422.
15. Kurtschiev D, Subat S, Adler D et al. Immunomodulating effect of ursodeoxycholic acid therapy in patients with primary biliary cirrhosis. J Hepatol. 1993;18:373–377.
16. Calmus Y, Gane P, Rouger P, Poupon R. Hepatic expression of class I and class II major histocompatibility complex molecules in primary biliary cirrhosis: effect of ursodeoxycholic acid. Hepatology. 1990;11:12–15.
17. Terasaki S, Nakunuma Y, Ogino H, Unora M, Kobayashi K. Hepatocellular and biliary expression of HLA antigens in primary biliary cirrhosis before and after ursodeoxycholic acid therapy. Am J Gastroenterol. 1991;86:1194–1199.
18. Calmus Y, Arvieux C, Gane P et al. Cholestasis induces major histocompatibility complex class I expression in hepatocytes. Gastroenterology. 1992;102:1371–1377.
19. Gianni L, Di Padova F, Zuin M, Podda M. Bile acid induced inhibition of the lymphoproliferative response to phytohaemaglutinin and pokeweed mitogen: an in vitro study. Gastroenterology. 1980;78:231–235.

20. Keane RM, Gadacz TR, Munster AM et al. Impairment of human lymphocyte function by bile salts. Surgery 1984;95:439–443.
21. Calmus Y, Guechot J, Podevin P et al. Differential effects of chenodeoxycholic acid and ursodeoxycholic acids on interleukin 1, interleukin 6 and tumour necrosis factor α production by monocytes. Hepatology. 1992;16:719–723.
22. Lacaille F, Paradis K. The immunosuppressive effect of ursodeoxycholic acid: a comparative in vitro study on human peripheral blood mononuclear cells. Hepatology. 1993;18:165–172.
23. Angulo P, Neuman MG, Jorgensen RA et al. Serum cytokines in patients with primary biliary cirrhosis: effect of treatment with ursodeoxycholic acid. Presented at Digestive Diseases Week, 1999, abstract L259.

Section III
Clinical trials

6
Primary biliary cirrhosis: long-term management with ursodeoxycholic acid

J. HEATHCOTE

PBC – THE DISEASE

Primary biliary cirrhosis (PBC) is a presumed autoimmune disease which causes slowly progressive destruction of the interlobular and septal bile ducts giving rise to progressive cholestasis, fibrosis and eventual liver failure.

Currently patients are most often diagnosed when they are asymptomatic and a recent study indicates that histological disease may already be present in subjects who carry the hallmark serum antimitochondrial antibody (AMA), but who have entirely normal liver biochemistry[1]. The survival of patients with PBC, whether symptomatic or asymptomatic, is less than that of age- and gender-matched populations. To date, there are no markers which predict which asymptomatic patients will develop symptomatic disease and which will not[2].

Once symptomatic, the height of the serum bilirubin is an excellent prognostic marker for survival[3]. The Mayo risk score has also been developed as a more sophisticated tool to predict outcome[4] and hence is now used to predict the appropriate time for intervention with liver transplantation. The benefit of the Mayo risk score and the serum bilirubin as surrogate markers for survival is that neither requires invasive tests. Although liver histology is helpful in the diagnosis of PBC, the presence or absence of cirrhosis at baseline correlates poorly with subsequent outcome. The major complication of PBC is portal hypertension, which is often present prior to the development of cirrhosis: nodular regenerative hyperplasia can be found in PBC patients with significant portal tract disease but without fibrosis[5]. Another major complication of PBC is osteoporosis[6]. Clinically silent osteoporosis is found in up to one-third of all PBC patients, regardless of gender and menopausal status.

Other autoimmune diseases are frequently observed in PBC patients, both at the time of diagnosis and noted later during follow-up[7]. More recently features of autoimmune hepatitis have been described in approximately 10% of patients who have been diagnosed with PBC[8,9]. Such features include five-fold or more elevation in serum aminotransferase levels, two-fold or more elevation in IgG levels and liver biopsy features of piecemeal necrosis. In addition, non-organ specific antibodies such as SMA and ANA may frequently be found in patients thought otherwise to have PBC. The natural history of patients with PBC with overlapping features of autoimmune hepatitis is less certain.

THE USE OF URSODEOXYCHOLIC ACID (UDCA) IN THE TREATMENT OF PBC

Leuschner was the first to report improvement in liver biochemistry in patients with chronic hepatitis complicated by gallstones who were treated with ursodeoxycholic acid[10]. Subsequently, Fisher noted that patients with PBC treated with UDCA had symptomatic improvement in pruritus as well as in liver biochemical tests[11]. The pilot study reported by Poupon in 15 patients with PBC treated with UDCA 13–15 mg/kg per day for 2 years clearly showed that the beneficial effect of UDCA was maintained throughout treatment. A sustained fall in serum bilirubin was seen in one-third[12].

MECHANISM OF ACTION OF UDCA

The mechanisms of action of UDCA in patients with chronic liver disease are multiple and include the enhancement of transhepatic and canalicular secretion of retained hydrophobic bile acids[13] and inhibition of terminal ileal uptake of hydrophobic bile acids[14]. Setchell et al.[15] have recently measured intracellular concentrations of bile acids and have shown UDCA treatment to significantly reduce hydrophobic bile acid levels. In an in vitro hepatocyte cell culture model where bile acids may induce apoptosis, this can be significantly inhibited by introducing UDCA into the medium[16].

CLINICAL TRIALS OF UDCA IN PBC

Effect on survival

There have been many randomized control trials of therapy employing UDCA in patients with primary biliary cirrhosis[17–26]; all have shown that even short term treatment leads to a marked improvement in the serum markers of chronic cholestasis, such as serum bilirubin, alkaline phosphatase, γ-glutamyl-trans-pepidase, serum cholesterol and IgM levels (Table 1). An improvement in aminotransferase levels is also reported following the introduction of UDCA therapy. The combined data from three of the largest clinical trials (which in total recruited over 500 patients) has shown that the level of serum bilirubin remains a valid indicator of outcome – normalization of the serum bilirubin upon introduction of treatment was associated with an improved, cumulative survival free of liver transplant (Figure 1) compared with that seen in patients whose serum bilirubin did not normalize on introduction of UDCA therapy[27]. In a somewhat smaller study it has also been shown that the Mayo risk score also

Table 1. Median percentage change in serum biochemistry from baseline to final follow-up in the 2-year Canadian randomized controlled trial of ursodeoxycholic acid[24]

Parameter	UDCA ($n = 106$)	Placebo ($n = 106$)	p
Bilirubin	–17.12	+20.00	< 0.001
Alkaline phosphatase	–42.43	+2.78	< 0.001
AST	–40.54	+5.71	< 0.001
ALT	–47.61	–5.69	< 0.001
Cholesterol	–13.61	+3.37	< 0.001
IgM	–18.47	–0.13	< 0.001

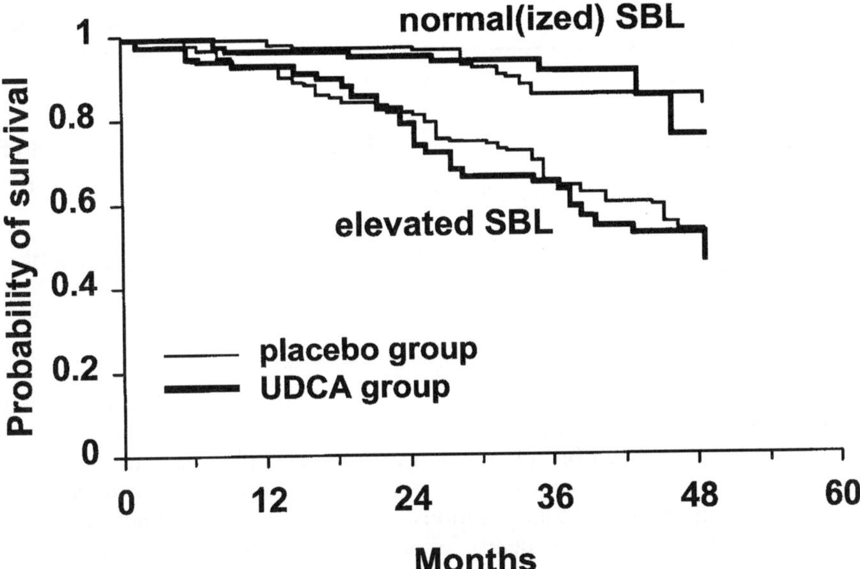

Figure 1. Time to liver transplantation in PBC patients according to bilirubin level following the introduction of UDCA.

remains valid in PBC patients taking UDCA at least in the short term, i.e. within 6 months of the introduction of therapy[28]. Overall, the combined analysis data showed that in patients treated with up to 4 years of UDCA survival free of transplantation was significantly improved compared with those initially randomized to placebo[29] (Figure 2). This significant improvement in survival was observed despite at least 50% of those patients who were initially randomized to placebo switching to UDCA for the last 2 years of the study. This suggests that the true benefit of UDCA on PBC survival may be even greater.

Although most patients with PBC show a marked improvement of the serum markers of cholestasis upon the introduction of UDCA, only about 20% of patients showed complete normalization of their biochemical tests[30]. There

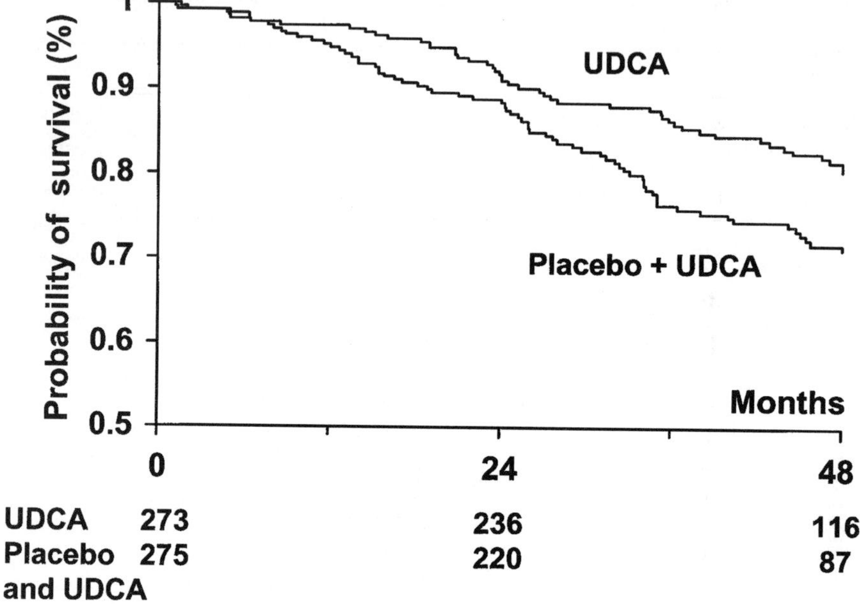

Figure 2. Time free of liver transplantation in PBC patients treated with up to 4 years of UDCA versus placebo.

appears to be no correlation between normalization of liver biochemistry with age, gender, prior biochemical findings or histological stage of disease; however, patients with the highest bilirubin and/or alkaline phosphatase activity tend not to normalize. Those patients whose serum biochemistry is seen to return to normal had higher biliary concentrations of UDCA. It remains unclear whether these patients have a greater degree of absorption or are more compliant than their counterparts whose serum biochemistry did not normalize. UDCA is poorly absorbed and efforts to increase intestinal absorption could possibly enhance overall effectiveness of this particular therapy in PBC. Longer follow-up studies are needed to show whether those patients whose serum biochemistry normalizes upon the introduction of UDCA therapy have an improved overall prognosis.

Effect on symptoms of PBC

The benefit of UDCA on the symptoms associated with PBC is less certain. No study has shown that UDCA therapy influences fatigue and the effect of therapy on pruritus is extremely variable. Occasionally pruritus may be significantly worsened after the introduction of UDCA but many patients experience relief from pruritus upon introduction of therapy. On average, treatment appears to have little overall beneficial effect on this sometimes distressing symptom.

Table 2. Transition of histological stage after 5 years of ursodeoxycholic acid therapy in PBC patients[31]

Histological stage	UDCA ($n = 16$)	Control ($n = 51$)	p
No change/improve	8 (50%)	15 (29%)	0.1
Worse	8 (50%)	36 (71%)	0.1
Cirrhosis (stage 4)	2 (13%)	25 (49%)	0.009

Effect on histology of PBC

The effect of UDCA treatment on the histology of PBC is conflicting. Two studies have shown that treatment appears to significantly reduce the degree of inflammation, suggesting an immunoregulatory effect of UDCA[21,26]. However, this was not noted in either the Mayo[23] or Canadian[24] studies. The latter showed a reduction in cholestasis and bile ductular proliferation in patients randomized to UDCA. Scores of fibrosis following 2 years of therapy have not shown a marked benefit of treatment; however, a recent study employing a 5 year follow-up implies that UDCA treatment reduces the rate of fibrosis in treated patients[31], but is never seen to reverse the baseline fibrosis (Table 2).

Effect on diseases associated with PBC

UDCA treatment does not appear to affect the osteoporosis associated with primary biliary cirrhosis, suggesting that osteoporosis may not be secondary to some 'toxic' effect of cholestasis on bone metabolism[32]. Although studies indicate UDCA may have an immunoregulatory effect and serum levels of IgM fall markedly upon the introduction of UDCA therapy, AMA titres are inconsistently influenced by this treatment although falls in titres have been reported[33]. UDCA therapy appears to have no effect on the rate of development of autoimmune diseases seen in association with PBC[34].

Effect on portal hypertension

A small study of sinusoidal pressure before and after the introduction of UDCA in PBC suggested therapy reduced the rate of rise in portal pressure over 2 years[35]. In another study, UDCA did not cause a reduction in the rate of bleeding varices, but did reduce the rate of development of oesophageal varices[36].

Effect on outcome following liver transplant

The need for liver transplantation and/or death is only delayed, not abolished, by treatment with UDCA. Although UDCA therapy delays the need for transplant, and hence patients live longer with their disease, it does not appear to adversely effect post-transplant outcome[37] (Table 3). Primary biliary cirrhosis may recur after transplantation; no factors have been identified which predict PBC recurrence[38]. Recurrence does not appear to have an overall detrimental effect on post-transplant outcome.

Table 3. Post liver transplantation outcome in PBC patients given ursodeoxycholic acid[37]

	UDCA ($n = 37$)	Placebo ($n = 53$)
Alive at 1 month	93.9%	88.4%
Alive at 1 year	90.3%	78.4%
Rejection at 1 month	31.3%	43.2%
Rejection at 1 year*	42.9%	68.8%
Infection at 1 month	31.3%	35.3%
Infection at 1 year	53.9%	58.1%

*$p = 0.04$

COST-EFFECTIVENESS OF UDCA IN PBC

Follow-up data from two large randomized controlled trials of ursodeoxycholic acid in PBC indicate that the number of events, such as development of ascites, varices, variceal haemorrhage, encephalopathy and death or need for liver transplantation is higher in patients receiving placebo than in those randomized to ursodeoxycholic acid[39]. These data have been used to assess the cost-effectiveness of UDCA in the treatment of primary biliary cirrhosis. As the cost of hepatic decompensation is high, and often requires hospitalization, UDCA treatment was determined not only to be cost effective but actually to be cost saving (Table 4).

In summary, the introduction of treatment with the dihydroxy hydrophilic bile acid, ursodeoxycholic acid has led to an improvement in survival of patients with primary biliary cirrhosis. This benefit is most obvious in patients with more severe disease, i.e. baseline bilirubin > 1.4 mg/dl and/or stage III and IV liver histology, simply because the number of events in such patients randomized to placebo is considerable. Although a benefit of UDCA therapy is likely in those

ble 4. Annual morbidity cost estimates and estimated annual cost savings per 100 patients[39]

Events	Events (100/year)		Estimated cost per event ($)	Estimated cost savings/100 ($)
	UDCA	Placebo		
Ascites	1.54	2.66	2 883	3 229
Varices	3.61	11.21	744	5 654
Variceal bleed	1.32	1.64	10 744	3 438
Encephalopathy	0.75	1.81	7 004	7 424
Orthotopic liver transplant	2.57	5.02	150 000	367 500
Death	2.57	4.40	—	
Total events	12.36	26.74		387 246

with mild liver disease (baseline bilirubin < 1.4 and/or stage I or II disease), such a benefit is impossible to demonstrate in terms of survival as the survival of untreated patients with such mild disease is excellent over many years. No trial will be large enough or conducted for long enough to clearly show a benefit of any therapy on the course of mild, often asymptomatic PBC.

REFERENCES

1. Mitchison HC, Bassendine MF, Hendrick A et al. Positive antimitochondrial antibody but normal alkaline phosphatase: is this primary biliary cirrhosis? Hepatology. 1986;6:1279–1284.
2. Springer J, Cauch-Dudek K, O'Rourke K, Wanless IR, Heathcote EJ. Asymptomatic primary biliary cirrhosis: A study of its natural history and prognosis. Am J Gastroenterol. 1999;94:47–53.
3. Shapiro JM, Smith H, Schaffner F. Serum bilirubin: A prognostic factor in primary biliary cirrhosis. Gut. 1979;20:137–140.
4. Dickson E, Grambsch PM, Fleming TR et al. Prognosis in primary biliary cirrhosis: model for decision making. Hepatology. 1989;10:1–7.
5. Colina F, Pinedo F, Solis JA et al. Nodular regenerative hyperplasia of the liver in early histological stages of primary biliary cirrhosis. Gastroenterology. 1992;102:1319–1324.
6. Hay JE. Bone disease in cholestatic liver disease. Gastroenterology. 1995;108:276–283.
7. Inoue K, Hirohara J, Nakano T et al. Prediction of prognosis of primary biliary cirrhosis in Japan. Liver. 1995;15:70–77.
8. Chazouilleres O, Wendum D, Serfaaty L, Montembault S, Rosmorduc O, Poupon R. Primary biliary cirrhosis – autoimmune hepatitis overlap syndrome: clinical features and response to therapy. Hepatology. 1998;28:296–301.
9. Czaja AJ. The frequency and nature of the variant syndromes of autoimmune liver disease. Hepatology. 1998;28:360–365.
10. Leuschner U, Leuschner M, Sieratzki J, Kurtz W, Hubner K. Gallstone dissolution with ursodeoxycholic acid in patients with chronic active hepatitis and two years follow-up. A pilot study. Dig Dis Sci. 1985;30:642–649.
11. Fisher MM, Paradine ME. Influence of ursodeoxycholic acid on biochemical parameters in cholestatic liver disease. Gastroenterology. 1986;90:1725.
12. Poupon R, Poupon RE, Calmus Y et al. Is ursodeoxycholic acid an effective treatment for primary biliary cirrhosis? Lancet. 1987;1:834–836.
13. Jazrawi RP, Caestecker JS, Goggin PM et al. Kinetics of hepatic bile acid handling in cholestatic liver disease: effect of ursodeoxycholic acid. Gastroenterology. 1994;106:134–142.
14. Stiehl A, Raedsch R, Rudolph G. Acute effects of ursodeoxycholic and chenodeoxycholic acid on the small intestinal absorption of bile acids. Gastroenterology. 1990;98:424–428.
15. Setchell KDR, Rodrigues CMP, Clerici C et al. Bile acid concentrations in human and rat liver tissue and in hepatocyte nuclei. Gastroenterology. 1997;112:226–235.
16. Rodrigues CM, Fan G, Ma X, Kren BT, Steer CJ. A novel role for ursodeoxycholic acid in inhibiting apoptosis by modulating mitochondrial membrane perturbation. J Clin Invest. 1998;101:2790–2799.
17. Leuschner U, Fischer H, Kurtz W et al. Ursodeoxycholic acid in primary biliary cirrhosis: results of a controlled double-blind trial. Gastroenterology. 1989;97:1268–1274.
18. Oka H, Toda G, Ikeda Y et al. A multi-centre double-blind controlled trial of ursodeoxycholic acid for primary biliary cirrhosis. Gastroenterol Jpn. 1990;25:774–780.
19. Battezati PM, Podda M, Bianchi FB et al. Ursodeoxycholic acid for symptomatic primary biliary cirrhosis. Preliminary analysis of a double-blind multicentre trial. J Hepatol. 1993;17: 332–338.
20. Eriksson LS, Olsson R, Glauman H et al. Ursodeoxycholic acid treatment in patients with primary biliary cirrhosis. A Swedish multi-centre, double-blind, randomized controlled study. Scand J Gastroenterol. 1997;32:179–186.
21. Poupon RE, Balkau B, Eschwege E, Poupon R et al. A multicentre controlled trial of ursodiol for the treatment of primary biliary cirrhosis. N Engl J Med. 1991;324:1548–1554.

22. Hadziyannis SJ, Hadziyannis ES, Makris A. A randomized controlled trial of ursodeoxycholic acid (UDCA) in primary biliary cirrhosis (PBC). Hepatology. 1989;10:580.
23. Lindor KD, Dickson ER, Baldus WP et al. Ursodeoxycholic acid in the treatment of primary biliary cirrhosis. Gastroenterology. 1994;106:1284–1290.
24. Heathcote EJ, Cauch-Dudek K, Walker V et al. The Canadian multicentre double-blind randomized controlled trial of ursodeoxycholic acid in primary biliary cirrhosis. Hepatology. 1994;19:1149–1156.
25. Turner IB, Myszor M, Mitchison HC et al. A two year controlled trial examining the effectiveness of UDCA in PBC. J Gastroenterol Hepatol. 1994;9:162–168.
26. Combes B, Carithers RL, Maddrey WC et al. A randomized, double-blind, placebo-controlled trial of ursodeoxycholic acid in primary biliary cirrhosis. Hepatology. 1995;22:759–766.
27. Bonnand A-M, Heathcote EJ, Lindor KD, Poupon RE. Clinical significance of serum bilirubin levels under ursodeoxycholic acid therapy in patients with primary biliary cirrhosis. Hepatology. 1999;29:39–43.
28. Kilmurry M, Heathcote EJ, Cauch-Dudek K et al. Is the Mayo model for predicting survival useful after the introduction of ursodeoxycholic acid treatment for primary biliary cirrhosis? Hepatology. 1996;23:1148–1153.
29. Poupon RE, Lindor KD, Cauch-Dudek K, Dickson ER, Poupon R, Heathcote EJ. Combined analysis of randomized controlled trials of ursodeoxycholic acid in primary biliary cirrhosis. Gastroenterology. 1997;113:884–890.
30. Jorgensen RA, Dickson ER, Hofmann AF et al. Characterization of patients with a complete biochemical response to ursodeoxycholic acid. Gut. 1995;36:935–938.
31. Angulo P, Batts KP, Therneau TM, Jorgensen RA, Dickson ER, Lindor KD. Long-term ursodeoxycholic acid delays histological progression in primary biliary cirrhosis. Hepatology. 1999;29:644–647.
32. Lindor KD, Janes CH, Crippen JS et al. Bone disease in primary biliary cirrhosis: does ursodeoxycholic acid make a difference? Hepatology. 1995;21:389–392.
33. Kisand KE, Karvonene AL, Vuoristo M et al. Ursodeoxycholic acid treatment lowers the serum levels of antibodies against pyruvate dehydrogenase and influences their inhibitory capacity for the enzyme complex in patient with primary biliary cirrhosis. J Mol Med. 1996;74:269–274.
34. Zukowski TH, Jorgensen RA, Dickson ER, Lindor KD. Autoimmune conditions associated with primary biliary cirrhosis: response to ursodeoxycholic acid therapy. Am J Gastroenterol. 1998;93:958–961.
35. Huet PM, Huet J, Deslauriers J. Portal hypertension in patients with primary biliary cirrhosis. In: Lindor KD, Heathcote EJ, Poupon R, eds. Primary biliary cirrhosis: From pathogenesis to treatment. London: Kluwer Academic Publishers, 1998:87–91.
36. Lindor KD, Jorgensen RA, Dickson ER. Ursodeoxycholic acid delays the onset of esophageal varices in primary biliary cirrhosis. Mayo Clin Proc. 1997;72:1137–1140.
37. Heathcote EJ, Stone J, Cauch-Dudek K et al. The effect of pre-transplant ursodeoxycholic acid therapy on outcome of liver transplantation in patients with primary biliary cirrhosis. Liver Transpl Surg. 1999; in press.
38. Balan V, Batts KP, Porayko MK et al. Histological evidence for recurrence of primary biliary cirrhosis after liver transplantation. Hepatology. 1993;18:1392–1398.
39. Pasha T, Heathcote J, Gabriel S et al. Cost-effectiveness of ursodeoxycholic acid therapy in primary biliary cirrhosis. Hepatology. 1999;29:21–26.

7
Management of patients with primary sclerosing cholangitis

A. STIEHL, C. BENZ and P. SAUER

CLINICAL FEATURES

Primary sclerosing cholangitis is characterized by progressive fibrosing inflammation of the bile ducts, leading to cholestasis and finally to cirrhosis of the liver. Its cause is unknown. The symptoms of the disease are nonspecific and include jaundice, pruritus and fatigue. Patients with dominant stenoses tend to have repeated episodes of bacterial cholangitis, requiring antibiotic treatment. The diagnosis of PSC is made by endoscopic retrograde cholangiography (ERCP). The disease is frequently associated with ulcerative colitis, and with an increased incidence of cholangial and colonic carcinomas. In a large multicentre study from Sweden of 305 PSC patients, a bile duct carcinoma was observed in 8% of patients over a median follow up of 63 months[1]. Very high rates of bile duct carcinoma have repeatedly been reported in the very selected groups of patients seen in transplantation centres.

ENDOSCOPIC TREATMENT

Dominant stenoses of the bile ducts are common at the time of presentation in PSC and may occlude the major bile ducts. Such stenoses cannot be expected to respond to medical treatment and need early endoscopic dilatation[2-10]. Repeat cholangiography in patients with narrowing of major bile ducts seems essential to detect stenosis early[2] and should be performed under antibiotic prophylaxis. Repeated dilatation is usually necessary till the duct remains open[2]. Intermittent stenting also has been used[2-10] but the stents tend to occlude early with inflammatory material shed from the bile ducts. Since occlusion of the stent leads to bacterial infection of the proximal biliary tree, stents should in general be removed or replaced within 2 weeks. In our hands, dilatation is by far the more effective form of endoscopic treatment.

MEDICAL TREATMENT

The treatment of PSC with immunosuppressive, anti-inflammatory or anti-fibrotic agents has not proved successful, and immunosuppressive treatment may even be harmful because of the frequency of bacterial cholangitis. Reports of the beneficial effect of methotrexate in one trial need confirmation in controlled trials. The observation that UDCA has a beneficial effect in patients with primary biliary cirrhosis (PBC) was a major breakthrough. Subsequently, patients with various cholestatic liver diseases including primary sclerosing cholangitis have been treated with UDCA.

EFFECTS OF URSODEOXYCHOLIC ACID

Treatment with UDCA 15–20 mg/kg has significantly reduced elevated serum levels of alkaline phosphatase (AP), γ-glutamyl transpeptidase (GGT), alanine and aspartate transaminase (ALT and AST) and cholesterol in all controlled studies[11,12,14,15], and serum bilirubin improved in three of four controlled studies[12,14,15]. Changes in IgA, IgM, and IgG were not significant. The relatively low dose of 600 mg/day produced no improvement in laboratory parameters in one trial[13]. Symptoms such as pruritus and fatigue improved in some patients but, in comparison to placebo, the effect was not significant[2].

Changes in liver histology were evaluated in four studies. Cellular infiltration of the portal triads decreased significantly in three studies[11,12,15], and histological stage in only one study using high dose therapy (20 mg/kg)[15]; no effect on liver histology was noted in the Mayo study[14]. The effect of high dose therapy (20 mg/kg)[15] is of particular interest. It is unclear whether the decrease in periductal inflammation with UDCA in PSC will influence the development of bile duct carcinomas in this disease. It is obvious that UDCA can have little or no effect on liver histology when dominant stenoses are present, and the number of patients with dominant stenoses must be considered when interpreting a trial. In a prospective trial of the effect of UDCA on bile duct disease using repeated cholangiography[2], 28/96 patients developed a progressive stenosis of major bile ducts over 12 years. It is evident that UDCA cannot treat obstruction of major bile ducts effectively, and that endoscopy is an essential part of conservative treatment.

Table 1. Ursodeoxycholic acid in primary sclerosing cholangitis: results of placebo controlled studies[a]

Author (Ref)	N	AP,GCiT, ALT or AST	Bilirubin	Histology
Stiehl[11]	20	improved	unchanged	favourable[b]
Beuers[12]	14	improved	improved	favourable
Lindor[14]	105	improved	improved	unchanged
Mitchell[15]	24	improved	improved	favourable

[a] Studies with UDCA doses > 10 mg/kg.
[b] Favourable effect in comparison to pretreatment histology.

In one controlled study none of 52 patients with PSC on UDCA developed a bile duct carcinoma, compared with three of 53 patients in the control group[14]. In a prospective study which is currently in progress in our institution, only two of 96 (2.3%) on UDCA have developed a bile duct carcinoma over almost 12 years[2]. It seems possible that the reduced inflammation around the bile ducts observed on UDCA[11,12,15] may reduce the incidence of bile duct carcinomas, but definite proof for this is lacking. PSC is a progressive disease with reduced survival, particularly in symptomatic patients. In a recent controlled study[14] in which endoscopic treatment of major duct stenoses did not play a role, UDCA treatment did not improve transplant-free survival over 2 years. In our prospective non-randomized study, by contrast, the actuarial Kaplan Meier estimate of survival after treatment with UDCA and dilatation of major duct stenoses was significantly more than the predicted survival ($p < 0.001$)[2]. The 5 year survival rate after liver transplantation for PSC is approximately 72% (European Transplant Registry). In centres where early transplantation is recommended, the 5 year survival rate of patients with colitis and PSC is approximately 80%, and the 8 year survival rate is approximately 70%[16]. Since the incidence of bile duct carcinoma is much lower than the incidence of death after transplantation, prophylactic transplantation (in precirrhotic stages of the disease) to prevent the development of bile duct carcinomas cannot be recommended.

CONCLUSION

We conclude that PSC may be treated conservatively by UDCA, with benefit in terms of liver function tests and probably histology. Transplant-free survival is prolonged only if patients who develop major duct stenoses are recognized and treated early by endoscopic dilatation. Liver transplantation is indicated in end-stage disease.

REFERENCES

1. Broome U, Olson R, Loof L et al. Natural history and prognostic factors in 305 Swedish patients with primary sclerosing cholangitis. Gut. 1996;38:610–615.
2. Stiehl A, Rudolph G, Sauer P et al. Efficacy of ursodeoxycholic acid and endoscopic dilation of major duct stenoses in primary sclerosing cholangitis. An 8-year prospective study. J Hepatol. 1997;26:560–566.
3. Grijm R, Huibregtse K, Bartelsman J et al. Therapeutic investigations in primary sclerosing cholangitis. Dig Dis Sci. 1986;31:792–798.
4. Johnson GK, Geenen JE, Venu RP, Hogan WJ. Endoscopic treatment of biliary duct strictures in sclerosing cholangitis: Follow up assessment of a new therapeutic approach. Gastrointest Endosc. 1987;33:9–12.
5. Huitbregtse K. Therapeutic investigations in primary sclerosing cholangitis. In: Huitbregtse K, ed., Endoscopic biliary and pancreatic drainage. Stuttgart: Georg Thieme 1988:78–85.
6. Cotton PB, Nickl N. Endoscopic and radiologic approaches to therapy in primary sclerosing cholangitis. Semin Liver Dis. 1991;11:40–48.
7. Craig PI, Hatfield RW. Endoscopic therapy in primary sclerosing cholangitis. Eur J Gastroenterol Hepatol. 1992;4:284–287.
8. Gaing AA, Geders JM, Cohen SA, Siegel JH. Endoscopic management of primary sclerosing cholangitis: review, and report of an open series. Am J Gastroenterol. 1993;88:2000–2008.

9. Lee JG, Schutz SM, England RE, Leung JW, Cotton PB. Endoscopic therapy of sclerosing cholangitis. Hepatology. 1995;21:661–667.
10. van Milligen AWM, van Bracht J, Rauws EAJ et al.. Endoscopic stent therapy for dominant extrahepatic bile duct strictures in primary sclerosing cholangitis. Gastrointest Endosc. 1996;44:293–299.
11. Stiehl A, Walker S, Stiehl L et al. Effects of ursodeoxycholic acid on liver and bile duct disease in primary sclerosing cholangitis. A 3 year pilot study with a placebo-controlled study period. J Hepatol. 1994;20:57–64.
12. Beuers U, Spengler U, Kruis W et al. Ursodeoxycholic acid for treatment of primary sclerosing cholangitis: a placebo controlled trial. Hepatology. 1992;16:707–714.
13. De Flaria N, Colantoni A, Rosenblom E, Van Thiel DH. Ursodeoxycholic acid does not improve the clinical course of primary sclerosing cholangitis over a 2-year period. Hepato-Gastroenterology. 1996;43:1472–1479.
14. Lindor KD and the Mayo PSC/UDCA study group: Ursodiol for the treatment of primary sclerosing cholangitis. N Engl J Med. 1997;336:691–695.
15. Blitchell SA, Bansi D, Hunt N et al. High dose ursodeoxycholic acid (UDCA) in primary sclerosing cholangitis (PSC): results after two years of a randomized double-blind, placebo-controlled trial. Gut. 1997;40(Suppl.1):TH 115.
16. Loftus EV, Aguzilar HI, Sandborn WJ et al. Risk of colorectal neoplasia in patients with primary sclerosing cholangitis and ulcerative colitis following orthotopic liver transplantation. Hepatology. 1998;27:685–690.

Section IV
Other cholestatic conditions

8
The genetics of bile acid transport

R. THOMPSON

ENTEROHEPATIC CIRCULATION OF BILE ACIDS

Cholesterol is a dirty word in the western world. However, cholesterol is of such biological importance that the human body not only efficiently extracts it from our diet, but also has the capacity to synthesize it de novo. Whilst most of the body's cholesterol is in cell membranes, it is an essential precursor of several physiologically important compounds. The list of cholesterol derivatives includes the steroid hormones, vitamin D and bile acids. Daily losses of all these compounds are themselves small. Bile acids appear to serve at least two physiological roles, both of which are dependent on their enterohepatic circulation. Bile acid flux is the major driving force of bile production and they are essential for the normal absorption of fats from the gastrointestinal tract.

There is no doubt that the liver cannot function without adequate bile flow. The true physiological purpose of bile flow, however, is less clear. Bile is a mixture of waste products, notably bilirubin and other conjugates, along with bile acids, lipids and inorganic ions, most of which are reabsorbed. While bile acids are an essential component of bile, they are themselves toxic. The main function of other constituents, notably phospholipids, may be to protect against the harmful effects of bile acids. The enterohepatic circulation of bile acids involves transport across two epithelial surfaces, as well as passage through the gut and portal blood. Given the importance of bile acid circulation, together with its toxicity, it is not surprising that a set of genes has evolved which appear to encode the proteins responsible for effecting these transport processes.

ILEAL TRANSPORT OF BILE ACIDS

Only about 2% of the bile acids excreted daily into the GI tract are lost in the stool. A single transporter appears to be responsible for this conservation through uptake in the distal ileum. The apical sodium-dependent bile salt transporter (ASBT)[1,2] is a transmembrane protein similar to the sodium-dependent bile acid transporter found in hepatocytes (NTCP)[3], which is discussed below. The gene is located on chromosome 13q33 and is referred to as *SLC10A2*[4]. The protein, when expressed in vitro, has Ki values in the range of 3.3 μM (cheno-deoxycholate) to 41.5 μM (cholate) for bile acids, but very high Ki values for a number of other organic anions[5]. This contrasts with NTCP, which appears to have a much broader specificity. The total daily bile acid loss in urine is three orders of magnitude less than that through stool. ASBT is also expressed in the kidney and is probably responsible for reclamation of bile acids from glomerular filtrate[5]. Recessive loss of function mutations in the ASBT gene have been found in patients with primary bile acid malabsorption[4].

The intracellular transport of hydrophobic molecules is less well characterized than that at membranes. However, a member of the fatty acid binding protein family was identified in the mouse and subsequently in humans, which binds conjugated and unconjugated bile acids[6]. The human protein, ileal lipid-binding protein 3 (ILBP3), is encoded by the *FABP6* gene on chromosome 5q23-q35[1].

There has to be an enterocyte export mechanism. Functionally, this seems to be an anion exchanger. A strong candidate has recently been identified, in rat, by low stringency PCR and library screening. This appears to be a member of the OATP family with approximately 80% homology with rat oatp 1 and 2. However, its subcellular location is not yet confirmed.

HEPATIC TRANSPORT OF BILE ACIDS

Bile acids are removed from the portal circulation by hepatocytes. This is achieved with such efficiency that despite a daily flux of ~50 mmol of bile acids, the concentration in the systemic circulation is generally <10 μmol/l. The major bile acid transporter in the basolateral membrane is the sodium taurocholate co-transporting polypeptide (NTCP)[3]. As mentioned above, this protein is 35% identical with ASBT and shares a similar predicted structure with seven transmembrane spans. Despite its name it does, however, have a broader substrate specificity. When expressed in vitro, human NTCP has a Km of ~6 μM for taurocholate[7]. This is consistent with the levels of bile acids present in the systemic circulation. The organic anion transporting polypeptides are capable of transporting bile acids, along with many amphipathic compounds[8]. Human OATP is encoded by the *SLC21A3* gene, located on chromosome 12p12. Whether OATP plays a physiologically significant role in bile acid transport is not clear. The nature of the hepatocytic intracellular bile acid carrier is equally unclear. However, fatty acid binding proteins and possibly glutathione S-transferase are likely to be involved.

Bile acid export from hepatocytes operates against a steep concentration gradient. The biliary bile acid concentration is at least 1000-fold higher than that in hepatocytes. It is not surprising, therefore, that the transport of bile acids across this membrane has been shown to be an energy dependent process. The protein responsible has proved elusive. A fragment of the *spgp* gene was first identified from a pig cDNA library during a search for members of the p-glycoprotein family[9]. This is the origin of the name sister of p-glycoprotein. The full length rat cDNA when expressed in vitro is an effective ATP-dependent bile acid transporter with a Km for taurocholate of ~5 μM[10]. The protein has, therefore, been named the bile salt export pump. The physiological role of this protein is supported by the finding of mutations in the human orthologue (*BSEP*) in patients with cholestatic liver disease[11]. The patients all have a progressive intrahepatic cholestasis with normal levels of serum γGT. In those where it has been measured, they also have low levels of biliary bile acids; this correlates well with the low γGT. The gene has been mapped to the same region of human chromosome 2 to which the disease had previously been linked[12]. BSEP is a member of the p-glycoprotein (or multi-drug resistance – MDR) subfamily of the ATP-binding cassette (ABC) family of proteins. It is predicted to have the same membrane topology as the other MDRs, with two transmembrane domains, each with six spans, and two nucleotide binding domains. It is exclusively expressed in the liver.

THE TRANSPORT OF BILE ACIDS BY CHOLANGIOCYTES

The concept of the cholehepatic shunt is attractive[13]. If bile acids are reabsorbed by cholangiocytes, they would be expected to re-enter portal blood and return to the hepatocyte basolateral membrane. This would have the effect of increasing the volume of bile flow for a given amount of bile acid excreted in mature bile. The ileal/renal sodium-dependent bile acid transporter, ASBT, is expressed in the cholangiocyte apical membrane and may well contribute to this cholehepatic shunting[14]. Further evidence for significant cholangiocyte bile acid transport comes from another human cholestatic disorder. *FIC1* has been shown to be mutated in some patients with progressive intrahepatic cholestasis, with different mutations present in patients with benign recurrent intrahepatic cholestasis[15]. These patients all have low serum γGT levels and very low levels of biliary bile acids. The *FIC1* gene is, however, not expressed in hepatocytes, but in cholangiocytes. The FIC1 protein is a P-type ATPase, and a member of a family of proteins which have been implicated in aminophospholipid transport[16]; this has, however, been refuted[17]. The mechanism by which this gene/protein, when mutated, leads to low biliary bile acid levels and cholestasis is unknown, but may shed important light on the handling of bile acids by cholangiocytes.

CONCLUSIONS

Most of the major bile acid transporter genes have now been cloned. The intracellular transport of bile acids is less well understood. Several new challenges now present themselves. How is the expression of the genes regulated? How are the proteins themselves transported to the correct cellular domains? Are they subject to other controlling factors once there? Once these questions are answered then significant therapeutic progress will be possible. In the meantime many of the genetic cholestases are very good candidates for gene therapy.

REFERENCES

1. Oelkers P, Dawson PA. Cloning and chromosomal localization of the human ileal lipid-binding protein. Biochim Biophys Acta. 1995;1257:199–202.
2. Wong MH, Oelkers P, Craddock AL, Dawson PA. Expression cloning and characterization of the hamster ileal sodium-dependent bile acid transporter. J Biol Chem. 1994;269:1340–1347.

3. Hagenbuch B, Stieger B, Foguet M, Lubbert H, Meier PJ. Functional expression cloning and characterization of the hepatocyte Na+/bile acid cotransport system. Proc Natl Acad Sci USA. 1991;88:10629–10633.

4. Oelkers P, Kirby LC, Heubi JE, Dawson PA. Primary bile acid malabsorption caused by mutations in the ileal sodium-dependent bile acid transporter gene (SLC10A2). J Clin Invest. 1997;99:1880–1887.

5. Craddock AL, Love MW, Daniel RW et al. Expression and transport properties of the human ileal and renal sodium-dependent bile acid transporter. Am J Physiol. 1998;274:G157–G169.

6. Birkenmeier EH, Rowe LB, Crossman MW, Gordon JI. Ileal lipid-binding protein (Illbp) gene maps to mouse chromosome 11. Mammalian Genome. 1994;5:805–806.

7. Hagenbuch B, Meier PJ. Molecular cloning, chromosomal localization, and functional characterization of a human liver Na+/bile acid cotransporter. J Clin Invest. 1994;93:1326–1331.

8. Bossuyt X, Muller M, Meier PJ. Multispecific amphipathic substrate transport by an organic anion transporter of human liver. J Hepatol. 1996;25:733–738.

9. Childs S, Yeh RL, Georges E, Ling V. Identification of a sister gene to P-glycoprotein. Cancer Res. 1995;55:2029–2034.

10. Gerloff T, Stieger B, Hagenbuch B et al. The sister of P-glycoprotein represents the canalicular bile salt export pump of mammalian liver. J Biol Chem. 1998;273:10046–10050.

11. Strautnieks SS, Bull LN, Knisely AS et al. A gene encoding a liver-specific ABC transporter is mutated in progressive familial intrahepatic cholestasis. Nature Genet. 1998;20:233–238.

12. Strautnieks SS, Kagalwalla AF, Tanner MS et al. Identification of a locus for progressive familial intrahepatic cholestasis PFIC2 on chromosome 2q24. Am J Hum Genet. 1997;61:630–633.

13. Yoon YB, Hagey LR, Hofmann AF, Gurantz D, Michelotti EL, Steinbach JH. Effect of side-chain shortening on the physiologic properties of bile acids: hepatic transport and effect on biliary secretion of 23-nor-ursodeoxycholate in rodents. Gastroenterology. 1986;90:837–852.

14. Lazaridis KN, Pham L, Tietz P et al. Rat cholangiocytes absorb bile acids at their apical domain via the ileal sodium-dependent bile acid transporter. J Clin Invest. 1997;100:2714–2721.

15. Bull LN, van Eijk MJ, Pawlikowska L et al. A gene encoding a P-type ATPase mutated in two forms of hereditary cholestasis. Nature Genet. 1998;18:219–224.

16. Tang X, Halleck MS, Schlegel RA, Williamson P. A subfamily of P-type ATPases with aminophospholipid transporting activity (published erratum appears in Science 1996;274:1597). Science 1996;272:1495–1497.

17. Siegmund A, Grant A, Angeletti C, Malone L, Nichols JW, Rudolph HK. Loss of Drs2p does not abolish transfer of fluorescence-labelled phospholipids across the plasma membrane of Saccharomyces cerevisiae. J Biol Chem 1998;273:34399–34405.

9
Congenital defects in bile acid synthesis cause a spectrum of diseases manifest as severe cholestasis, neurological disease, and fat-soluble vitamin malabsorption

K.D.R. SETCHELL, N.C. O'CONNELL, R.H. SQUIRES and J.E. HEUBI

INTRODUCTION

In humans, hepatic synthesis of the primary bile acids, cholic and chenodeoxycholic acids, is critical to the development and maintenance of the enterohepatic circulation and for lipid absorption from the intestine[1]. Synthesis from cholesterol proceeds via two independent pathways: the classical *neutral* pathway involving a cholesterol 7α-hydroxylase, and the *acidic* pathway which utilizes a developmentally regulated and distinct microsomal oxysterol 7α-hydroxylase[2–4]. Both pathways are complex and share common reactions catalysed by at least 15 enzymes located within different subcellular compartments of the hepatocyte. The final steps in bile acid synthesis involve conjugation with the amino acids glycine and taurine, so that very small proportions of unconjugated bile acids are normally secreted in bile[5].

The biosynthetic pathway for bile acids was elucidated many decades ago, and the first recognized genetic defect was a 27-hydroxylase deficiency accounting for the rare lipid storage disease of cerebrotendinous xanthomatosis[6]. Further biochemical defects have since been identified, in which the activities of the enzymes catalysing reactions affecting the steroid nucleus and the side-chain are deficient.

All defects can be identified from urinary bile acid analysis by fast atom bombardment ionization mass spectrometry (FAB-MS). This relatively simple technique involves spotting a few microlitres of urine or a urine extract onto a glycerol matrix that is bombarded by a beam of fast atoms upon introduction of

"

the probe into the mass spectrometer. Mass spectra are characterized by an absence or markedly reduced concentration of primary bile acids and concomitant increases in atypical bile acids having structural features resembling the substrates for the deficient enzymes. Inborn errors in bile acid synthesis account for at least 2% of cases of liver disease in infants and children, and should be considered an important category of metabolic liver disease[7–10].

DEFECTS INVOLVING REACTIONS TO THE STEROID NUCLEUS

Three well defined defects have been identified involving enzymes catalysing reactions that modify the AB rings of the steroid nucleus[11–13]. The structural position of these defects is indicated in Figure 1. In addition, a 12α-hydroxylase defect was proposed some years ago but never definitively confirmed[14]. The clinical presentation of all of these metabolic defects is variable[9,10], but in general, progressive cholestatic liver disease is the main manifestation of patients presenting with markedly impaired primary bile acid synthesis due to steroid nuclear defects. Typical biochemical abnormalities are elevations in serum liver enzymes, a conjugated hyperbilirubinaemia and evidence of fat-soluble vitamin malabsorption. In the early years, subnormal levels of serum fat-soluble vitamins, and in some cases rickets, often precede any evidence of liver dysfunction[15]. These abnormalities are generally corrected by oral vitamin supplementation, but patients eventually present later in life with hepatosplenomegaly and elevated serum liver enzymes. The 3β-hydroxy-C$_{27}$-steroid dehydrogenase/isomerase deficiency is the most common of the bile acid synthetic defects accounting for late-onset chronic cholestatic syndromes. A normal

3β-Hydroxy-C$_{27}$-steroid dehydrogenase/isomerase deficiency
(Clayton P.T. et al J. Clin Invest. 1997;79:1031–9) involving carbon atoms C-5 and C-6
Δ^4-3-oxosteroid 5β-reductase deficiency
(Setchell K.D.R. et al J. Clin Invest. 1988;82:2148–57) involving carbon atoms C-4 and C-5 and the C-3 hydroxyl
oxysterol 7α-hydroxylase deficiency
(Setchell K.D.R. et al J. Clin Invest. 1988;102:1690–1703) involving hydroxy at C-7

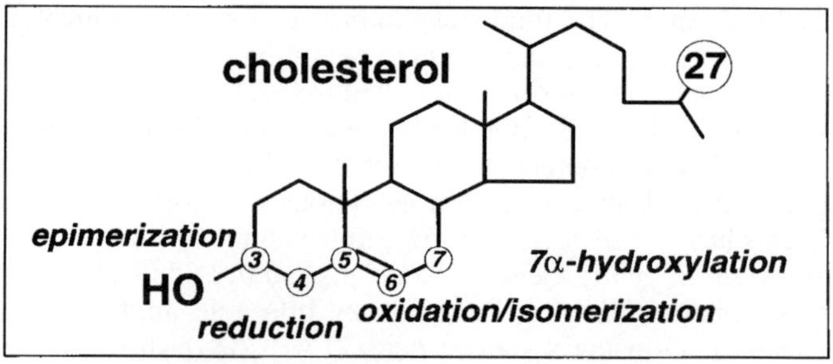

Figure 1. Metabolic defects involving changes to the steroid rings are clinically manifest as familial intrahepatic cholestatic (PFIC) syndromes.

gamma-glutamyltranspeptidase (GGT) is strongly associated with, although not an exclusive feature of, all of these bile acid synthetic defects.

Bile acid synthetic defects are a cause of progressive familial intrahepatic cholestasis (PFIC), and should be classified as a distinct entity of the PFIC syndrome, separate from the defects in canalicular transport proteins[16]. PFIC was initially identified in an Amish family named Byler, thus the designation of Byler's disease[17]. Byler's disease has been genetically mapped to the same chromosomal region as that of benign recurrent intrahepatic cholestasis (BRIC) even though these two cholestatic syndromes are phenotypically different[18,19]. It has become evident that PFIC syndromes can be caused by defects in several canalicular transporters, including the BSEP (bile salt export pump) deficiency and MDR1 and MDR3 (multidrug resistant protein) mutations[16], but these can be differentially diagnosed. A shared feature of Byler's disease (designated PFIC Type 1), and the bile salt exporter defect (designated PFIC Type 2)[20] with inborn errors in bile acid synthesis, is a consistently low serum GGT level, but the diagnoses can be distinguished by bile acid analysis (Table 1). PFIC Type 1 and 2 patients have high serum bile acid concentrations, whereas primary bile acids are absent or negligible in bile acid synthetic defects. PFIC Type 3, on the other hand, is characterized by a high GGT level and defective phospholipid secretion[21]. All of these defects can be recognized by a combination of molecular and analytical studies. Bile acid and phospholipid analysis of bile facilitates the differential diagnosis.

There are several key differences in the clinical presentation and prognosis of bile acid synthetic defects and of Byler's disease (Table 1). The prognosis for patients with bile acid synthetic defects is excellent when oral bile acid therapy is initiated before there is significant loss of quantitative liver function. In several patients the need for orthotopic liver transplantation has been avoided once a

Table 1. Comparative features of patients with intrahepatic cholestasis due to bile acid synthetic defects and Byler's syndrome, recently separated into PFIC-1 and PFIC-2

Feature	Bile acid defects	PFIC-1* and PFIC-2[†]
Age at presentation	Variable, late onset	< 1 year*[†]
Prognosis	Excellent	Fatal in first[†] to second* decade
Liver	Hepatosplenomegaly	Hepatosplenomegaly*[†]
Pruritus	Usually absent	Severe*[†]
Growth failure	Mild	Severe*[†]
Jaundice	+/–	Mild/severe*[†]
Serum transaminases	Elevated	Slight* to substantial[†] elevations
Serum GGT	Generally normal	Normal*[†]
Serum cholesterol	Normal or low	Low*[†]
Fat-soluble vitamins	Malabsorption	Malabsorption*[†]
Bile acids	No primary bile acids	Primary bile acids*[†]
Treatment	Bile acid therapy	Transplantation*[†]

* caused by *FIC1* mutations
[†] caused by *BSEP* mutations

diagnosis was made, and we would suggest that all patients awaiting transplantation should be screened for these bile acid synthetic defects. By contrast, patients with Byler's disease have severe growth failure and often die before 3 years of age without transplantation.

A more recently described defect, an oxysterol 7α-hydroxylase deficiency, has been found in only one patient thus far[13] but has provided insight into the developmental importance of the acidic pathway for bile acid synthesis in early life. The index case was a patient from a consanguineous marriage who presented with jaundice, elevated transaminases but a normal GGT, and eventually died of sepsis following orthotopic liver transplantation. The urine fast atom bombardment-MS mass spectrum revealed the lack of any primary bile acids, with a predominance of unsaturated monohydroxy-C_{24} bile acids conjugated with sulphate and glycosulphate moieties. Upon further analysis by gas chromatography-mass spectrometry, > 95% of the bile acids in urine and serum were confirmed to be 3β-hydroxy-Δ^5-cholenoic acids, and there was complete lack of any 7α-hydroxylated compounds. In addition, the neutral sterol profiles of urine and serum had 27-hydroxycholesterol levels that were > 4500-fold greater than normal, and there was no evidence of any 7α-hydroxycholesterol. At the time of transplantation of the patient with the oxysterol 7α-hydroxylase deficiency, the liver was obtained and showed portal fibrosis, multinucleated giant-cell transformation, and bile duct proliferation. Liver tissue was devoid of oxysterol 7α-hydroxylase activity and mRNA, and analysis of the structure of the *CYP7B1* gene revealed a cytosine to thymidine transition mutation at position 388, providing unambiguous confirmation of the genetic defect. These combined findings supported a defect in oxysterol 7α-hydroxylase. This enzyme is active on 27-hydroxycholesterol and is essential for protecting the liver from hepatotoxic and cholestatic 3β-hydroxy-Δ^5-monohydroxy bile acids that would otherwise accumulate from synthesis in this acidic pathway[13].

DEFECTS INVOLVING REACTIONS LEADING TO SIDE-CHAIN MODIFICATION

Those defects involving side-chain hydroxylation and oxidation (Figure 2) tend to present with a wide spectrum of neurological disease, failure to thrive, and fat-soluble vitamin malabsorption[22,23]. The final step in bile acid synthesis couples the amino acids, glycine and taurine to cholic and chenodeoxycholic acids, and this is a two step reaction involving a bile acid-CoA ligase[24] and a bile acid-CoA:amino acid N-acyltransferase[25]. The capacity of the human liver for conjugation is high and consequently the proportion of unconjugated bile acids in bile is typically < 2%[26]. Conjugation of bile acids ensures conservation of the pool, stimulates bile flow and lipid secretion and promotes lipid and fat-soluble vitamin absorption[1]. Defective amidation has been described recently in several patients, and is manifest clinically as a syndrome of severe fat-soluble vitamin malabsorption and rickets. Three patients have now been diagnosed with an amidation defect after a failure to identify any glycine or taurine conjugated bile acids in their urine, serum, bile, or faeces: these fluids contained exclusively unconjugated deoxycholic and cholic acids, and sulphate and glucuronide con-

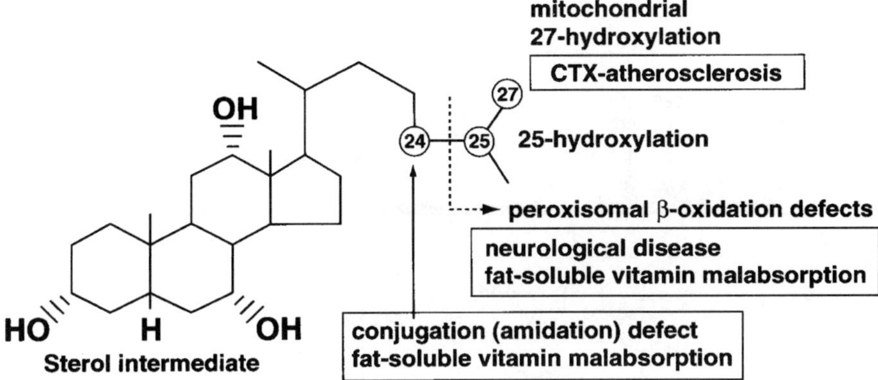

Figure 2. Metabolic defects involving changes to the side-chain.

jugates. The absence of intraluminal bile acid conjugates and the rapid passive absorption of unconjugated cholic acid from the proximal small intestine leads to a lack of mixed micelles necessary for the absorption of fat-soluble vitamins, and accounts for the rickets in these patients[27]. The recent finding of conjugation defects in three patients indicates that screening for bile acid synthetic defects should be extended to conditions of unexplained fat-soluble vitamin malabsorption[27].

The peroxisome is an essential organelle for bile acid synthesis, because it packages the enzymes responsible for β-oxidation of the side-chain of the bile acid intermediates, dihydroxy- and trihydroxy-cholestanoic acid[22,28]. Complete absence of peroxisomes, as in the condition of Zellweger syndrome, or deficiencies of a single peroxisomal enzyme have a profound effect on primary bile acid synthesis, resulting in a heterogeneous clinical phenotype[8]. Most notably, there is often a significant liver involvement, especially in the more severely affected patients, and as a result of diminished primary bile acid synthesis, fat-soluble vitamin absorption is usually impaired. Zellweger patients generally have elevated liver enzymes, and although bile acid therapy with cholic acid has proved effective in treating the liver involvement[23], the prognosis for such patients is poor due to multi-organ abnormalities. Bile acid therapy, however, can be helpful in those patients having single enzyme defects because it will increase intraluminal concentrations of bile acids to assist in the absorption of fats and fat-soluble vitamins while preventing the onset of liver disease.

IDENTIFICATION OF A THCA-CoA OXIDASE DEFICIENCY

Several years ago we identified a unique patient who presented at the Children's Hospital in Dallas at 3 weeks of age with a mild elevation in serum transaminases (AST 114 IU/l, ALT 59 IU/l, GGT 273 IU/l) and very low concentrations of fat-soluble vitamins. Her serum 25-hydroxy-vitamin D was 5 ng/ml (normal > 15 ng/ml) and vitamin E was 2.2 ng/ml (normal range 3–15 ng/ml).

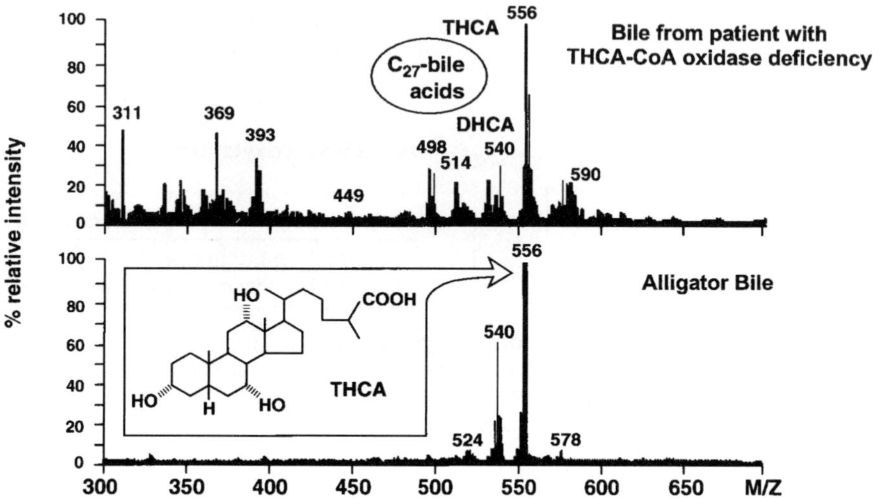

Figure 3. FAB-MS analysis of bile from a patient with a THCA-CoA oxidase deficiency and an alligator (*Alligator mississippiensis*).

Physical examination of this African-American female was unremarkable. At 2.5 months of age, on the suspicion of a bile acid synthetic defect, urine from this patient was analysed by FAB-MS and found to have a mass spectrum typical of patients with Zellweger syndrome[29]. The major ion in the mass spectrum was at m/z 572, reflecting the excretion of taurine-conjugated tetrahydroxy-cholestanoic (C_{27}) acid isomers characteristic of peroxisomal dysfunction. Confirmation of these bile acids was established from subsequent GC-MS analysis. Trihydroxy-cholestanoic acid (THCA) alone accounted for 10%, 28%, and 27% of the bile acids in urine, plasma and bile respectively. C_{27}-bile acids are the major bile acids of the alligator and other reptiles and amphibians[30,31], and a bile sample obtained from an alligator (*Alligator mississippiensis*) in Florida interestingly showed an almost identical FAB-MS spectrum to that of the patient (Figure 3), having intense ions at m/z 556 and m/z 540 consistent with the pseudomolecular ions for taurine conjugated trihydroxy- and dihydroxy-cholestanoic acids, respectively.

The FAB-MS and GC-MS analyses of the urine, bile and serum were consistent with that seen in cerebrohepatorenal syndrome of Zellweger[29,32]; but the patient had none of the physical signs or clinical symptoms of Zellweger syndrome. Plasma very long chain fatty acids (VLCFA) and other peroxisomal enzyme markers were all normal. At 10 weeks of age the patient was admitted to the Children's Hospital in Cincinnati for further clinical investigation and then started on fat-soluble vitamin supplements, and cholic acid therapy (15 mg/kg/day). The patient is neurologically and developmentally normal at age 3.5 years. Her LFTs have normalized on therapy. The family history of this patient was also remarkable: a previous sibling who was healthy until 5.5 months of age died suddenly following an intracranial bleed secondary to vitamin K deficiency. The liver of this sibling, apparently with the same bile acid synthetic defect, was transplanted, and the recipient is in good health 5 years later but receiving oral bile acid therapy.

The biochemical presentation of this patient is consistent with a deficiency in the peroxisomal enzyme, THCA-CoA oxidase. The finding of significant levels of C_{29}-dicarboxylic acid would rule out a defect in THCA-CoA synthetase enzyme, although it is still possible that there may be defective delivery of THCA-CoA into the peroxisome, which could explain the biochemical presentation. The finding of normal VLCFA rules out a disorder in the peroxisomal trifunctional protein or the thiolase, since these enzymes share common substrates in bile acids and VLCFA. Two distinct acyl-CoA oxidases have been identified in humans[33], while the rat has three isozymes[34]. The human acyl-CoA oxidase active on bile acid C_{27}-cholestanoic acid intermediates has been found in the human to be the same enzyme that catalyses the oxidation of 2-methyl branched chain fatty acids[33]. The cDNA of the gene encoding this human enzyme has now been cloned[35]. There have been several case reports of presumed THCA-CoA oxidase deficiencies, and phytanic acid and pristanic acid, when measured, have been elevated in these patients[36–40].

Based on very limited descriptions of the clinical history of four patients[36–38], and on detailed information on a fifth patient[40], it appears that the infant we describe exhibits quite a different phenotype. All of the previously reported patients showed ataxia as a primary feature of the disease, its onset occurring at about 3.5 years of age. The patient we describe here has no evidence of a neurological disorder and has developed normally, albeit while on bile acid therapy. There has been no history of ataxia and the primary clinical presentation is one of severe fat-soluble vitamin malabsorption. The family history is marked by the transplantation of apparently the same biochemical disorder. The phenotype of disorders in peroxisomal β-oxidation of bile acids is extremely heterogeneous and difficult to predict.

Our findings again exemplify the important role that bile acids play in the intraluminal solubilization of fat-soluble vitamins. We propose that screening for a bile acid synthetic defect should be considered for patients presenting with unexplained fat-soluble vitamin malabsorption or rickets. Compromised vitamin status in the very young infant can be fatal, as was the case for the sibling of our patient. Early diagnosis of a bile acid synthetic disorder will allow the maximum benefit to be gained from a regimen of primary bile acid therapy in combination with fat-soluble vitamin supplementation.

Acknowledgements

The work described herein was supported in part by grants from the Department of Health and Human Services, Food and Drug Administration grant number FD-R-000995 and the National Institutes of Health, General Clinical Research Center grant number RR08084. We are grateful to Dr. Alex Knisely for helpful discussions relating to PFIC syndromes.

REFERENCES

1. Hofmann AF. Chemistry and enterohepatic circulation of bile acids. Hepatology. 1984;4:4S–14S.
2. Javitt NB. Bile acid synthesis from cholesterol: regulatory and auxiliary pathways. Fed Am Soc Exp Biol J. 1994;8:1308–1311.

3. Cooper AD. Bile acid biosynthesis: An alternate synthetic pathway joins the mainstream. Gastroenterology. 1997;113:2005–2008.

4. Vlahcevic ZR, Stravitz RT, Heuman DM, Hylemon PB, Pandak WM. Quantitative estimations of the contribution of different bile acid pathways to total bile acid synthesis in the rat. Gastroenterology. 1997;113:1949–1957.

5. Russell DW, Setchell KDR. Bile acid biosynthesis. Biochemistry. 1992;31:4737–4739.

6. Setoguchi T, Salen G, Tint GS, Mosbach EH. A biochemical abnormality in cerebrotendinous xanthomatosis. Impairment of bile acid biosynthesis associated with incomplete degradation of the cholesterol side chain. J Clin Invest. 1974;53:1393–1401.

7. Setchell KD, Street JM. Inborn errors of bile acid synthesis. Semin Liver Dis. 1987;7:85–99.

8. Clayton PT. Inborn errors of bile acid metabolism. J Inherit Metab Dis. 1991;14:478–496.

9. Setchell KDR, O'Connell NC. Inborn errors of bile acid metabolism. In: Suchy F, ed. Liver Disease in Children. St. Louis, MO: Mosby-Yearbook, Inc.; 1994:835–851.

10. Setchell KDR. Disorders of bile acid synthesis and metabolism. In: Walker W, Durie P, Hamilton J, Walker-Smith J, Watkins J, eds. Pediatric Gastrointestinal Disease. Pathophysiology, Diagnosis, Management. Toronto/Philadelphia: B.C. Decker, Inc.; 1996.

11. Clayton PT, Leonard JV, Lawson AM et al. Familial giant cell hepatitis associated with synthesis of $3\beta,7\alpha$-dihydroxy- and $3\beta,7\alpha,12\alpha$-trihydroxy-5-cholenoic acids. J Clin Invest. 1987;79:1031–1038.

12. Setchell KDR, Suchy FJ, Welsh MB, Zimmer-Nechemias L, Heubi J, Balistreri WF. Δ^4-3-Oxosteroid 5β-reductase deficiency described in identical twins with neonatal hepatitis. A new inborn error in bile acid synthesis. J Clin Invest. 1988;82:2148–2157.

13. Setchell KDR, Schwarz M, O'Connell NC et al. Identification of a new inborn error in bile acid synthesis: Mutation of the oxysterol 7α-hydroxylase gene causes severe neonatal liver disease. J Clin Invest. 1998;102:1690–1703.

14. Iser JH, Dowling RH, Murphy GM. Congenital bile salt deficiency associated with 28 years of intractable constipation. In: Paumgartner G, Stiehl A, eds. Bile Acid Metabolism in Health and Disease. Lancaster: MTP Press, 1977:231–234.

15. Loomes KM, Setchell KDR, Rheingold SR, Piccoli DA. Bile acid synthetic disorder in a symptomatic patient with normal liver enzymes. J Pediatr Gastroenterol Nutr. 1998;26:579.

16. Trauner M, Meier PJ, Boyer JL. Molecular pathogenesis of cholestasis. N Engl J Med. 1998;339:1217–1227.

17. Clayton RJ, Iber FL, Ruebner BH, McKusick VA. Byler disease. Fatal familial intrahepatic cholestasis in an Amish kindred. Am J Dis Child. 1969;117:112–124.

18. Bull LN, van Eijk MJT, Pawlikowska L et al. A gene encoding a P-type ATPase mutated in two forms of hereditary cholestasis. Nat Genet. 1998;18:219–223.

19. Bull LN, Carlton VE, Stricker NL et al. Genetic and morphological findings in progressive familial intrahepatic cholestasis (Byler disease [PFIC-1] and Byler syndrome): evidence for heterogeneity. Hepatology. 1997;26:155–164.

20. Strautnieks SS, Bull LN, Knisely AS et al. A gene encoding a liver-specific ABC transporter is mutated in progressive familial intrahepatic cholestasis. Nature Genet. 1998;20:233–238.

21. De Vree JML, Jacquemin E, Sturm E et al. Mutations in the *MDR3* gene cause progressive familial intrahepatic cholestasis. Proc Natl Acad Sci USA. 1998;95:282–287.

22. Wanders RJA, van Roermund CWT, Schutgens RBH et al. The inborn errors of peroxisomal β-oxidation: A review. J Inher Metab Dis. 1990;13:4–36.

23. Setchell KDR, Bragetti P, Zimmer-Nechemias L et al. Oral bile acid treatment and the patient with Zellweger syndrome. Hepatology. 1992;15:198–207.

24. Wheeler JB, Shaw DR, Barnes S. Purification and characterization of a rat liver bile acid coenzyme A ligase from rat liver microsomes. Arch Biochem Biophys. 1997;348:15–24.

25. Falany CN, Johnson MR, Barnes S, Diasio RB. Glycine and taurine conjugation of bile acids by a single enzyme. Molecular cloning and expression of human liver bile acid CoA:amino acid N-acyltransferase. J Biol Chem. 1994;269:19375–19379.

26. Matoba N, Une M, Hoshita T. Identification of unconjugated bile acids in human bile. J Lipid Res. 1986;27:1154–1162.

27. Setchell KDR, Heubi JE, O'Connell NC, Hofmann AF, Lavine JE. Identification of a unique inborn error in bile acid conjugation involving a deficiency in amidation. In: Paumgartner G, Stiehl A, Gerok W, eds. Bile Acids in Hepatobiliary Diseases: Basic Research and Clinical Application. Dordrecht: Kluwer Academic Publishers. 1997:43–47.

28. Bjorkhem I, Kase BF, Pedersen JI. Role of peroxisomes in the biosynthesis of bile acids. Scand J Clin Lab Invest Suppl. 1985;177:23–31.
29. Lawson AM, Madigan MJ, Shortland D, Clayton PT. Rapid diagnosis of Zellweger syndrome and infantile Refsum's disease by fast atom bombardment–mass spectrometry of urine bile salts. Clin Chim Acta. 1986;161:221–231.
30. Haslewood GA. Bile salt evolution. J Lipid Res. 1967;8:535–550.
31. Kuramoto T, Kikuchi H, Sanemori H, Hoshita T. Bile salts of anura. Chem Pharm Bull (Tokyo). 1973;21:952–959.
32. Clayton PT, Lake BD, Hall NA, Shortland DB, Carruthers RA, Lawson AM. Plasma bile acids in patients with peroxisomal dysfunction syndromes: analysis by capillary gas chromatography-mass spectrometry. Eur J Pediatr. 1987;146:166–173.
33. Vanhove GF, Van Veldhoven PP, Fransen M et al. The CoA esters of 2-methyl-branched chain fatty acids and of the bile acid intermediates di- and trihydroxycoprostanic acids are oxidized by one single peroxisomal branched chain acyl-CoA oxidase in human liver and kidney. J Biol Chem. 1993;268:10335–10344.
34. Van Veldhoven PP, Vanhove G, Assselberghs S, Eyssen HJ, Mannaerts GP. Substrate specificities of rat liver peroxisomal acyl-CoA oxidases: palmitoyl-CoA oxidase (inducible acyl-CoA oxidase), pristanoyl-CoA oxidase (non-inducible acyl-CoA oxidase), and trihydroxyco-prostanoyl- CoA oxidase. J Biol Chem. 1992;267:20065–20074.
35. Baumgart E, Vanhooren JC, Fransen M et al. Molecular characterization of the human peroxisomal branched-chain acyl-CoA oxidase: cDNA cloning, chromosomal assignment, tissue distribution, and evidence for the absence of the protein in Zellweger syndrome. Proc Natl Acad Sci USA. 1996;93:13748–13753.
36. Christensen E, Van Eldere J, Brandt NJ, Schutgens RB, Wanders RJ, Eyssen HJ. A new peroxisomal disorder: di- and trihydroxycholestanaemia due to a presumed trihydroxy-cholestanoyl-CoA oxidase deficiency. J Inherit Metab Dis. 1990;13:363–366.
37. Przyrembel H, Wanders RJ, van Roermund CW, Schutgens RB, Mannaerts GP, Casteels M. Di- and trihydroxycholestanoic acidaemia with hepatic failure. J Inherit Metab Dis. 1990;13:367–370.
38. Wanders RJ, Casteels M, Mannaerts GP et al. Accumulation and impaired in vivo metabolism of di- and trihydroxycholestanoic acid in two patients. Clin Chim Acta. 1991;202:123–132.
39. ten Brink HJ, Wanders RJA, Christensen E, Brandt NJ, Jakobs C. Heterogeneity in di/trihydroxy-cholestanoic acidaemia. Ann Clin Biochem. 1994;31:195–197.
40. Clayton PT, Johnson AW, Mills KA et al. Ataxia associated with increased plasma concentrations of pristanic acid, phytanic acid and C27 bile acids but normal fibroblast branched-chain fatty acid oxidation. J Inherit Metab Dis. 1996;19:761–768.

10
The liver in cystic fibrosis

C. COLOMBO, S. COMI and N. BETTINARDI

INTRODUCTION

Cystic fibrosis (CF) is the most common potentially lethal genetic disorder of the Caucasian population, affecting between 1 in 2000 and 1 in 4500 newborns in different ethnic groups[1]. The clinical manifestations of this disease are related to a specific secretory defect which affects epithelial cells in different organs and which causes an inability to maintain the luminal hydration of secretions and progressive duct obstruction. Sweat glands, pancreas, lungs and, in males, the Wolffian ducts are the most commonly affected organs and progressive pulmonary disease is responsible for more than 90% of deaths in CF patients.

Since liver involvement in CF is much less frequent than pulmonary and pancreatic disease and was until recently considered untreatable, it has received little attention for many years. Only recently, due to the improved survival and longer follow-up of CF patients, whose median survival age now exceeds 30 years[2], has there been increasing interest in liver disease since clinically relevant hepatic problems are more frequently observed. According to the American Cystic Fibrosis Foundation Patient Registry, liver disease is now one of the major causes of death in CF patients. Data collected during 1996 on over 19 000 patients revealed that liver disease and liver failure were the third cause of death after cardiorespiratory and transplantation complications, accounting for 2.3% of overall CF mortality[3].

A variety of liver disease occurs in CF (Table 1), including neonatal cholestasis, hepatic steatosis, and hepatic congestion from right-side congestive heart failure. Focal biliary cirrhosis is considered the specific hepatic lesion of CF,

Table 1. Hepatic manifestations of CF

Asymptomatic elevations of serum liver enzymes	10–35%
Neonatal cholestasis	< 2%
Hepatic steatosis, steatohepatitis	20–60%
Focal biliary cirrhosis	11–70%
Multilobular biliary cirrhosis	5–15%

and is the most clinically relevant CF-associated hepatic problem, since progression of the fibrogenic process may result in multilobular biliary cirrhosis, portal hypertension and related complications[4].

As in other liver disease characterized by initial involvement of bile ducts and not of hepatocytes, liver failure is a late event. By contrast, the haemodynamic consequences of cirrhosis are often prominent and severe, favouring early development of portal hypertension and related complications[4]. In a recent retrospective study spanning a 26-year period, of 44 children with CF investigated for liver cirrhosis, oesophageal varices developed in 38 (86%), 50% of whom ultimately bled early in their second decade. Liver failure occurred later in 36% of patients at a mean age of 15 years[5].

PREVALENCE AND INCIDENCE OF LIVER DISEASE IN CF

The prevalence and incidence of focal biliary cirrhosis in CF patients are not clearly defined, mainly because this condition is generally asymptomatic and often associated with normal liver biochemistry[4]. In the absence of sensitive and specific diagnostic markers, focal biliary cirrhosis may not be detected without invasive investigations which are unsuitable for studies in large patient populations. Data derived from autopsy studies indicate a progressive increase in prevalence with age, from 10% in infants[6] to 72% in adults[7].

Prevalence figures obtained by retrospective analyses of clinical records of CF patients are much lower, ranging between 4%[8] and 7%[9]. These studies have also reported a preponderance of male patients among those with liver disease and an incidence peak in adolescence, with a subsequent decrease during the third decade of life[8,9]. On the other hand, studies in which liver disease was actively searched for in large series of CF patients, using biochemical and ultrasonographic assessment, have reported prevalence figures ranging from 18 to 37%[4].

Only two studies have prospectively evaluated the incidence and outcome of liver involvement in CF patients[4,10] and both have provided substantial evidence that liver disease is a relatively early complication of CF, which may be therefore suitable for prophylactic strategies. In fact, in both these cohorts of Swedish[10] and Italian[4] CF patients, who had been followed up for about 10 years, liver disease developed before adolescence, had a slow rate of progression and did not influence nutritional status and severity of pulmonary involvement until the most advanced stage of the disease.

In the Swedish study, liver biopsy performed in 41 patients, 15 of whom had had a previous biopsy, showed that the histological changes also progressed slowly[10]. In the Italian study, CF patients who had a history of neonatal meconium ileus were about six times as likely to develop liver disease as those who did not. This finding is in agreement with data obtained by a necropsy study[11], and suggests that liver disease in CF preferentially develops in patients who have already suffered intestinal obstruction due to inspissated gut content.

PATHOGENESIS OF CF-ASSOCIATED LIVER DISEASE

After the discovery of the CF gene in 1989, it became clear that the CF gene product, CFTR (cystic fibrosis transmembrane regulator), is a cAMP-dependent chloride channel located in the apical membrane of secretory epithelial cells, whose function is to regulate not only transmembrane efflux of chloride ions, but also other ion channels (outward rectifying chloride and basolateral potassium channels) and to operate in parallel with different anion exchangers (Cl^-/ HCO_3^- and Na^+/H^+ exchangers). CFTR is therefore involved in multiple epithelial transport functions, including HCO_3^- secretion, Na^+ reabsorption, exocytosis and mucin secretion[12]. Studies of tissue localization of CFTR have indicated that its expression at the hepatobiliary level occurs exclusively at the apical domain of epithelial cells lining intra and extra-hepatic bile ducts and gallbladder. CFTR is not expressed in hepatocytes and other liver cells and its main role is to participate in the first step of ductal secretion[13].

Absence or dysfunction of CFTR-associated chloride channel in the apical membrane of bile duct cells in CF patients would impair chloride efflux, a process which is essential in the generation of a negative intraluminal potential, paracellular movement of sodium and water, HCO_3^- extrusion via Cl^-/HCO_3^- exchange and ultimately dilution and alkalinization of bile. It should be noted, however, that studies directly assessing the effects of mutated CFTR in cholangiocytes (which may be relevant also to explain the variable severity of liver disease in CF) are not yet available, and that no relationship has been found between liver disease and specific CFTR mutations[14,15]. Abnormalities in mucin secretion may also increase bile viscosity in CF patients[12]. Obstruction of intrahepatic bile ductules by dehydrated secretions may then occur and lead to abnormalities in biliary drainage and, eventually, focal biliary cirrhosis[4]. The biliary epithelium may be then predisposed to damage by cytotoxic compounds excreted into the bile such as bile acids, and to aggression by infectious agents. Light- and electron-microscopic investigations of liver biopsies in CF patients have shown that abnormalities of cholangiocytes, with irregular shapes, necrosis and increased collagen deposition are a consistent finding, and may represent the anatomical expression of a long-standing impairment of ductular bile flow[16].

TREATMENT OF CF-ASSOCIATED LIVER DISEASE

With better knowledge of the pathophysiology of the disease, a number of therapeutic strategies are under study, including pharmacological correction of the defective ion transport function and transfer of the normal CF gene into epithelial cells, which may become applicable to liver disease[17].

At present, oral bile acid therapy, aimed at improving biliary secretion in terms of bile viscosity and bile acid composition, is the most promising therapeutic approach and is virtually devoid of serious side effects[4]. Several open studies and a few controlled studies have documented the beneficial effects of ursodeoxycholic acid (UDCA) treatment in CF patients with liver disease. Biochemical improvement has been a consistent finding, and dose–response studies have established that the optimal dose of UDCA in CF patients is 20 mg/kg body weight/day. This dose is higher than that conventionally used in other cholestatic liver diseases, so as to compensate for poor intestinal absorption[18]. Improvement in hepatic excretory function and biliary drainage has been documented by hepatobiliary scintigraphy, suggesting that a flushing effect of UDCA due to its cholerectic properties may be important in CF patients whose bile ducts are plugged by inspissated secretions[19,20].

The effects of UDCA treatment on liver morphology have recently been described in 10 CF patients with cirrhosis aged 8–28 years, who were treated with a relatively dose of UDCA (10 mg/kg/day) for 2 years[21]. Liver biopsy was performed before, and after 12 and 24 months of treatment, and evaluated blindly using a scoring system focused on portal changes. Liver morphology improved and in some patients there was also amelioration in some electron microscopic features, including bile duct dilatation and blebbing, number and shape of microvilli.

Improvement in essential fatty acid status has been also documented in a placebo-controlled crossover study and may have important extrahepatic implications[22]. Essential fatty acid deficiency occurs in a substantial proportion of patients with CF, and is not corrected by essential fatty acid supplementation[23]. It may have a negative impact on the progression of pulmonary disease by altering eicosanoid production and immune function.

These data are extremely important, but information on the long-term effects of treatment is urgently needed. None of the three placebo-controlled trials of UDCA so far available has been large or long enough (maximum follow-up 12 months) adequately to assess the effects of treatment on clinically relevant endpoints such as need for liver transplantation and death[24–26]. However, the dramatic improvement of biochemical and scintigraphic parameters of cholestasis suggests that long-term, placebo-controlled trials of UDCA can no longer be considered feasible or ethically justifiable. Data on long-term treatment should be obtained by careful monitoring and follow-up of patients.

In our CF patients with liver disease, the clinical and biochemical response to long-term UDCA administration was much better in those who showed impairment of biliary drainage, as indicated by prolonged time of intestinal appearance of the tracer on hepatobiliary scintigraphy; patients presenting with similar biochemical abnormalities but no scintigraphic abnormality did not seem to benefit from treatment[27]. It is likely that different pathogenetic mechanisms are involved in CF patients with liver disease and that in some UDCA may be ineffective.

CONCLUSIONS

UDCA is usually administered to CF patients only after signs and symptoms of liver disease become evident, but at this stage liver disease has usually progressed. It is likely that effectiveness of bile acid therapy is greatest in patients with early stage liver disease, before symptoms have become evident. Early diagnosis and identification of CF patients who are more liable to development of liver disease should be actively pursued. Prospective studies evaluating the effects of early treatment with UDCA should be carried out.

REFERENCES

1. Welsh MJ, Tsui L, Boat TF et al. Cystic fibrosis. In: Scriver CR, Beaudet AL, Sly WS et al., eds. The metabolic and molecular bases of inherited disease. 7th ed. New York: McGraw-Hill, 1995: 3799–3876.
2. FitzSimmons SC. The changing epidemiology of cystic fibrosis. J Pediatr. 1993;122:1–9.
3. FitzSimmons SC. Cystic Fibrosis Foundation, Patent Registry 1996 Annual Data Report, Bethesda, Maryland, August 1997.
4. Colombo C, Battezzati PM, Strazzabosco M, Podda M. Liver and biliary problems in cystic fibrosis. Semin Liver Dis. 1998;18:227–235.
5. Debray D, Lykavieris P, Gauthier F et al. Outcomes of liver cirrhosis in cystic fibrosis. Management of portal hypertension. J Hepatol. 1999 in press.
6. Oppenheimer EH, Esterly JR. Hepatic changes in young infants with cystic fibrosis: possible relation to focal biliary cirrhosis. J Pediatr. 1975;86:683–689.
7. Vawter GF, Shwachman H. Cystic fibrosis in adults: an autopsy study. Pathol Ann. 1979;14:357–382.
8. Scott-Jupp R, Lama M, Tanner MS. Prevalence of liver disease in cystic fibrosis. Arch Dis Child. 1991;66:698–701.
9. Feigelson J, Anagnostopoulos C, Pouquet M, Pecau Y, Munck A, Navarro J. Liver cirrhosis in cystic fibrosis. Therapeutic implications and long-term followup. Arch Dis Child. 1993;68:653–657.
10. Lindblad A, Glaumann H, Strandvik B. CF-associated liver disease – a prospective study for 15 years. Proceedings of the 22nd European Cystic Fibrosis Conference. Berlin, June 1998, p. 109.
11. Maurage C, Lenaerts C, Weber AM, Brochu P, Yousef I, Roy CC. Meconium ileus and its equivalent as a risk factor for the development of cirrhosis: an autopsy study in cystic fibrosis. J Pediatr Gastroenterol Nutr. 1989;9:17–20.
12. Stutts MJ, Boucher RC. Cystic fibrosis gene and functions of CFTR. Implications of dysfunctional ion transport for pulmonary pathogenesis. In: Yankaskas JR, Knowles MR, eds. Cystic Fibrosis in Adults. Philadelphia: Lippincott-Raven Publishers,1999:3–25.
13. Cohn JA, Strong TV, Picciotto MEt, Nairn AC, Collins FS, Fitz JG. Localization of the cystic fibrosis transmembrane conductance regulator in human bile duct epithelial cells. Gastroenterology. 1993;105:1857–1864.
14. Duthie A, Doherty DG, Williams C et al. Genotype analysis for DF 508, G551D and R553X mutations in children and young adults with cystic fibrosis with and without liver disease. Hepatology. 1992;15:660–664.
15. Colombo C, Apostolo MG, Ferrari M et al. Analysis of risk factors for the development of liver disease in CF. J Pediatr. 1994;124:393–399.
16. Lindblad A, Hultcrantz ET, Strandvik B. Bile duct destruction and collagen deposition: a prominent ultrastructural feature of the liver in cystic fibrosis. Hepatology. 1992;16:372–381.
17. Yang Y, Raper SE, Cohn LA, Engelhardt JF, Wilson JM. An approach for treating the hepatobiliary disease of cystic fibrosis by somatic gene transfer. Proc Natl Acad Sci USA. 1993;90:4601–4605.
18. Colombo C, Crosignani A, Assaisso ML et al. Ursodeoxycholic acid therapy in Cystic Fibrosis associated liver disease: a dose-response study. Hepatology. 1992;16:924–930.
19. Colombo C, Castellani MR, Balistreri WF, Seregni E, Assaisso ML, Giunta A. Scintigraphic documentation of an improvement in hepatobiliary excretory function after treatment with ursodeoxycholic acid in patients with cystic fibrosis and associated liver disease. Hepatology. 1992;15:677–684.
20. O'Connor PJ, Southern KW, Bowler IM, Irving HC, Robinson PJ, Littlewood JM. The role of hepatobiliary scintigraphy in cystic fibrosis. Hepatology. 1996;23:281–287.
21. Lindblad A, Aaumann H, Strandvik B. A two-year prospective study of the effect of ursodeoxycholic acid on urinary bile acid excretion and liver morphology in cystic fibrosis. Hepatology. 1998;23:166–174.

22. Lepage G, Paradis K, Lacaille F et al. Ursodeoxycholic acid improves the hepatic metabolism of essential fatty acids and retinol in children with cystic fibrosis. J Pediatr. 1997;130:52–58.
23. Dodge JA, Custance JM, Goodchild MC, Laing SC, Vaughan M. Paradoxical effects of essential fatty acid supplementation on lipid profiles and sweat electrolytes in cystic fibrosis. Br J Nutr. 1990;63:259–271.
24. O'Brien S, Fitzgerald MX, Hegarty JE. A controlled trial of ursodeoxycholic acid treatment in cystic fibrosis-related liver disease. Eur J Gastroenterol Hepatol. 1992;4:857–863.
25. Merli M, Bertasi S, Servi R et al. Effect of a medium dose of ursodeoxycholic acid with or without taurine supplementation on the nutritional status of patients with cystic fibrosis: a randomized, placebo-controlled, crossover trial. J Pediatr Gastroenterol Nutr. 1994;19:198–203.
26. Colombo C, Battezzati PM, Podda M, Betffnardi, Giunta A and the Italian Group for the Study of Ursodeoxycholic acid in Cystic Fibrosis. Ursodeoxycholic acid for liver disease associated with cystic fibrosis: a double-blind multicenter trial. Hepatology. 1996;23:1484–1490.
27. Colombo C, Crosignani A, Battezzati PM et al. Delayed intestinal visualization at hepatobiliary scintigraphy is associated with response to long-term treatment with ursodeoxycholic acid in patients with cystic fibrosis-associated liver disease. J Hepatol. 1999;31:672–677.

11
Canalicular secretion of lysyl-fluorescein conjugated bile acids in 17β-estradiol glucuronide (17βEG) induced cholestasis: protective effect of s-adenosyl-L-methionine (SAMe)

P. MILKIEWICZ, C.O. MILLS, M.G. ROMA,
J. AHMED-CHOUDHURY, R. COLEMAN and E. ELIAS

INTRODUCTION

Lysyl-fluorescein conjugated bile acid analogues (LFCBAA)

These represent a group of fluorescein-labelled congeners of naturally occurring bile acids. All these compounds are soluble in water and have several physico-chemical and biological properties similar to their natural equivalents[1-4]. In this study we applied three different LFCBAA: cholyl-lysyl-fluorescein (CLF), an analogue of cholyl-glycine; ursodeoxycholyl-lysyl-fluorescein (UDCLF), an analogue of ursodeoxycholyl-glycine; and sulpholithocholyl-lysyl-fluorescein (sLLF), an analogue of sulpholithocholyl-glycine. Molecular structures of these LFCBAA are given in Figure 1. Previous work showed that these compounds are taken up by the liver and secreted into bile in a fashion similar to their natural congeners[4]. Moreover, our recent study in mutant TR-/GY (Groningen Yellow) rats[5] clearly showed that biliary secretion of sLLF is impaired to an extent similar to that of sulpholithocholyl-glycine, suggesting that sLLF, like its parent compound, is a substrate of the multidrug resistant protein 2 (mrp2) localized to the canalicular membrane of the hepatocyte[6,7].

Oestrogen cholestasis

Although the cholestatic properties of oestrogens have been documented in several studies, the mechanisms by which they impair bile flow are still debated.

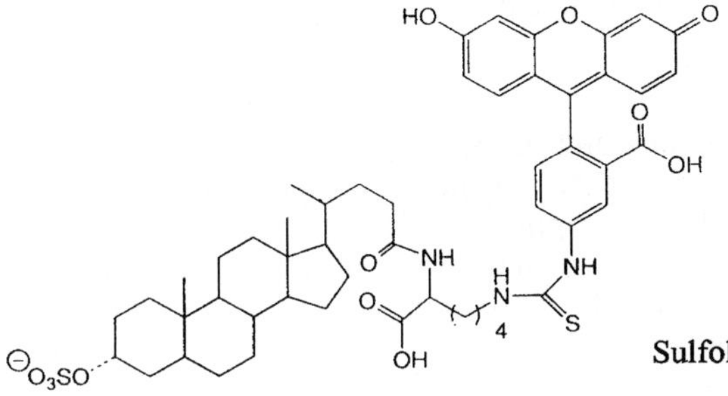

Figure 1. Molecular structures of the LFCBAAs used in this study.

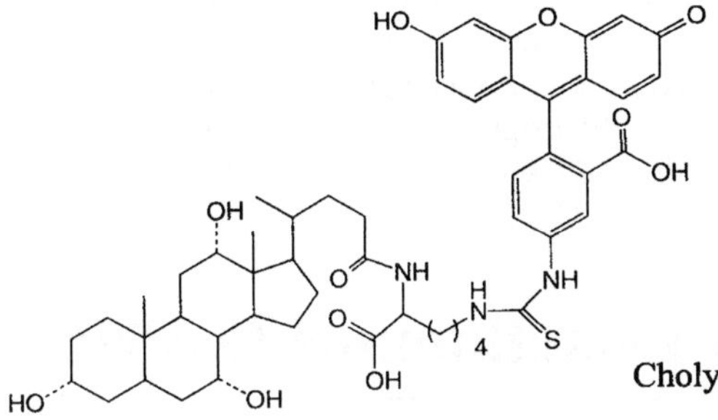

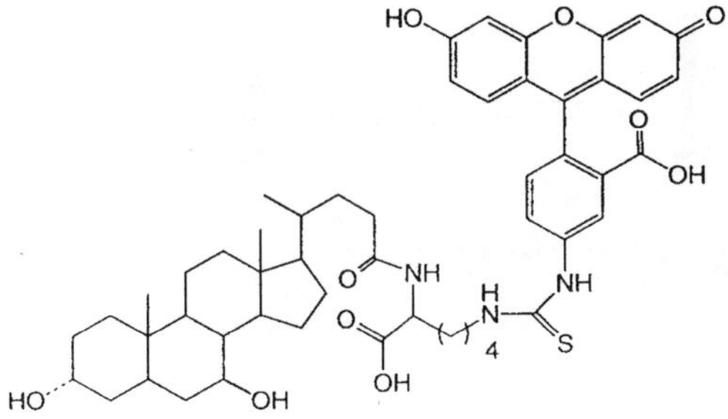

Several mechanisms potentially involved in oestrogen-induced cholestasis have been postulated, including impairment of the fluidity of the sinusoidal membrane[8], increased permeability of tight junctions[9,10], decreased sinusoidal uptake of bile acids[11] or decreased expression of mrp2[11–13]. The cholestatic effect of naturally occurring oestrogens may be mediated by 17β-estradiol glucuronide (17βEG), the oestrogen metabolite with greatest cholestatic potential[14,15].

S-adenosyl-L-methionine

SAMe is a naturally occurring compound participating in several biochemical processes. It is a major methyl donor in mammalian cells, and transmethylation by SAMe is an important mechanism applied by hepatocytes to detoxify a variety of substances. It is also an intermediary metabolite in the synthesis of cysteine and glutathione, and may also be a provider of sulphate[16,17] (Figure 2). Liver glutathione, which is derived from SAMe through the trans-sulphuration pathway, plays a crucial role in the maintenance of the normal redox potential[18]. Chronic liver disease may cause depletion of SAMe, which may lead to a potentially significant impairment of detoxifying processes mediated by this compound or its metabolites. Some studies have suggested that supplementation with SAMe in ethinyl oestradiol (EE)-induced cholestasis increases membrane fluidity and function of Na$^+$/K$^+$ATPase[19]. It has also been postulated that SAMe may be involved in methylation of oestrogen metabolites[20]. Stramentinoli et al. have also suggested that SAMe may enhance sulphation of putative toxic

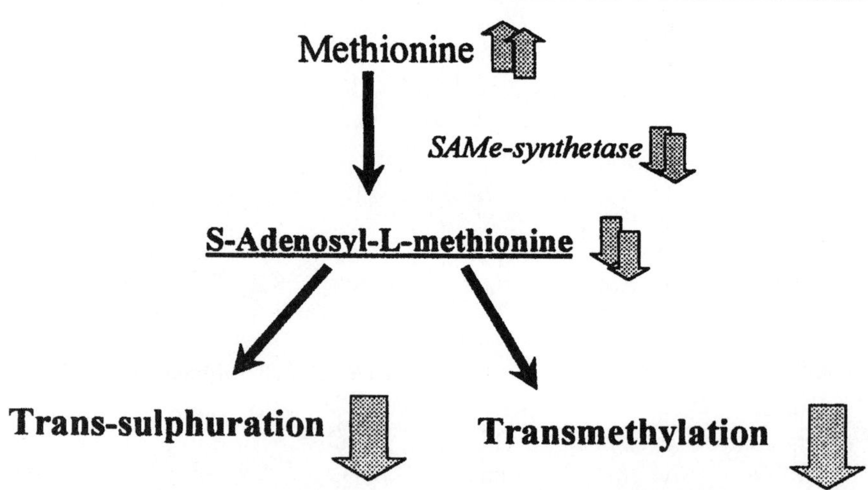

Figure 2. Proposed mechanisms involved in SAMe deficiency-induced hepatic damage. Decreased synthesis of SAMe impairs two crucial detoxifying processes: trans-methylation and trans-sulphuration. It may lead to disturbance of intracellular redox potential and impaired metabolism and elimination of several toxic compounds including hydrophobic bile acids and oestrogen metabolites.

metabolites of oestrogen[21]. Possible consequences of impaired synthesis of SAMe are shown in Figure 2.

Hepatocyte couplets

In these in vitro studies we used hepatocyte couplets, which have proved to be a useful and reproducible model for the study of intrahepatic cholestasis[22].

The aim of this work was to study the canalicular secretion of CLF, UDCLF, and sLLF, the substrate of multidrug resistant protein (mrp2), in 17βEG induced cholestasis. Both CLF and UDCLF are bile salt export pump (BSEP) substrates, but may take different transcellular pathways across the hepatocyte[23]. We also wanted to find out whether SAMe exerts any protective effect on any putative impairment of canalicular accumulation of the fluorescent bile acids caused by 17βEG.

MATERIALS AND METHODS

Materials

Cholyl-lysyl-fluorescein (CLF), ursodeoxycholyl-lysyl-fluorescein (UDCLF) and sulpholithocholyl-lysyl-fluorescein (sLLF) were synthesized according to the method of Mills et al.[1]. The synthetic procedure gave a high yield of all the compounds which appeared as a single spot after high-performance thin layer chromatography. SAMe, in the form of the stable disulfate-di-p-toluene-sulfonate, was provided by Knoll Farmaceutici Spa, Milan, Italy. Collagenase (type A) was obtained from *Clostridium histolyticum* (Boehringer Mannheim, Lewes, Sussex, England). Leibovitz-15 tissue culture medium (L-15) was purchased from Gibco (Paisley, Scotland) and bovine serum albumin was obtained from Winlab (Maidenhead, Berkshire, England); 17βEG and other fine chemicals were obtained from Sigma (Poole, Dorset, England).

Animals

All experimental protocols were approved according to the Animals Scientific Procedures Act 1986. Male Wistar rats (230–240 g body weight) were allowed free access to standard laboratory diet and tap water ad libitum. Surgery was performed between 8 am and 9 am to minimize circadian variations. Anaesthesia was achieved using ketamine hydrochloride, 7 mg/100 body wt with medetomidine, 25 μg/100 g body wt.

Hepatocyte couplet preparation

An initial preparation of hepatocyte couplets was obtained from rat liver according to the two-step collagenase perfusion technique described by Wilton et al.[24], adapted from Gautam et al.[25]. In summary, the procedure involved perfusion of the liver with a Ca^{2+}- and Mg^{2+}- free Hanks balanced salt solution into the portal vein followed by infusion with collagenase (approximately 0.02% according to batch) in Hanks balanced salt solution. The liver was then removed, chopped and agitated in ice-cold Krebs-Henseleit solution. The final suspension was filtered through nylon gauze and the remaining tissue reincubated in the collagenase solution at 37°C to liberate a second cell preparation with high overall viability, as estimated by trypan blue exclusion (using an improved Neubauer haemocytometer). This initial preparation contained 20–30% couplets with viability > 90%. Couplet content was further enriched using centrifugal elutriation as described by Wilton et al.[24]. The final preparation contained 65–80% of couplets, with viability > 95%, which were plated in L-15 medium containing 50 U/ml penicillin and 50 μg/ml streptomycin into 35 mm plastic culture dishes (2 ml/dish) at a density of 0.5×10^6 units/ml, and incubated at 37°C for 4.5 h prior to experimentation. The experimental design for the couplets preparation is presented in Figure 3.

Assessment of canalicular vacuolar accumulation (cVA)

Couplets were incubated for 30 min at 37°C with 2 μM final concentration CLF and UDCLF and for 60 min with sLLF. The cells were then washed twice with 2 ml L-15 medium, and examined using an inverted fluorescence microscope (Olympus IMT2-RFL, Olympus, London, England). The number of couplets accumulating LFCBAA into their canalicular vacuoles as a proportion of the total couplets analysed (100–250 in each experiment) was then determined. This parameter is referred to as cVA of CLF, UDCLF or sLLF.

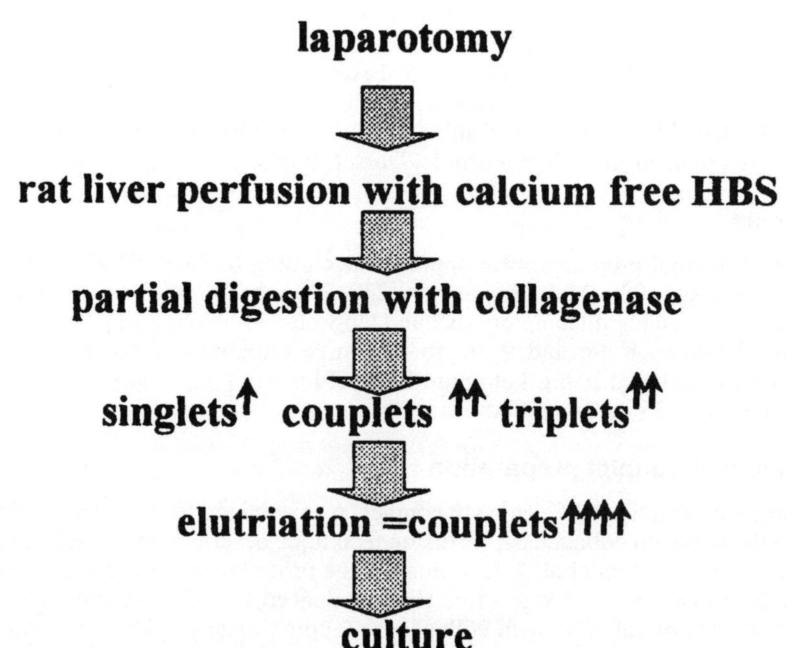

Figure 3. Methodology of hepatocyte couplets preparation.

Effects of 17βEG on cVA of CLF

17βEG was dissolved in dimethyl-sulphoxide (DMSO) and added in increasing concentrations into culture dishes to reach final concentrations of 25, 50, 100, 150 μmol/l. After 30 min incubation at 37°C with 17βEG the culture medium was replaced with fresh L-15 medium and then CLF (to 2 μmol/l final concentration) was added to each plate and incubated at 37°C for 30 min. The couplets were then washed twice with 2 ml L-15 and the accumulating couplets counted as above. On the basis of this experiment a concentration of 17βEG of 50 μmol/l was selected for further studies.

Effect of 17βEG on cVA of UDCLF and sLLF

Couplets were incubated for 30 min with 17βEG. The medium was then replaced with fresh L-15 medium and the couplets were subsequently incubated with UDCLF (2 μmol/final concentration, 30 min) or sLLF (2 μmol/l final concentration, 60 min) and subsequently washed twice with L-15 medium. cVA of CLF was analysed as described above.

Protection against 17βEG-induced cholestasis with SAMe

Couplets were incubated for 30 min at 37°C with 50 μM 17βEG or 17βEG + SAMe (100 μM final concentration). The culture medium was then replaced with L-15 medium and the couplets were subsequently incubated with either CLF, or UDCLF (2 μm mol/l final concentration, 30 min) or sLLF (2 μmol/l final concentration, 60 min). The cVA values with these bile acids were then assessed and compared to those in controls (couplets untreated with 17βEG, incubated with each LFCBAA).

Statistical analysis

Results are expressed as mean or mean ± SE. Statistical comparisons were made using ANOVA factorial using a computing program (Stat View). Differences were considered significant when $p < 0.05$.

RESULTS

Incubation of cells with increasing doses of 17βEG caused a dose dependent decrease of cVA of CLF (Figure 4). On the basis of this curve a concentration of 17βEG of 50 μM was selected for further experiments.

This concentration caused a significant decrease in the cVA of all analysed LFCBAAs (Figures 5–7), with most pronounced effect on cVA of sLLF: p values were < 0.01 for CLF; < 0.05 or UDCLF and < 0.0001 for sLLF respectively (Figures 5–7).

The impairment in the cVA of CLF caused by 17βEG was completely abolished by SAMe, which caused significant improvement in the cVAs of CLF ($p < 0.01$) and UDCLF ($p < 0.05$) (Figures 5, 6), but not sLLF (cVA increase 3–9%, NS: Figure 7).

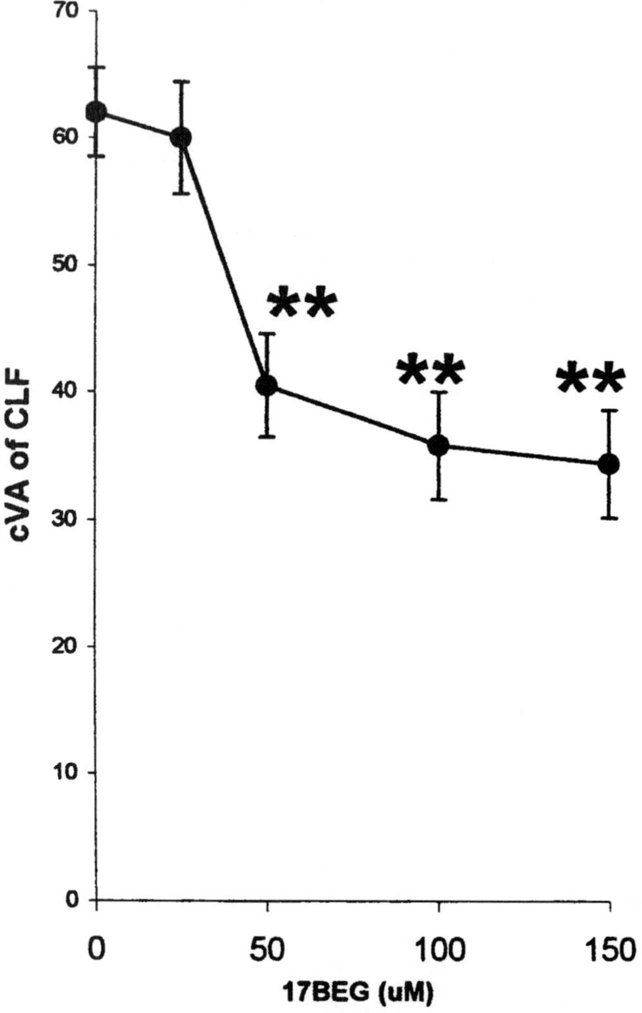

Figure 4. Dose dependent impairment of cVA of CLF induced by 17βEG. On the basis of this curve a 50 μM concentration of 17βEG has been chosen for further experiments. Data expressed as mean ± SE; n = 4–5; **p < 0.01.

DISCUSSION

Fluorescent bile acids have been found to be a useful tool for the study of physiology and pathophysiology of processes involved in the uptake, intracellular transport and canalicular secretion of bile acids. LFCBAA, in particular CLF, have been used extensively in both in vivo and in vitro studies of the physiological and toxicological aspects of hepatocellular function[26–31].

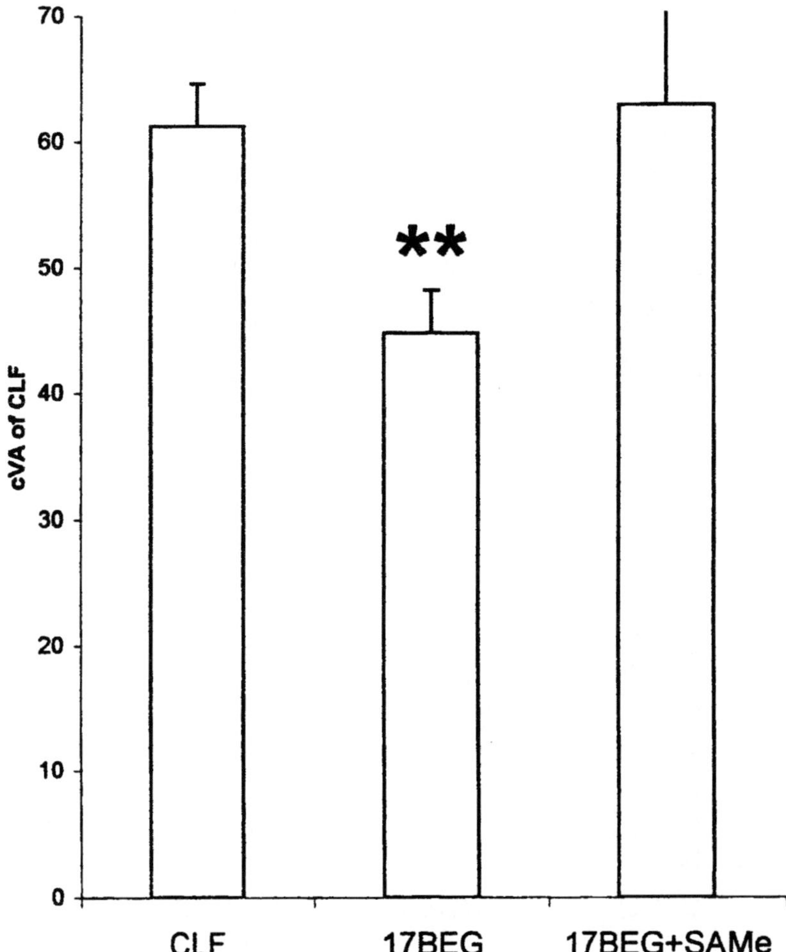

Figure 5. Effect of 17βEG and 17βEG + SAMe on cVA of CLF. 17βEG caused significant decrease of cVA of CLF ($p < 0.01$); SAMe protected against this effect and caused complete restoration of cVA of CLF ($p < 0.01$). Data presented as mean ± SE; $n = 7$; **$p < 0.01$.

In the present work we have demonstrated the canalicular accumulation of three LFCBAA, with different properties in terms of transport, in hepatocyte couplets. All three applied LFCBAA were taken by the couplets and secreted into the canalicular vacuole. Using whole animals or isolated perfused livers, the kinetic parameters of CLF such as K_m or V_{max}, biliary secretion and stimulation of biliary output are close to those of natural cholyl-glycine[1–4]. In other studies, it was shown that UDCLF is comparable to glycoursodeoxycholate (GUDCA) in its hepatocyte transport and biliary secretion and its ability to protect erythrocyte membranes from damage done by taurodeoxycholate[32]. Both CLF and UDCLF are substrates for bile salt transporters in the sinusoidal

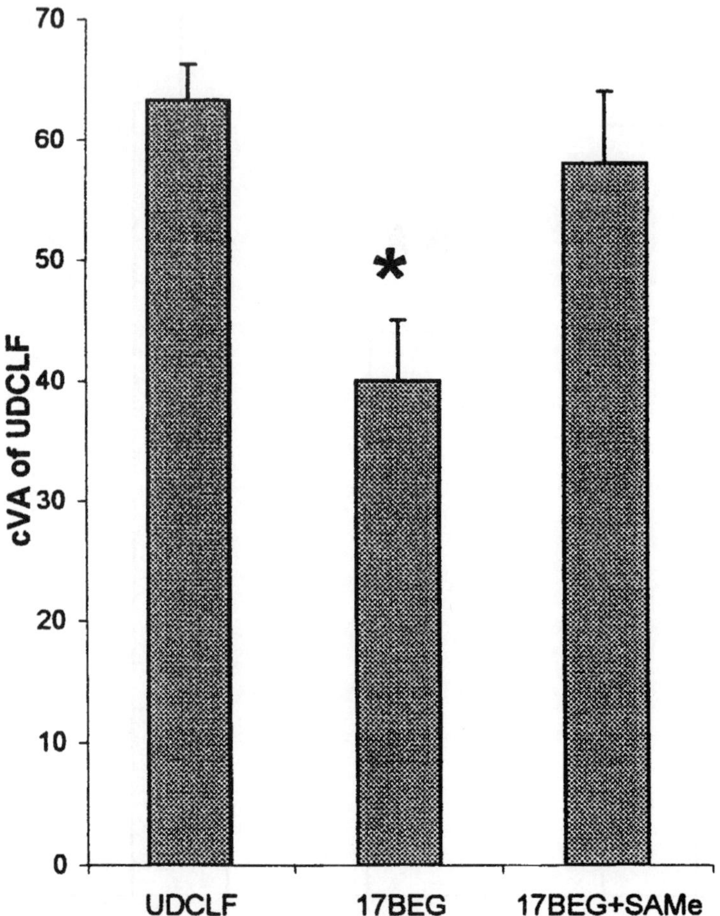

Figure 6. Effect of 17βEG and 17βEG + SAMe on cVA of UDCLF. cVA of UDCLF was significantly reduced by 17βEG ($p < 0.05$) and protected by SAMe ($p < 0.05$). Data presented as mean ± SE; $n = 4$; *$p < 0.05$.

membrane of the hepatocyte and are likely to be substrates for BSEP on the canalicular domain. sLLF has been shown to be secreted into rat bile[5], but with different kinetics from the above two LFCBAA. Its biliary accumulation in TR-/GY rats is, moreover, significantly impaired and, in in vitro studies, the kinetics of sLLF resembles that of mrp2 substrates and suggest that this bile acid may be secreted into the canaliculus via mrp2 rather than BSEP[5].

17βEG causes an impairment of bile flow in rats and disturbance of bile excretory function in the rhesus monkey[33] but the exact mechanisms of the hepatocellular dysfunction caused by 17βEG have not yet been fully elucidated. It has been shown that 17βEG may increase tight junctional permeability[34]; reduce the microvilli at the canalicular pole of the hepatocyte and thicken the peri-

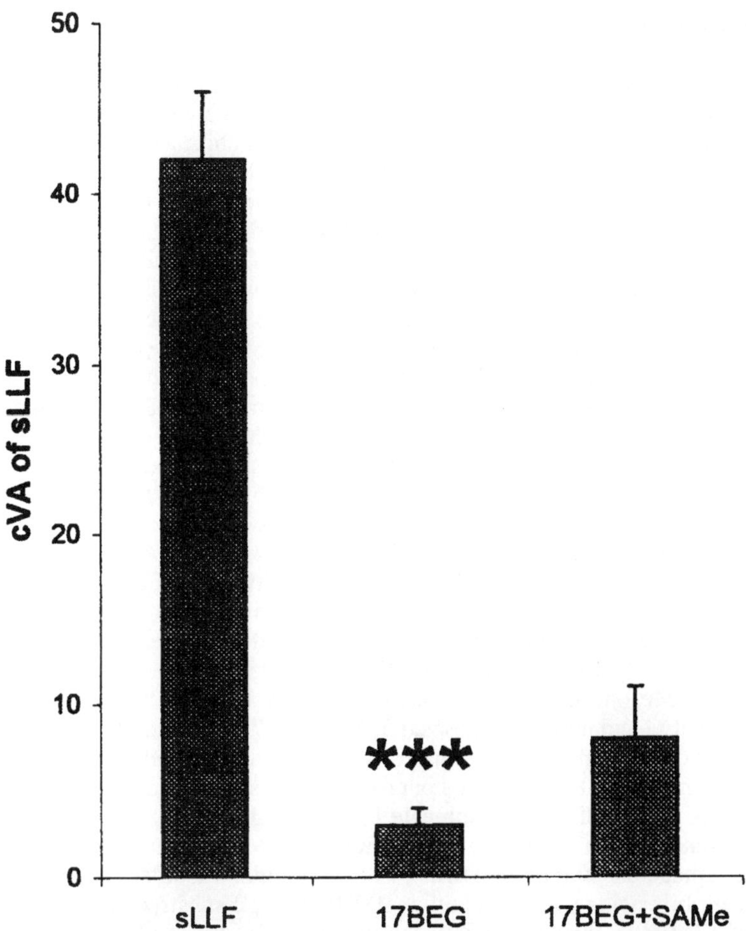

Figure 7. Effect of 17βEG and 17βEG + SAMe on cVA of UDCLF. 17βEG caused a more significant decrease in cVA of sLLF when compared to CLF or UDCLF. Coincubation of the couplets with 17βEG + SAMe did not significantly abolish the effect, despite a clear trend towards a higher cVA of sLLF when SAMe was co-administered. (p = NS). Data presented as mean ± SE; n = 4; ***$p < 0.0001$.

canalicular cytoplasm[35]; and specifically inhibit the function of bile salt transporter(s) due to the structural similarity between D-ring steroidal glucuronides and bile acids[14].

In a recent study, Takikawa et al. demonstrated that 17βEG is secreted into bile, and that biliary secretion of 17βEG was significantly impaired in mutant EHBR rats which, similarly to TR-/GY, do not express functional mrp2[36]. Impaired biliary excretion of 17βEG in mutant EHBR rats, lacking functional mrp2, strongly suggests that 17βEG is an mrp2 substrate. However, if 17βEG is used in cholestatic doses, its uptake at these doses by rat canalicular membrane vesicles has been shown to be inhibited by MDR1 substrates[36], suggesting that at these higher doses it may also become a MDR1 substrate.

Our study showed that 17βEG, at a dose of 50 μM, caused significant impairment of cVA of all analysed LFCBAA. This effect could involve impairment of the accumulation at a number of sites, but the fact that its cholestatic effect was much more pronounced for sLLF may indicate that 17βEG, at cholestatic doses, causes more specific impairment of mrp2 than of BSEP. If we assume that 17βEG participates in the cholestatic effect of oestrogens this finding could complement a recent in vivo study which showed decreased expression of mrp2 and its mRNA in rats chronically treated with ethinyl oestradiol[12]. Although decreased expression of mrp2 seems to be unlikely in the present experiments due to the much shorter time scale used, acute changes in localization of mrp2 may be involved. It has been recently shown, in support of this, that short term perfusion of the rat liver with phalloidin caused dramatic reduction of the presence of mrp2 in the canalicular membrane due to relocalization of mrp2 to intracellular membrane structures[38]. On the other hand, the significant decrease in the cVA of sLLF caused by 17βEG could be also explained by substrate competition for mrp2 by both 17βEG and sLLF.

The impairment of cVA of CLF and UDCLF was almost completely abolished by SAMe. Our preliminary data suggest that SAMe, by acting as a precursor of cysteine and sulphate, may protect against the toxicity of 17βEG by promoting its sulphation in position 3 of the steroid ring. Interestingly, the protective effect of SAMe on canalicular accumulation of sLLF seemed to be weak, despite the fact that it more than doubled the cVA of CLF. We speculate that the apparently weaker effect of SAMe on sLLF may be artificially low because of the competition between 17βEG and newly synthesized 3-sulphate 17-β oestradiol glucuronide for sLLF transport through mrp2, compared with sLLF transport alone through mrp2. Both CLF and UDCLF are pumped out of the cell via BSEP and therefore they do not compete with 17βEG and 3-sulphate 17-β oestradiol glucuronide for mrp2.

In summary, we have shown that 17βEG exerted a cholestatic effect on hepatocyte couplets, causing an impairment of canalicular vacuolar accumulation of fluorescent bile acids which are either BSEP or mrp2 substrates. The inhibitory effect of 17βEG on the canalicular accumulation of sLLF, is likely to be due to a combination of both transporter defect and competition for the canalicular carrier between the cholestatic agent and sLLF. SAMe protects against the cholestasis caused by 17βEG by mechanisms which are under active investigation by ourselves at the present time.

Acknowledgements

We thank the following for support of various aspects of this work: The Sir Jules Thorn Trust (R.C.), EASL/The Sir Samuel Scott of Yews Trust (P.M.), The Wellcome Trust (M.G.R)

REFERENCES

1. Mills CO, Rahman K, Coleman R, Elias E. Cholyl-lysylfluorescein: synthesis, biliary excretion in vivo and during single-pass perfusion of isolated perfused rat liver. Biochim Biophys Acta. 1991;1115:151–156.

2. Baxter DJ, Rahman K, Bushell AJ, Mills CO, Elias E, Billington D. Biliary lipid output by isolated perfused rat livers in response to cholyl-lysylfluorescein. Biochim Biophys Acta. 1995;1256:374–380.
3. Mills CO, Milkiewicz P, Molloy DP, Baxter DJ, Elias E. Synthesis, physical and biological properties of lithocholyllysylfluorescein: a fluorescent bile salt analogue with cholestatic properties. Biochim Biophys Acta. 1997;1336:485–496.
4. Mills CO, Milkiewicz P, Saraswat V, Elias E. Cholyllysylfluorescein and related lysyl fluorescein conjugated bile acid analogues. Yale J Biol Med. 1997;70:447–457.
5. Mills CO, Milkiewicz P, Muller M et al. Different pathways of canalicular secretion of sulfated and non-sulfated fluorescent bile acids: a study in isolated hepatocyte couplets and TR⁻ rats. J Hepatol. 1999;31:678–684.
6. Oude Elferink RPJ, Meijer DKF, Kuipers F, Jansen PLM, Groen AK, Groothuis GM. Hepatobiliary secretion of organic compounds; molecular mechanisms of membrane transport. Biochim Biophys Acta. 1995;1241:215–268.
7. Paulusma CC, Bosma PJ, Zaman GJ et al. Congenital jaundice in rats with a mutation in a multidrug resistance-associated protein gene. Science. 1996;271:1126–1128.
8. Adinolfi LE, Utili R, Gaeta GB, Abernathy CO, Zimmerman HJ. Cholestasis induced by estradiol 17Beta-D-glucuronide: mechanisms and prevention by sodium taurocholate. Hepatology 1984;1:30–37.
9. Elias E, Iqbal S, Knutton S, Hickey A, Coleman R. Increased tight junction permeability: a possible mechanism of oestrogen cholestasis. Eur J Clin Invest. 1983;13:383–390.
10. Iqbal S, Mills CO, Elias E. Biliary permeability during ethinyl estradiol induced cholestasis studied by segmented retrograde intrabiliary injections in rats. J Hepatol. 1985;1:211–219.
11. Bossard R, Stieger B, O'Neil B, Fricker G, Meier PJ. Ethinylestradiol induces multiple canalicular membrane transport alterations in rat liver. J Clin Invest. 1993;91:2714–2720.
12. Trauner M, Arrese M, Soroka GL et al. The rat canalicular conjugate export pump (mrp2) is downregulated in intrahepatic and obstructive cholestasis. Gastroenterology. 1997;113:255–264.
13. Koopen NR, Wolters H, Havinga R, Vonk RJ, Jansen PLM, Muller M, Kuipers F. Impaired activity of the bile canalicular organic anion transporter (Mrp2/cmoat) is not a main cause of ethinylestradiol-induced cholestasis in the rat. Hepatology. 1998;27:537–545.
14. Meyers M, Slikker W, Pascoe G, Vore M. Characterization of cholestasis induced by estradiol-17beta-D-glucuronide in the rat. J Pharmacol Exp Ther. 1980;214:887–893.
15. Vore M. Estrogen cholestasis: membranes, metabolites or receptors? Gastroenterology. 1987;93:643–649.
16. Friedel H, Goa KL, Benfield P. S-adenosyl-L-methionine. A review of its pharmacological properties and therapeutic potential in liver dysfunction and disorders in relation to into physiological role in cell metabolism. Drugs. 1989;38:389–416.
17. Owen JS, Rafique S, Osman E, Burroughs AK. Ability of S-adenosyl-L-methionine to ameliorate lipoprotein induced membrane lipid abnormalities and cellular dysfunction in human liver disease. Drug Invest. 1992;Suppl 4:22–40.
18. Corrales F, Ochoa P, Rivas C, Martin-Lomas M, Mato JM. Inhibition of glutathione synthesis leads to S-adenosyl-L-methionine synthetase reduction. Hepatology. 1991;14:528–533.
19. Boelsterli UA, Rakhit G, Balazs T. Modulation by S-adenosyl-L-methionine of hepatic Na/K-ATPase, membrane fluidity and bile flow in rats with ethynyl estradiol induced cholestasis. Hepatology. 1983;3:12–17.
20. Giulidori P, Galli-Kienle M, Catto E, Stramentinoli G. Transmethylation, transsulphuration, and aminopropylation reactions of S-adenosyl-L-methionine in vivo. J Biol Chem. 1984;259: 4205–4211.
21. Stramentinoli G, Di Padova C, Gualano M, Ethynyl estradiol induced impairment of bile secretion in the rat: protective effect of S-adenosyl-L-methionine and its implication in estrogen metabolism. Gastroenterology. 1981;80:154–158.
22. Coleman R, Wilton JC, Stone V, Chipman JK. Hepatobiliary function and toxicity in vitro using isolated hepatocyte couplets. Gen Pharmacol. 1995;26:1445–1453.
23. Wilton JC, Matthews GM, Burgoyne RD, Mills CO, Chipman JK, Coleman R. Fluorescent choleretic and cholestatic bile salts take different paths across the hepatocyte: transcytosis of glycolithocholate leads to an extensive redistribution of annexin II. J Cell Biol. 1994;127: 401–410.
24. Wilton JC, Williams DE, Strain AJ, Parslow RA, Chipman JK, Coleman R. Purification of hepatocyte couplets by centrifugal elutriation. Hepatology. 1991;14:180–183.

25. Gautam A, Ng OC, Boyer JL. Isolated rat hepatocyte couplets in short term culture: structural characteristics and plasma membrane reorganisation. Hepatology. 1987;7:216–223.
26. El-Saidy AZ, Mills CO, Elias E, Crawford JM. Lack of evidence for vesicle trafficking of fluorescent bile salts in rat hepatocyte couplets Am J Physiol 1997;272 (Gastrointest Liver Physiol. 35):G298–G309.
27. Ahmed-Choudhury J, Orsler DJ, Coleman R. Hepatobiliary effect of tertiary-buthyloperoxide in isolated rat hepatocyte couplets. Toxicol Appl Pharmacol. 1999 in press
28. Roman I, Johnson GD, Coleman R. S-adenosyl-L-methionine prevents disruption of canalicular function and pericanalicular cytoskeleton integrity caused by cyclosporin A in isolated rat hepatocytes couplets. Hepatology. 1996;24:134–140.
29. Milkiewicz P, Baiocchi L, Mills CO et al. Plasma clearance of cholyl-lysyl-fluorescein: a pilot study in humans. J Hepatol. 1997;27:1106–1109.
30. Roma MG, Stone V, Shaw R, Coleman R. Vasopressin-induced disruption of actin cytoskeletal organisation and canalicular function in isolated rat hepatocyte couplets: possible investment of protein kinase C. Hepatology. 1998;28:1031–1041.
31. Milkiewicz P, Mills CO, Roma MG, Ahmed-Choudhury J, Elias E, Coleman R. Tauro-ursodeoxycholate and S-adenosyl-L-methionine exert an additive ameliorating effect on tauro-lithocholate-induced cholestasis: a study in isolated rat hepatocyte couplets. Hepatology. 1999;29:471–476.
32. Cardenas T, Milkiewicz P, Elias E, Mills CO. Effects of lysyl fluorescein conjugated bile acid analogues on human erythrocytes: ursodeoxycholyl lysyl fluorescein inhibits taurodeoxycholate toxicity. Hepatology. 1998;4:631A.
33. Sikker W, Vore M, Bailey JR, Montgomery C. Hepatotoxic effect of estradiol-17beta-D-glucuronide in the rat and monkey. J Pharmacol Exp Ther. 1983;225:138–143.
34. Kan KS, Monte MJ, Parslow RA, Coleman R. Oestradiol 17-beta-glucuronide increases tight-junctional permeability in rat liver. Biochem J. 1989;261:297–300.
35. Alvaro D, Angelico M, Cantafora A et al. Improvement of estradiol 17-beta-D-glucuronide cholestasis by intravenous administration of dimethylethanolamine in the rat. Hepatology. 1991;13:1158–1172.
36. Liu Y, Huang L, Hoffman T, Gosland M, Vore M. MDR1 substrates/modulators protect against beta-estradiol-17β-D-glucuronide cholestasis in rat liver. Cancer Res. 1996;56:4992–4997.
37. Takikawa H, Yamazaki R, Sano N, Yamanaka M. Biliary excretion of estradiol-17-beta-glucuronide in the rat. Hepatology. 1996;23:607–613.
38. Rost D, Kartenbeck J, Keppler D. Changes in the localisation of the rat canalicular conjugate export pump mrp2 in phalloidin induced cholestasis. Hepatology. 1999;29:814–821.

Section V
Alcoholic and other liver diseases

12
Ethanol metabolism

T.J. PETERS and V.R. PREEDY

All the effects of alcohol ingestion, beneficial or detrimental, are directly or indirectly related to ethanol itself or to the products of ethanol metabolism. The claims during the 1940s and 1950s of Best, Daft, Himsworth and others that the toxic effects of chronic alcohol misuse on the liver related to an associated nutritional impairment were disproven by the seminal studies of Charles Lieber during the 1960s. A caveat, however, remains that specific vitamin deficiency syndromes, such as Wernicke-Korsakoff psychosis, niacin deficiency encephalopathy and alcohol–tobacco vitamin B_{12} amblyopia, may complement this metabolic toxicity, affecting especially the nervous system. The toxic consequences of ethanol ingestion may relate to the ethanol itself (Table 1). High levels of ethanol have a fluidizing effect on cell membranes, and this has direct effects on intrinsic membrane proteins including enzymes, receptors and cytoskeletal elements. The fluidizing effects of exposure to ethanol are counteracted by compensatory changes in membrane lipid components: increased cholesterol content and a higher proportion of more-saturated fatty acids in the phospholipid components oppose the fluidizing effects of chronic ethanol exposure, thus stabilizing the membranes in the presence of alcohol.

The basic pathway of alcohol metabolism is straightforward, with the progressive oxidation of ethanol to acetate via acetaldehyde. The major site of this oxidation is the liver parenchymal cells but other potential sites include the gastrointestinal tract (colonic bacteria), vascular tissue and brain. The initial oxidation is catalysed by a cytosolic NAD-linked alcohol dehydrogenase

Table 1. Metabolic consequences of alcohol ingestion

1. Direct cellular effects

2. Increased membrane fluidity

3. Indirect effects of membrane fluidity changes, including alterations in properties of extrinsic and intrinsic proteins

4. Formation of fatty acid ethyl esters

5. Endocrine responses, including increased adrenal activity

(ADH). It is now clear that there are at least six classes of ADH. The hepatic ADH2 enzymes exhibit genetic polymorphism. This polymorphism may contribute to inter-individual variations in rates of ethanol metabolism.

The primary product of all ADH activities is acetaldehyde, a highly reactive intermediate which has potent vasoactive properties. It has also been implicated, directly and indirectly, in several aspects of the alcohol misuse syndrome ranging from alcohol dependency via the formation of opioid-like isoquinolines, tissue changes by direct toxicity (particularly to thiol groups), reactive oxygen species generation, to the formation of acetaldehyde adducts and immunological reactions (Table 2). The further oxidation of acetaldehyde to acetate is catalysed by acetaldehyde dehydrogenase, predominantly the low K_m mitochondrial enzyme. Aldehyde dehydrogenases are widely distributed and thus the plasma levels of acetaldehyde are in the 1–2 μM range, compared with millimolar levels of ethanol and acetate. An exception occurs in Oriental subjects who have a genetic defect in their mitochondrial acetaldehyde dehydrogenase, rendering the enzyme almost completely catalytically inactive. These individuals generally metabolize ethanol at normal rates but show very reduced rates of acetaldehyde oxidation. After a relatively small dose of ethanol they have very high levels of blood and tissue acetaldehyde with toxic and aversive consequences particularly affecting the cardiovascular and gastrointestinal systems.

An important consequence of ethanol and acetaldehyde oxidation is the increase in both cytosolic and mitochondrial NADH/NAD$^+$ ratios. Many of the metabolic consequences of alcohol ingestion are a result of this redox change (Table 3). Thus the increase in the cytosolic NADH/NAD$^+$ ratio causes an increase in the lactate/pyruvate ratio mediated via lactate dehydrogenase. This increase in lactate has been implicated in such alterations as hyper-uricaemia, collagen deposition, impaired gluconeogenesis and, via an increased NADPH/NADP$^+$ ratio, increased fatty acid synthesis[1]. The increased NADH/NAD$^+$ ratio in mitochondria increases the β-hydroxy-butyrate/acetoacetate ratio with development of ketoacidosis, impaired citric acid cycle activity and decreased fatty acid oxidation. Attractive as the redox hypothesis is, it may have

Table 2. Metabolic and toxic effects of acetaldehyde

1. Alteration of biogenic amine metabolism

2. Formation of proaddictive isoquinoline opioid-like substances

3. Inhibition of mitochondrial oxidative phosphorylation

4. Inhibition of protein synthesis

5. Formation of adducts with thiol and amine groups in amino acids and peptides

6. Formation of autoantibodies to acetaldehyde neoantigen adducts

7. Generation of free radicals and reactive oxygen species

8. Lipid peroxidation

9. Microtubule disruption

10. Enhanced vitamin metabolism

Table 3.   Metabolic consequences of alcohol

Redox Effects – $\dfrac{NADH}{NAD} \rightleftharpoons \dfrac{Lactate}{pyruvate}$ (cytosol)

Increased lipid synthesis

Enhanced collagen formation

Hyperuricaemia

Impaired protein synthesis

Hypoglycaemia

Hormonal changes: cortisol $\uparrow$, androgens $\downarrow$

---

been overemphasized. Thus pre-treatment of rats with methylene blue, which dissipates the increased NADH/NAD+ ratio, does not prevent hepatic lipid accumulation in rats fed alcohol[2]. Similarly, direct measurement of human hepatic fatty acid synthesis in vitro shows no direct effect of ethanol on synthesis rates: tissues from alcoholics show base line rates of fatty acid synthesis below that of normal tissue with no change on the direct addition of ethanol[3,4].

Although alcohol dehydrogenase is the major catalyst of acetaldehyde formation, alternate pathways are important. The peroxidative activity of catalase, a cytosolic and a peroxisomal enzyme, can lead to the formation of acetaldehyde. However, the rate is low and is limited by the supply of H_2O_2, and probably accounts for no more than 5% of the ethanol oxidation by the body, although recent studies suggest this mechanism may be important in the brain[5]. A more important non-ADH pathway is MEOS (microsomal ethanol oxidizing system), located predominantly in the smooth endoplasmic reticulum. This cytochrome P_{450}-2E1 has several important characteristics: a higher K_m for ethanol than ADH, its induction by chronic ethanol ingestion and other enzyme-inducing drugs, the concomitant oxidation of NADPH, and the generation of free radicals during its activity. Its contribution to overall ethanol oxidation is small at low blood ethanol levels (about 10%), but increases with increasing blood ethanol levels, particularly in chronic alcoholics where the MEOS system may contribute up to 50% of the ethanol oxidation rate. The adaptive responses to chronic ethanol oxidation, including induction of MEOS and mitochondrial, endoplasmic reticulum and peroxisomal proliferation, all contribute to the hepatomegaly of chronic alcoholics, who overall show a two-fold increase in ethanol oxidation rates. It should, however, be noted that all these enhanced oxidation rates lead to increased acetaldehyde formation.

A relatively recent series of studies[6] have highlighted the possible role of fatty acid esters in ethanol-induced organ damage. This includes toxic effects on cardiac mitochondria[7], pancreatic lysosomes[8] and altered neuronal functions[9]. As well as mediating cellular damage, these fatty acid ethyl esters may form useful markers of chronic ethanol abuse.

In conclusion[10], it is clear that there are many possible metabolic consequences of ethanol ingestion, both local and systemic, direct and indirect. These include ethanol oxidation and esterification, redox (NADH/NAD) changes, acetaldehyde and acetate formation, free radical and reactive oxygen species formation and enzyme induction and inhibition. The relative contribution of these various effects is determined by the ethanol load, chronicity of intake, concomitant drug ingestion, nutritional status and the genetic make up of the individual. The relative importance of these individual effects still remains to be determined in specific individuals in spite of the increasing research efforts over the past 30 years.

REFERENCES

1. Lieber CS. Alcohol and the liver: metabolism of ethanol, metabolic effects and pathogenesis of injury. Acta Med Scand Suppl. 1985;703:11–55.
2. Ryle PR. Hepatic redox state alteration as a mechanism of fatty liver production after ethanol: fact or fiction. Alcohol Alcoholism 1986;21:131–135.
3. Venkatesan S, Leung NWY, Peters TJ. Fatty acid synthesis in vitro by liver tissue from control subjects and patients with alcoholic liver disease. Clin Sci. 1986;71:723–728.
4. Simpson KJ, Venkatesan S, Peters TJ. Fatty acid synthesis by rat liver after chronic alcohol feeding with a low fat diet. Clin Sci. 1994;87:441–446.
5. Smith BK, Aragon CMG, Amit Z. Catalase and the production of brain acetaldehyde: a possible mediator of the psychopharmacological effects of ethanol. Add Biol. 1997;2:277–289.
6. Laposta M. Fatty acid ethyl esters: non-oxidative metabolites of ethanol. Add Biol. 1998;3:5–14.
7. Lange LG, Sobel BE. Mitochondrial dysfunction induced by fatty and ethyl esters: myocardial metabolites of ethanol. J Clin Invest. 1983;72:724–731.
8. Haber PS, Wilson JS, Apte MV, Pirola RC. Fatty acid ethyl esters increase rat pancreatic lysosomal fragility. J Lab Clin Med. 1993;121:759–764.
9. Zheng Z, Hungund BL. Effects of acute and chronic ethanol exposure on fatty acid ethyl ester synthesis in mouse cerebellar membranes. Add Biol. 1998;3:85–90.
10. Peters TJ, Preedy VR. Metabolite consequences of alcohol ingestion. In: Alcohol and Cardiovascular Diseases. Chapman D, ed. Novartis Foundation Symposium 216. John Wiley, Chichester, 1998;19–34.

13
Alcohol abuse: treatment and prevention

H. GHODSE and C. DRUMMOND

INTRODUCTION

Alcohol occupies a unique place in contemporary society, both socially and economically, as a legally available psychoactive substance. Many people enjoy drinking alcohol and many do so in a sensible way, with low risk to their health, while the alcohol industry makes a significant contribution to the economy in terms of employment and tax revenue. At the same time alcohol, used excessively and inappropriately, can cause severe physical and psychological damage to the individual, as well as significant public health problems. Thus, in alcohol, we have a potent psychoactive substance, which has become part of the social fabric of society, and which is legally available, over the counter – not the pharmacist's counter, like most drugs, but from the off-licence, supermarket or bar. It is a psychoactive substance that is used comparatively safely by most, but dangerously by many.

POPULATION DRINKING LEVELS

The visible public consequences of alcohol abuse, such as drink/driving accidents and public disorder, provoke disquiet and there is a perception that the UK, with its unusual licensing regulations, somehow manages alcohol less well than other European countries. It is therefore interesting to compare alcohol consumption in the UK with consumption in other European countries, although it should be noted that obtaining accurate information is not simple because, in addition to 'recorded' consumption, usually for the purpose of taxation, there may be high levels of 'unrecorded' consumption, usually for domestically produced alcohol, brewed for personal use or for wider, often illicit, distribution[1]. Many East European countries, for example, estimate very high levels of unrecorded consumption.

Notwithstanding such limitations, it is immediately apparent that there are wide variations in recorded consumption between different countries, from Turkey where annual consumption is 0.87 l per capita to Luxembourg with 12.7 l per capita, with Germany, France and Portugal close behind. UK consumption is about 8.0 L per capita, putting it at 20th position in Europe (out of 41)[2].

From a public health perspective, trends in consumption are probably of more interest than absolute levels at a fixed point and there are quite different trends in different countries. For example, in France, Italy and Spain there have been very marked reductions in consumption since the early 1980s, with smaller reductions in Iceland, Netherlands, Norway, Portugal, Slovakia and Switzerland. However, there is increasing consumption in 21 other countries including Greece, Iceland, Luxembourg (already at the top of the graph for highest recorded consumption), Macedonia and the Czech Republic. Although reduced levels of recorded consumption have been reported in several other countries which have recently undergone major political and economic change, estimates for unrecorded consumption have increased, suggesting an increasing rather than a decreasing overall trend. A third group of countries, including Denmark, Sweden, Turkey, Finland and the UK, has relatively stable consumption levels[3].

PATTERNS OF CONSUMPTION

In addition to variations in the levels of consumption by different populations, there are also differences in drinking habits and in the patterns of consumption. These are more difficult to describe because of a lack of standardization of consumption categories, and of the ways of measuring consumption. There are, for example, marked differences in the alcoholic beverage of choice, with some countries predominantly drinking wine (France, Greece, Portugal); some predominantly drinking beer (Denmark, Netherlands and Norway); and some predominantly drinking spirits (Iceland, Poland).

Despite these differences in favoured drink, it appears that, in general, patterns of consumption across the European Union are converging, and that the distribution of consumption in different drinking populations has a certain uniformity: the majority of the population drink moderately; the number of individuals decreases gradually as the volume of consumption increases; and, although heavy drinkers consume many times more than the majority, there is no sharp cut-off point between moderate and heavy drinkers. In other words, alcohol consumption embraces a continuous spectrum of drinking behaviours and this makes it more difficult to be specific about harmful drinking at an individual level.

In the UK, however, it is estimated that 1.4 million people drink at levels regarded as harmful to health (50 units per week for men; 35 units per week for women), while 7 million drink more than 'recommended sensible' limits (21 units for men; 14 units for women)[4-6].

Recently there has been increasing concern about drinking by young people. Data in this area is incomplete but, among 15-year-old boys, the percentage drinking at least once per week varies from 50% in Wales to 8.3% in Greece. There is also evidence from a long-term study in Ireland that more young people are drinking, more are drinking regularly and that more are getting drunk[2,6].

One worrying trend, seen in countries such as the Russian Federation, since the late 1980s and the break-up of the old Soviet Union, is that the proportion of spirits in total alcohol consumption has increased, as has the ratio of unrecorded to recorded consumption. When this unrecorded consumption, based on the reports of the countries themselves, is taken into account, they have the highest level of consumption in Europe[3]. Unrecorded consumption on this scale reflects large-scale illicit production and the increased possibility of harm due to toxic contaminants.

RELATIONSHIP BETWEEN PRICE OF ALCOHOL AND CONSUMPTION LEVELS

Studies carried out in a number of countries have demonstrated that, among many factors affecting alcohol consumption, the price of alcoholic beverages, relative to the level of income, is a major factor[1,3]. Interestingly, price also impacts on those who drink heavily and on young people, so that pricing policy can be used as one tool in alcohol control, and such an approach can reduce the problems of heavy drinking in vulnerable populations. Reflecting on problems of increased consumption in Eastern Europe and the former Soviet Union, it is worth noting that they have experienced rapid inflation which has made it difficult to adjust the price of alcohol relative to that of other consumer goods. Thus, in these countries, alcohol has become comparatively cheaper.

NATURE AND PREVALENCE OF ALCOHOL-RELATED HARM

The consequences for the individual of excessive alcohol consumption are well known, and it is fair to say that no system of the body remains undamaged if there is prolonged, excessive drinking. We propose to focus here, not just on the consequences to personal health of heavy drinking, but on the public health consequences, and on what we can learn about population alcohol consumption from studying the epidemiology of the associated morbidity and mortality.

Liver disease and cirrhosis

The death rate from cirrhosis is frequently used as a fairly reliable indicator of alcohol-related harm, because it tends to vary in tandem with consumption levels, albeit with a time lag. It is not a perfect indicator, because not all cirrhosis deaths are related to alcohol and the proportion that is alcohol-related varies from one country to another.

A related indicator is the standardized death rate (SDR) for chronic liver disease and cirrhosis, which shows considerable variation from one country to another, both in terms of its absolute level and its trend direction. For example, in Iceland, the SDR is 0.3/100 000 population, and this rate seems relatively stable. In contrast, in Hungary the rate is nearly 80/100 000 and is increasing. It is interesting that most of the countries with very high rates are in Eastern Europe and have experienced major political change and instability in recent years[2].

Alcoholic psychosis

Hospitalization rate for alcoholic psychosis is another frequently used indicator of alcohol-related harm, although figures from different countries have to be interpreted cautiously because some report rates of admission, some report rates of discharge and some report rates of treatment. Furthermore, diagnostic practices vary between countries. In Europe, eight countries report admission rates above 35/100 000 population per annum of which seven are in Eastern Europe/Russian Federation, and in most of these the rate is higher now than it was 15 years ago[3].

Injury and accidents

In addition to the personal harm caused by excessive alcohol consumption, demonstrated by the prevalence of liver disease and cirrhosis, there are also problems such as accidents and other injuries that affect the wider population. Again, there is a similar pattern, with Eastern European countries with high levels of consumption experiencing staggeringly high death rates of 233 deaths/100 000 population per annum in Latvia due to external causes of injury and poisoning, compared with only 30 in the UK. It is also possible to trace the sharply growing trend in injury and poisoning over the last decade in the Baltic states and the Russian Federation[2]. Alcohol-related road traffic accidents (RTA) are a cause of particular concern in the UK. It is difficult to use RTA rates as an international comparator because the rate of car ownership varies significantly and there are different official requirements for testing for blood alcohol levels after an accident. However, of the 30 European countries providing adequate information, France, with 297 alcohol-related RTAs per 100 000 population per annum overshadows all other European countries[3].

Other consequences of excessive consumption

Many statistics demonstrate the measurable types of harm caused by alcohol. Much more difficult to measure, and therefore often ignored, are the adverse consequences in areas such as friendships, general health, happiness, family life, studying and employment, and there is evidence that these adverse social consequences increase as alcohol consumption increases[7]. Certainly, the proportion with diagnosable (ICD10) alcohol dependence rises regularly with alcohol consumption.

ALCOHOL POLICY

Having outlined the scale of alcohol-related problems and the observable trends in Europe in recent years, it is interesting to turn to the ways in which different countries respond to these problems, in terms of control policies. Here it is worth emphasizing that alcohol policies are not just about dealing with alcoholics/ heavy drinkers but should also encompass the less severe problems that affect more people including the social and psychological aspects of alcohol-related harm. Given the clear relationships between alcohol consumption and harm, it follows that actions that might increase the availability of alcohol must be fully assessed in terms of public health and safety before they are introduced. Because drinking patterns and the associated problems form a continuous spectrum, policy measures that influence most drinkers will also impact on heavier drinkers and their more serious problems.

There are a number of different instruments available for governments aiming to control alcohol consumption.

Taxation

Because of the evidence that population consumption of alcohol is responsive to price, artificially adjusting the price by the selective imposition of taxes is an obvious mechanism for influencing consumption, and one which all governments employ. In Europe, for example, it has been estimated that a 10% increase in price leads to approximately a 5% reduction in beer consumption, 7.5% reduction in wine consumption and 10% reduction in spirits consumption, so the potential for benefit would seem to be great[3]. However, governments have to take some other factors into account: steep rises in excise taxes are inevitably unpopular and may have electoral consequences. If alcohol becomes too expensive, more people will make their own and/or resort to illicit sources. Revenue from alcohol taxation is/may become a significant source of income for a government. But it may be reluctant to increase taxation in case this results in a net reduction of revenue from this source. Because of considerations such as these, as well as the differing social context of alcohol, it is not surprising that there is great variation in the systems and level of taxation in different countries. Many set the tax level by pure alcohol content of the beverage, so that there are higher taxes on drinks with higher alcohol content and many have higher duties on imported alcohol. In Europe, Nordic countries, Ireland and the UK have higher alcohol taxes than Mediterranean countries.

Regulations aimed at consumers

There is a wide range of measures which influence access to and therefore the availability of alcohol and these can make a significant contribution to preventing alcohol problems. Such measures include age restrictions on the sale of alcohol, restrictions on the places where alcohol can be sold and/or consumed, restrictions on the time when alcohol can be sold and/or consumed (a British approach), restrictions on the type of activity permitted when alcohol has been consumed (drink driving regulations), and limits on the quantity of alcohol that can be brought into the country without paying duty.

Drink-driving regulations

These have attracted considerable public attention and are effective in reducing alcohol-related RTAs. Strict enforcement combined with high visibility random testing can lead to sustained reductions in RTAs, and there is scope for further refinement. For example, as young drinkers are particularly at risk because they are inexperienced at both drinking and driving, so there would be a logic in having lower permissible blood alcohol levels for young drivers. It is also possible in several countries to make the person serving alcohol to an already intoxicated driver legally responsible for the driver's subsequent behaviour.

Regulation of marketing

There is a number of different ways in which restrictions can be imposed on alcohol advertising including, of course, a total ban. Less draconian measures include restriction of the content, restrictions on the use of different media, restrictions on events used to promote alcohol, withdrawal of tax relief on marketing, and regulation of the way in which alcohol is portrayed in the mass media. There is some evidence that such restrictions are effective, with reduced consumption of alcohol and alcohol-related harm in countries with advertising restrictions.

Public education

The aim of the public education component of an alcohol policy is to influence individuals' knowledge of alcohol and its effect, their attitudes towards it and their drinking behaviour. This is notoriously difficult to achieve and certainly very difficult to measure. As yet there is no evidence to support the efficacy of public education campaigns, and therefore no justification for the commitment of major resources in this area. Specifically, there is no evidence that a public health strategy focusing on a 'safe' number of units of alcohol is worthwhile. Indeed, there is a fear that formally identifying a 'safe' limit may encourage those who would have formerly consumed less, to increase their consumption up to this limit.

Although there are reservations about the value of public education campaigns, this does not mean that alcohol should be ignored in the broader personal and social health curriculum in schools. Indeed it is essential that young people, as part of this curriculum, are provided with adequate information and are helped to develop appropriate skills to resist the social and marketing pressures to misuse alcohol and other substances.

Treatment interventions

Specialist inpatient units

For many years, the disease model of alcoholism prevailed, in which alcoholism was seen as a specific illness, affecting a small proportion of the population. This led to the establishment of specialized treatment centres and an emphasis on the development of intensive, often inpatient, treatment for a small group of patients with severe problems. Unfortunately, focusing on the needs of the few ignores the less severe problems of the many, and a more recent awareness that alcohol use disorders are a spectrum of disorders has led to a reappraisal of treatment interventions[8].

The importance of such an appraisal is emphasized by studies comparing specialist inpatient treatment with less intensive, outpatient approaches to detoxification, most of which have failed to demonstrate evidence of any extra benefit. However, before dismissing inpatient units as an unnecessary and expensive adjunct to treatment services, it is worth noting that better matching of patients to treatment (using specialist inpatient facilities only for the treatment of those with more severe or complex problems) may improve effectiveness[9].

Community-based services

The cost of maintaining inpatient units and doubts about their effectiveness has led to specialist teams (doctor/nurse/social worker) providing outreach services in community settings, often in conjunction with the primary care team. The patient can then be seen in the familiar and convenient environment of the general practitioner's surgery, and this greater accessibility, combined with less stigmatization, may encourage people with alcohol use disorders to seek help at an earlier stage, when treatment is more likely to be effective

Brief interventions

Because of the scale of alcohol-related problems, and the comparatively small number of specialist professionals, there is growing interest in developing primary care-led models shared between primary care and specialist teams. Some primary care teams are reluctant to become involved in this field, and if more are to do so further training and continuing support will undoubtedly be necessary. Nevertheless, so-called 'brief interventions', usually undertaken in primary care, and comprising an assessment of alcohol intake, information on hazardous drinking and clear advice to reduce consumption are becoming more popular. They offer a much less costly form of treatment, which is attractive when financial resources are limited, but still require further evaluation of their true cost-effectiveness[10].

It seems likely that the development of skills and expertise in primary care may lead to the identification of a considerable volume of previously un-diagnosed need. Some of these patients will be managed satisfactorily by the primary care team, but those with more severe problems may need intervention from a specialist team. Lacking at present, but definitely needed, are tools to match sub-groups of patients to the treatment services appropriate to their needs, to ensure maximum cost-effectiveness. In this context, it is worth emphasizing the particular needs of minority groups for access to appropriate alcohol services.

It is also important to note that the self help movement of AA, which was founded in the US in 1935, is a major provider of help and support for people with AUDs, with more than 73 000 groups worldwide[11]. Indeed a higher pro-portion of problem drinkers attend AA than formal alcohol treatment programmes[12]. Although this approach is largely unevaluated, because of the difficulty of using conventional randomized controlled trials in this setting, there is evidence that regular AA attendance is associated with better outcomes in those with a high level of alcohol dependence[13,14]. Regular AA attenders are, of course, self-selected.

Supportive environments

It can be seen that brief interventions, provided within a local and familiar envir-onment and with a strong educational component, could play an important role within a public education policy. But there is scope for much wider initiatives to develop an environment and social climate that promote and reward modera-tion as the norm, rather than a culture in which getting drunk is considered a desirable goal. Measures could include: encouraging public houses to become more café-like and family oriented, with a far greater range of low and non-alcoholic drinks; training bar-tenders to detect and control alcohol misuse; restricting the availability of alcohol in public places; introducing unit labelling to inform consumers and to encourage self-monitoring; and including health warnings on alcohol.

The similarities between some of these proposals and measures already introduced in the UK against cigarettes are apparent, and useful lessons can indeed be drawn from this source. Because of the change in public attitudes towards smoking, far more draconian measures have been introduced to reduce smoking than could have been contemplated twenty years ago. The beginnings of a similar change in public attitude towards alcohol are perhaps just germinating now: there is, for example, far less tolerance of drink driving now than previously and this behaviour is increasingly stigmatized. The time seems ripe therefore to press for policy initiatives that build on and reinforce the public mood.

Alcohol and the economy

While firmly advocating such changes, it would be naive to ignore the wider role of alcohol within any country's economy. The alcohol industry creates jobs, income and revenue, and the scale of this is enormous: 2 million people in 12 EU states work in the alcohol industry, equivalent to 2% of civilian employment. Tax revenue from alcoholic beverages is about 2.4% of all tax revenue in the EU[3]. These figures highlight the problems that arise when any commodity becomes embedded within the economy, making it much more difficult to take action to reduce consumption. It is worth pointing out that these lessons should not be forgotten when demands are made to legalize other substances of abuse.

National and European policies

The scale of alcohol consumption and alcohol use disorders across Europe is such that most governments have developed or are developing alcohol policies, albeit of varying degrees of comprehensiveness. Thus, by 1995 only eight out of 39 countries assessed their own national policy as comprehensive, and five of these eight were the Nordic countries. Issues given most priority were developing specialized treatment services, working in particular settings (usually schools), dealing with drink driving and developing mass media campaigns. Reducing the availability of alcohol and using pricing policy to reduce demand figured somewhat less often. In the UK, the publication of Health of the Nation was a landmark for the development of public policy in relation to alcohol because it set targets for improving public health in five specific areas, in all of which alcohol consumption was a significant factor[15].

Evaluating the effectiveness of alcohol policies is clearly not a simple task and the Rudimentary Scale of Alcohol control has been developed for this purpose. It is a 30-item scale, measuring the presence/absence of 30 possible control mechanisms covering production, distribution, social and environmental measures and price and fiscal measures. Given the levels of alcohol consumption and the demonstrable trends in consumption currently being seen in some parts of

Europe, it seems likely that evaluation of newly developed policies will be of increasing importance.

REFERENCES

1. Edwards G et al. Alcohol Policy and the Public Good. Oxford University Press 1994.
2. Harkin AM, Anderson P, Goos C. Smoking, drinking and drug taking in the European Region. Alcohol, Drugs and Tobacco Programme. WHO Regional Office for Europe, Copenhagen, Denmark, 1997.
3. Harkin AM, Anderson P, Lehto J. Alcohol in Europe – a health perspective. WHO Regional Office for Europe, Copenhagen, Denmark, 1995.
4. Alcohol Concern. Proposals for a national strategy for England. London: Alcohol Concern; 1999.
5. Office of National Statistics. Living in Britain. Results from the 1996 General Household Survey: A survey carried out by the Social Survey Division. London: HMSO; 1998.
6. Lord President's Report on Action Against Alcohol Misuse. HMSO. London. 1991.
7. Ghodse AH. Living with an alcoholic. Postgrad Med J. 1982;58:636–640.
8. Drummond DC, Thom B, Brown C, Edwards G, Mullan MJ. Specialist versus general practitioner treatment of problem drinkers. Lancet. 1990;336:915–918.
9. Walsh DC, Hingson RW, Merrigan DM et al. A randomised trial of treatment options for alcohol-abusing workers. New Engl J Med. 1991;325:775–782.
10. Chick J. Brief interventions for alcohol misuse. Br Med J. 1993;307:1374.
11. Makela K. Social and cultural preconditions of Alcoholics Anonymous (AA) and factors associated with the strength of AA. Br J Addic. 1991;86:1405–1413.
12. Weisner C, Greenfield T, Room, R. Trends in the treatment of alcohol problems in the US general population, 1979 through 1990. Am J Public Health. 1995;85:55–60.
13. Edwards G, Brown D, Duckitt A et al. Outcome of alcoholism: the structure of patient attributions as to what causes change. Br J Addic. 1987;82:533–545.
14. Emrick C. Alcoholics Anonymous: affiliation processes and effectiveness as treatment. Alcoholism: Clin Exp Res. 1987;112:416–423.
15. The Health of the Nation. HMSO, London. 1991.

14
Pathogenesis of alcoholic liver disease

C.S. LIEBER

INTRODUCTION

Alcoholism affects virtually all organs of the body but the most severe functional and structural alterations occur in the liver. Ethanol is readily absorbed from the gastrointestinal tract: only 2–10% of that absorbed is eliminated through the kidneys and lungs; the rest must be oxidized in the body, principally in the liver. This relative organ specificity probably explains why, despite the existence of intracellular mechanisms responsible for homeostasis, ethanol oxidation produces striking metabolic imbalances in the liver, especially since ethanol provides a large caloric load, sometimes in excess of all other nutrients. These effects are aggravated by lack of feedback mechanisms to adjust the rate of ethanol oxidation to the metabolic state of the hepatocyte, and the inability of ethanol, unlike other major sources of calories, to be stored or metabolized to a significant degree in peripheral tissues. The adverse effects of alcohol on the liver result from both indirect mechanisms (e.g. nutritional disorders) and more direct metabolic and toxic effects.

ROLE OF DIETARY DEFICIENCIES AND OF SELECTIVE SUPPLEMENTATION

Alcohol is rich in energy (7.1 kcal/g) and, in many societies, alcoholic beverages are considered part of the basic food supply, whereas in others alcohol is consumed mainly for its mood-altering effects. Under both circumstances, a large intake of alcohol has profound effects on nutritional status[1]. Such an intake may cause primary malnutrition by displacing other nutrients in the diet because of the high energy content of the alcoholic beverages (Figure 1) or because of associated socioeconomic and medical disorders. Secondary malnutrition (Figure 1) may result from either maldigestion or malabsorption of nutrients caused by gastrointestinal complications associated with alcoholism, involving especially the pancreas[2] and the small intestine[3]. These effects include malabsorption of

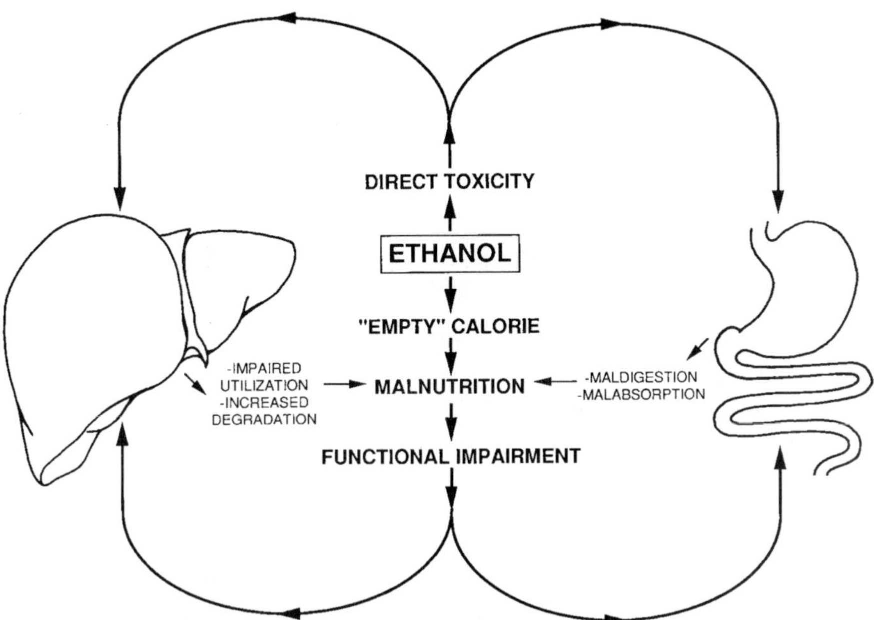

Figure 1. Interaction of direct toxicity of ethanol with malnutrition due to primary or secondary deficiencies. Secondary malnutrition may be caused by either maldigestion and malabsorption or impaired utilization (decreased activation and/or increased inactivation) of nutrients. Both direct toxicity of ethanol and malnutrition (whether primary or secondary) may affect function and structure of liver and gut[297].

thiamine and folate as well as maldigestion and malabsorption secondary to alcohol-induced pancreatic insufficiency and intestinal lactase deficiency[4]. Such primary and secondary malnutrition can affect virtually all nutrients, as described in detail elsewhere[1], and has been incriminated as a primary aetiological factor. Specifically, choline deficiency has been incriminated in the pathogenesis of liver injury for several decades. Its role as a lipotrope in humans was first considered because deficiencies in dietary protein and lipotropic factors (choline and methionine) can produce fatty liver in growing rats[5]. Furthermore, it has been reported that ethanol increases choline requirements in the rat[6], possibly by enhancing choline oxidation[7]. Primates, however, are far less susceptible to protein and lipotropic deficiency than rodents[8]. Clinically, choline treatment of patients suffering from alcoholic liver injury has been found to be ineffective in the face of continued alcohol abuse[9–12]. Furthermore, massive supplementation with choline failed to prevent the fatty liver produced by alcohol in volunteer subjects[13]. This is not surprising since, unlike rat liver, human liver contains very little choline oxidase activity, which may explain the species differences with regard to choline deficiency. In man, choline deficiency has been documented in only very limited circumstances of extremely restricted diets[14]. Moreover, fatty liver as well as fibrosis (including cirrhosis) developed in baboons despite liberal amounts of methionine[15] and massive supplementation with choline, even to the point of toxicity[16]. Some of the liver changes associated with the alcohol intake have been attributed to the overall decrease in food consumption when alcohol is given as part of a liquid diet[17]. However, energy restriction achieved through partial reduction of dietary carbohydrate[18] or an across-the-board restriction of nutrients[19] had no apparent ill effects in terms of liver morphology or fat content. Alcoholics who consume a poor diet are also lacking in a number of other nutrients, as reviewed in detail elsewhere[1,3].

DECREASED NUTRIENT ACTIVATION

Methionine and S-adenosylmethionine (SAMe)

Decreased activation of essential nutrients represents a mixed mechanism of pathogenesis, both nutritional and toxic. A case in point is methionine. Methionine deficiency has been invoked and its supplementation has been considered for the treatment of liver diseases, especially the alcoholic variety, but excess methionine was shown to have some adverse effects[20], including a decrease in hepatic ATP[21]. Whereas in some patients with alcoholic liver disease, circulating methionine levels are normal[22], in others elevated levels were observed[23–25]. Kinsell et al.[26] found a delay in the clearance of plasma methionine after its systemic administration to patients with liver damage. Similarly, Horowitz et al.[27] reported that the blood clearance of methionine after an oral load of this amino acid was slowed. Since about half the methionine is metabolized by the liver, these observations suggested impaired hepatic metabolism of

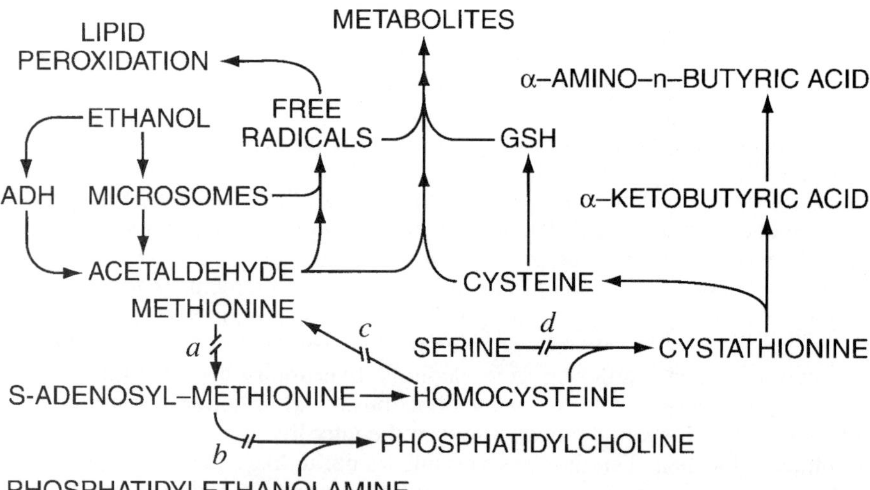

Figure 2. Increased free radical generation and acetaldehyde production by ethanol-induced microsomes, resulting in enhanced lipid peroxidation. Metabolic blocks caused by alcoholic liver disease (a,b), folate (c), B_{12} (c) or B_6 (d) deficiencies are illustrated, with the resulting depletion in S-adenosylmethionine, phosphatidylcholine and glutathione (GSH).

this amino acid in patients with alcoholic liver disease. Indeed, Duce et al.[28] reported a decrease in S-adenosylmethionine (SAMe) synthetase activity in cirrhotic livers (Figure 2). Long-term alcohol consumption was found to be associated with enhanced methionine utilization and depletion[29]. As a consequence, SAMe depletion, as well as its decreased availability, can be expected. Indeed, long term ethanol consumption is associated with a significant depletion of hepatic SAMe[30]. Potentially, such SAMe depletion may have a number of adverse effects. SAMe is the principal methylating agent in various vital transmethylation reactions which are important to nucleic acid and protein synthesis. Hirata and Axelrod[31] and Hirata et al.[32] also demonstrated the importance of methylation to cell membrane function, with regard to membrane fluidity and the transport of metabolites and transmission of signals across membranes. Thus, depletion of SAMe, by being detrimental to methyltransferase activity, may promote the membrane injury which has been documented in alcohol-induced liver damage[33]. Not only is SAMe the methyl donor in almost all transmethylation reactions, but it plays a key role in the synthesis of polyamines and provides a source of cysteine for glutathione production. Orally administered SAMe may play a precursor role for intracellular SAMe both as unchanged SAMe and also by the methionine it provides. Compared with methionine, administration of SAMe has the advantage of bypassing the deficit in SAMe synthesis from methionine referred to above. The role of methionine deficiency is not fully clarified but, since there is a deficit in tissue levels of SAMe, administration of the latter may be useful. Thus, a compound (in this case SAMe) can become essential in man because a disease process (i.e. cirrhosis), interferes with the in vivo production from its normal precursor (i.e. methionine) (Figure 2). Fundamentally, in healthy subjects, methionine is essential and therefore must be provided in the diet, whereas its product SAMe can be synthesized endogenously. By contrast, in patients with liver disease the converse pertains: methionine is often plentiful because of the impairment in its utilization, whereas SAMe must be provided exogenously since the capacity for its synthesis is affected by the disease process that reduces SAMe synthetase activity. The validity of this concept and its importance are illustrated by the fact that the consequences of the underlying defect can be alleviated by providing SAMe, the product of the reaction. SAMe deficiency results in a number of pathological consequences, which in cirrhotics appear to be associated with an increased mortality that can be attenuated by SAMe supplementation[34].

Polyenylphosphatidylcholine (PPC) and dilinoleoylphosphatidylcholine (DLPC)

In primates, ethanol also results in a decrease of liver phospholipids and of phosphatidylcholine (PC); both can be corrected by PC supplementation[35]. Specifically, the total phospholipid content of the mitochondrial membranes is decreased, with a significant reduction in the levels of phosphatidylcholine[36] and associated striking morphologic changes. The alterations in the phospholipid composition of the mitochondrial membranes appear responsible for some of the depression of cytochrome oxidase activity produced by chronic ethanol consumption[36]. This, in turn, may be the cause, at least in part, for the biochemical alterations observed in the hepatic mitochondria of baboons fed ethanol. Indeed, the impairment of the mitochondria after chronic ethanol consumption included a significant decrease in cytochrome oxidase activity, associated with a depletion in mitochondrial phosphatidylcholine due, in part, to increase phospholipase A2 activity[36]. Replenishment of phosphatidylcholine restored the cytochrome oxidase activity (in vitro)[36] and in vivo[37]. The mechanism whereby chronic ethanol consumption alters phospholipids has not been clarified but appears to be related, at least in part, to decreased phospholipid methyltransferase activity described in cirrhotic liver[28] (Figure 2). That this is not simply secondary to the cirrhosis but may in fact be a primary defect related to alcohol is suggested by the observation that the enzyme activity is decreased already prior to the development of cirrhosis[38]. Furthermore, administration of polyenylphosphatidylcholine (PPC), has shown promising results in the prevention of alcohol-induced fibrosis[35,39]. PPC contains choline, but it was found that choline, in amounts present in PPC, has no protective action against the fibrogenic effects of ethanol in the baboon[16]. Thus, the polyunsaturated phospholipids themselves appear to be responsible, perhaps because of their high bioavailability and selective incorporation into liver membranes[40]. Furthermore, PPC decreased the transformation of the hepatic lipocytes to collagen producing transitional cells[35,41]. Moreover PPC prevented the acetaldehyde-stimulated collagen accumulation in lipocytes in vitro and it stimulated collagenase activity 2–3 fold[42]. PPC also exerted striking antioxidant effects.

TOXIC INTERACTIONS WITH NUTRIENTS

Of practical importance are the interactions of ethanol with vitamin A and its precursor β carotene.

Interactions of ethanol with vitamin A

Role of nutritional factors and liver injury

This pathology again results from interactions of purely nutritional deficiencies with the effects of liver disease and direct toxic actions of ethanol.

It has been a longstanding observation that alcoholics with cirrhosis may suffer from night blindness[43], related to vitamin A deficiency[44]. Plasma vitamin A[45] as well as retinol-binding protein (RBP) levels[46] are decreased in patients with alcoholic cirrhosis. These complications have usually been attributed to malnutrition, since poor dietary intake is common in alcoholics with[1,46] or without[47] cirrhosis. It is also possible that these complications may result from hepatic injury because decreased plasma vitamin A and RBP levels have been reported in patients with liver disease without apparent alcohol intake[47]. These low plasma levels may be due to defective synthesis of RBP in the liver[47]. Alcoholic cirrhosis is often associated with zinc deficiency[45], which can decrease plasma RBP through impaired mobilization of RBP from the liver[48]. In addition to these classic aspects of vitamin A deficiency due to either poor dietary intake or severe liver disease, direct effects of alcohol on vitamin A metabolism, and resulting alterations in hepatic vitamin A levels, have been elucidated.

Direct effects of ethanol on hepatic vitamin A

Depletion of hepatic vitamin A by ethanol and its mechanism Patients with alcoholic liver disease have very low levels of hepatic vitamin A at all stages of their disease. Already with simple fatty livers, hepatic vitamin A concentration was found to be much lower than in normal livers (on the average 1/5th); it was also significantly lower than in patients with chronic persistent hepatitis, despite the fact that the degree of liver injury associated with the fatty liver was moderate and not more severe than in chronic persistent hepatitis, as judged by liver morphology and liver tests[49]. Furthermore, in both groups, blood levels of retinol binding protein and prealbumin were normal and there was no evidence of deficient vitamin A intake. In patients with alcoholic hepatitis, liver levels of vitamin A were depressed even further (to 1/10th normal or less). The lower hepatic vitamin A values were observed in patients with cirrhosis (30 times below normal). Thus, alcoholic liver disease is associated with severely decreased hepatic vitamin A levels, even when liver injury is moderate (fatty liver) and when blood values of vitamin A, RBP, and prealbumin are still unaffected. It is noteworthy that serum RBP, which has been considered as a good index of vitamin A deficiency and more sensitive even than dark adaptation[50], was in fact still normal in the subjects with alcoholic fatty liver.

Malnutrition, when present, can of course contribute to hepatic vitamin A depletion but the patients with low liver vitamin A in the study of Leo and Lieber[49] appeared well nourished, which suggested a more direct effect of alcohol. Indeed, under strictly controlled conditions, chronic ethanol consumption was found to decrease hepatic vitamin A in baboons pair-fed a nutritionally adequate liquid diet containing 50% of total energy either as ethanol or isocaloric carbohydrate. In these baboons, fatty liver developed after 4 months of ethanol feeding with a 59% decrease in hepatic vitamin A levels, and fibrosis or cirrhosis appeared after 24–84 months with a 95% decrease[51]. Similarly, hepatic vitamin A levels of rats fed ethanol (36% of total energy) were decreased after 3 weeks (by 42%) and continued to decline up to 9 weeks. In contrast, serum vitamin A and RBP levels were not significantly changed. When dietary vitamin A was increased 5-fold, hepatic vitamin A was again decreased in ethanol-fed rats relative to the corresponding controls, and sometimes even compared to the rats given five times less vitamin A (without ethanol)[51]. To avoid the confounding effect of dietary vitamin A, it was virtually eliminated in some experiments. Under those conditions, the depletion rate of vitamin A from endogenous hepatic storage was observed to be 2.5 times faster in ethanol-fed rats than in controls.

The observations summarized above suggested that the effects of ethanol on vitamin A were not due solely to alcohol-induced severe hepatic damage, since retinol depletion was already apparent at the early and relatively benign fatty liver stage. Furthermore, they showed that even when hepatic vitamin A storage is depressed, plasma vitamin A levels are not decreased. Therefore, plasma vitamin A is not necessarily a good marker for hepatic vitamin A storage in alcoholic patients. When dietary vitamin A intake was virtually eliminated, the difference in hepatic storage between ethanol-fed rats and controls was much greater than could be accounted for by the total vitamin A intake. Thus, malabsorption was not the only reason for the depletion of hepatic vitamin A. Two possible mechanisms other than malabsorption can be invoked: increased mobilization of vitamin A from the liver, and enhanced catabolism of vitamin A in the liver or in other organs. There is experimental evidence for both, with induction of hepatic microsomal cytochrome P450 dependent system by ethanol, contributing to the enhanced degradation and depletion of retinol as reviewed elsewhere[52].

Liver abnormalities associated with low vitamin A levels

In patients with severe as well as moderate depletion of hepatic vitamin A, multivesicular lysosome-like organelles were detected in increased numbers[53,54]. That a lowered vitamin A contributes to these lesions was verified experimentally in the rat: whereas multivesicular lysosomes were not seen in the rats fed a control diet, administration of a low vitamin A diet resulted in the appearance of such lesions[53,54]. Moreover, addition of ethanol to the low vitamin A diet increased the number of these structures. These vesicles seemed to be filled with numerous lipid-like particles suggesting that impaired lipoprotein secretion might be involved. Indirect evidence in favour of such a hypothesis was provided by the observation of lowered circulating VLDL lipoproteins in rats fed the low vitamin A diet compared to animals fed the normal vitamin A regimen.

Hepatic vitamin A depletion plays a key role in hepatic fibrosis, and both hepatocytes and stellate cells are involved. Hepatic stellate cells are the principal storage site of vitamin A. Dietary vitamin A is taken up by parenchymal cells and then transferred to stellate cells for storage. RBP is probably synthesized in the hepatocytes and is necessary for the intercellular transfer[55]. It is unclear whether ethanol decreased vitamin A content directly in stellate cells or whether it interferes with the uptake of vitamin A by parenchymal cells and its subsequent transfer to stellate cells. The activation of stellate cells into myofibroblast-like cells, which then synthesize collagen, is associated with a decrease in vitamin A storage in these cells[56]. Furthermore, retinoic acid, and to a lesser extent retinol, were shown to reduce stellate cell proliferation and collagen production in culture[56–58]. It is of interest that retinoic acid was also shown to decrease $\alpha_1(I)$ collagen transcription and message in cultured human lung fibroblasts[59]; conversely lack of retinoids could promote fibrosis in these tissues, especially in the liver, consistent with the associated activation of stellate cells[56]. It has also been shown that chronic alcohol intake, by reducing retinoic acid concentration, enhances AP-1 (c-Jun and c-Fos) expression in rat liver[60]. Increased AP-1 activity after the alcohol exposure could cause cell proliferation and promote the alcohol-induced cell injury, fibrosis and malignant transformation. Paradoxically, however, vitamin A excess may also promote fibrosis and carcinogenesis (*vide infra*).

Extra-hepatic manifestations of vitamin A deficiency and their potentiation by alcohol

Increasing evidence for a role of vitamin A in the proliferation and differentiation of a variety of human cells makes it apparent that reduction in vitamin A levels may be significant in the development of tumours. Accordingly, potentiation of vitamin A deficiency by alcohol may exacerbate this effect. A relatively high risk of squamous cell carcinoma of the lung was found in a Norwegian population that drank large amounts of alcohol and had a low dietary intake of vitamin A[61]. Furthermore, a positive association between alcohol consumption and lung cancer has been reported in Japanese men in Hawaii[62].

Abnormalities associated with vitamin A excess

An excess of vitamin A is known to be hepatotoxic[63,64]. Traditionally, vitamin A toxicity was reported following consumption of doses of the order of 100 000 IU/day for periods ranging from weeks to months[65]. Daily vitamin supplement of 2 capsules of 25 000 IU vitamin A for a couple of years was associated with severe vitamin A toxicity and a rise of the plasma vitamin A level to 10 times normal in a 16-year-old[66] and in health food users[67]. Minuk et al.[68] reported observations that suggest toxicity of vitamin A at an even lower level of intake (20 000–45 000 IU/day). The smallest daily supplement of vitamin A reported to be associated with liver cirrhosis is 7500 μg RE (25 000 IU) taken for 6 years[69]. These supplements fall well within common therapeutic dosages and amounts used prophylactically with over-the-counter preparations by the population at large.

It must be pointed out, however, that the relationship between vitamin A and fibrogenesis, is complex: in addition to vitamin A promoting fibrogenesis, under certain circumstances, the opposite effect has been described, for instance in isolated fibroblasts[70] in which retinoids were shown to down-regulate procollagen gene expression and in CCl_4-induced hepatic fibrosis reported to be suppressed by vitamin A[71].

The mechanism of retinoid toxicity is poorly understood[72] but, in recent years, the effect of alcohol abuse, one of the most common aggravating factors of vitamin A toxicity, has been elucidated. Potentiation of vitamin A hepatotoxicity by ethanol was first demonstrated in rats fed diets for 2 months with either normal or 5-fold increased vitamin A content, both with or without ethanol[73]. Whereas, under these conditions, ethanol alone produced only modest changes, and vitamin A supplementation at the dose used had no adverse effect, the combination resulted in striking lesions, with giant mitochondria containing 'paracrystalline' filamentous inclusions and depression of oxygen consumption in state 3 respiration with five different substrates. The potentiation of vitamin A toxicity by ethanol was also seen in patients treated with 10 000 IU vitamin A/day for sexual dysfunction attributable to excess alcohol consumption[74]. In addition to giant mitochondria, with a more than 1000-fold increase in volume, striking filamentous or crystalline-like inclusions were seen. Such inclusions were also described by others[68] in the liver mitochondria of patients with hypervitaminosis A, but the amount of vitamin A consumed in all of these previous cases was much higher than when vitamin A toxicity was potentiated by ethanol. The latter was most dramatically documented in another study in which rats were given a combination of vitamin A supplementation and ethanol for up to 9 months[75]: there was striking hepatic inflammation and necrosis, accompanied by a rise of liver enzymes in the serum (glutamic dehydrogenase and aspartate aminotransferase).

Alcohol may also act indirectly by causing liver disease which, in turn, might affect the capacity of this organ to export vitamin A, thereby enhancing its local toxicity. Indeed, in alcoholics, the carrying capacity of RBP was at times exceeded even with low serum retinol levels[76] and, in such cases, caution in the amount of vitamin A used for therapy is advised. Similarly, diets severely deficient in proteins may affect the export capacity of the liver for vitamin A and enhance its hepatotoxicity.

Vitamin A supplementation results in an increased number of stellate cells. By contrast, when vitamin A supplementation was combined with ethanol administration, both vitamin A levels in the liver and the number of stellate cells was decreased, with the appearance of numerous transitional cells (prevalent in the perisinusoidal spaces) and myofibroblasts (prevalent in the perivenular areas) in association with abundant collagen fibres. Promotion of the transformation of stellate cells to more fibroblastic transitional cells under the influence of alcohol has also been observed in the baboon[77]. The mechanism of these effects is not known. Retinol itself is not directly responsible for the enhanced toxicity after chronic ethanol consumption, since levels of vitamin A in the liver were in fact much lower than in the controls. Since retinol, retinal and retinoic acid can be further metabolized by liver microsomes, particularly when the latter system is induced by chronic ethanol consumption[78–81], one can postulate that some of these metabolites produced in increased amounts (possibly by some specific forms of cytochrome P-450) might also participate in the enhanced toxicity.

Interactions of ethanol with β-carotene

Interactions of alcohol and liver disease with β-carotene levels

There is a correlation between alcohol consumption and plasma β-carotene concentration[82]. Thus, whereas in general, alcoholics have low plasma β-carotene levels[82,83], presumably reflecting low intake, alcohol per se might in fact increase blood levels in man[82]. There was also an increase in women, with a dose as low as two drinks per day[84], and also in non-human primates[85]. Indeed, in baboons fed ethanol chronically, liver β-carotene was increased, in contrast with vitamin A, which was depleted. Similarly, plasma β-carotene levels were elevated in ethanol-fed baboons, with a striking delay in the clearance from the blood after a β-carotene load. Furthermore, whereas β-carotene administration increased hepatic vitamin A in control baboons, this effect was much less evident in alcohol-fed animals. The combination of an increase in β-carotene and a relative lack of a corresponding rise in vitamin A suggests a blockage in the conversion of β-carotene to vitamin A by ethanol.

The relationship between liver disease and hepatic carotenoids is complex. In most patients with liver disease, absolute levels of hepatic α- and β-carotene and retinoids were found to be very low, even in the presence of normal serum levels of lycopene α and/or β-carotene; in patients with cirrhosis, hepatic levels were particularly low[86]. However, even in these patients with very low liver α- and β-carotene concentrations, more than half had blood levels in the normal range, suggesting that liver disease interferes with the uptake, excretion or, perhaps, metabolism of α- and β-carotene. In only one-third of the subjects were α- and β-carotene serum levels low, probably reflecting poor dietary intake.

Beta-carotene, oxidative stress and liver injury

In the baboon, the administration of ethanol together with β-carotene resulted in a more striking hepatic injury than with either compound alone[85]. This toxic interaction in the baboon occurred at a total dose of β-carotene (30–45 mg/ 1000 kCal of diet) which is common in subjects taking supplements. As to the dose of alcohol administered to the baboons (50% of dietary energy), it was equivalent to that of the average alcoholic[87]. In the rat, the dose of alcohol was even lower (36% of total dietary energy). Nevertheless, the well-known hepatotoxicity of ethanol was potentiated by large amounts of β-carotene, and the concomitant administration of both resulted in striking liver lesions[88]. These were characterized at the biochemical level by increased activity of liver enzymes in the plasma, at the light microscopic level by an inflammatory response and, at the ultrastructural level, by striking autophagic vacuoles and alterations of the endoplasmic reticulum and the mitochondria[88]. In the latter study, β-carotene was administered in beadlets which enhanced its bioavailability. Beadlets resulted in proliferation of the smooth endoplasmic reticulum and in leakage of the mitochondrial glutamate dehydrogenase into the plasma, reflecting mitochondrial injury. The corresponding lesion was documented by electron microscopy[88]. The reason for this toxicity is not clear. The present composition of the beadlets is proprietary; of the known ingredients, none has been identified as toxic thus far.

Extra-hepatic side effects

The toxic effects of β-carotene and their interaction with ethanol also comprise an increased incidence of pulmonary cancer. Two epidemiological investigations, namely the ATBC[89] and the CARET[90] studies, revealed that β-carotene supplementation increases the incidence of pulmonary cancer in smokers. Because heavy smokers are commonly heavy drinkers, we raised the possibility that alcohol abuse was contributory[91], since alcohol is known to act as a carcinogen and to exacerbate the carcinogenicity of other xenobiotics, especially those of tobacco smoke[92]. Why this should be aggravated by β-carotene is not clear, but since pulmonary cells are exposed to relatively high oxygen pressures, and since at higher pressures β-carotene loses its antioxidant activity and shows an autocatalytic, pro-oxidant effect[93], such an interaction is at least plausible and deserves further study. Indeed, subsequently the data of the ATBC and CARET studies showed that the increased incidence of pulmonary cancer was related to the amount of alcohol consumed by the participants[94–96].

In the ATBC Study[89] and in the CARET Trial[90], it was noted that, in smokers, β-carotene supplementation increased the incidence of death from coronary heart disease. The mechanism involved has not been elucidated as yet. Since alcohol increases β-carotene levels and since cardiovascular complications are apparently related to β-carotene, this raises the question of cardiotoxicity of elevated β-carotene, a possibility which is still largely unexplored.

Therapeutic implications

Detrimental effects result from deficiency as well as from excess of retinoids and carotenoids and, paradoxically, both have similar adverse effects in terms of fibrosis and carcinogenesis[52]. Treatment efforts therefore must carefully respect the resulting narrow therapeutic window, especially in drinkers in whom alcohol narrows this therapeutic window even further by promoting the depletion of retinoids and by potentiating their toxicity.

Interactions with α-tocopherol

Bjøneboe et al.[97] reported a reduced hepatic α-tocopherol content after chronic ethanol feeding in rats receiving adequate amounts of vitamin E, as well as in the blood of alcoholics. Furthermore, hepatic lipid peroxidation was significantly increased after chronic ethanol feeding in rats receiving a low vitamin E diet[98], indicating that dietary vitamin E is an important determinant of hepatic lipid peroxidation induced by chronic ethanol feeding. The lowest hepatic α-tocopherol was found in rats receiving a combination of low vitamin E and ethanol: both low dietary vitamin E and ethanol feeding significantly reduced hepatic α-tocopherol content, the latter, in part, because of increased conversion of α-tocopherol to α-tocopherylquinone[98]. In patients with cirrhosis, diminished hepatic vitamin E levels have been observed[86], as also shown by von Herbay et al.[99]. At earlier stages of liver injury, however, hepatic vitamin E levels are usually normal[86].

DIRECT HEPATOTOXICITY OF ETHANOL

Hepatotoxicity of ethanol in rats

The initial assertion that ethyl alcohol was not more toxic to the liver than sugar[5], was based largely on experimental work in rats given ethanol in drinking water. With this technique, however, ethanol consumption does not usually exceed 10–20% of the total caloric intake of the animal. A comparable or even greater amount of alcohol, when given with an adequate diet, resulted in negligible ethanol levels in the blood[18,100]. Thus, the results of such studies may not be relevant to the conditions prevailing in the heavy drinkers in whom liver lesions develop in association with an alcohol intake that results in significant blood levels. By incorporating ethanol in a totally liquid diet, the amount of ethanol consumed by the rat was increased to 36% of total energy, an intake comparable to that of heavy drinkers. With these nutritionally adequate diets, isocaloric replacement of either carbohydrate or fat by ethanol consistently produces a 5- to 10-fold increase in hepatic triglycerides[18,100,101]. Ethanol-fed animals developed lesions that were not present in pair-fed controls, despite equal intake of either dietary carbohydrate or fat[18], thereby clearly incriminating ethanol itself and not simply a lack of carbohydrate. Similarly, when carbohydrate (36% of energy) was omitted from the control liquid diet, the effects that had been seen with alcohol were not reproduced. All these results, as well as the data obtained in primates (*vide supra*), clearly rule out a lack of carbohydrate as a significant aetiologic factor in that model of alcohol-induced liver injury which still provided 11% of energy as carbohydrates. Moreover, an across-the-board increase in the mineral and vitamin content of the liquid diet by 50% had no impact on the capacity of ethanol to affect the liver[102]. Thus it is clear, especially from the latter data, that rats fed minerals, vitamins and proteins in excess of the amount recommended still develop signs of liver toxicity when given relevant amounts of alcohol.

Liquid diets have also been administered to rats by continuous infusion[103]. This mode of administration allows for control of the rate of diet intake in the various groups of animals. Using this technique, lesions more severe than simply fatty liver have been produced, including some necrosis and fibrosis[103], even when alcohol was given with 'adequate' diets[104,105]. More recently, however, the role of carbohydrate deficiency in that model has been reevaluated and found to have a profound impact on the severity of liver injury. Indeed, Badger et al.[106] found no such severe lesions using continuous intragastric infusion of a diet containing an adequate carbohydrate content (at least 11% of total energy). They incriminated as the cause of the lesions observed by the former investigators the very low dietary carbohydrate (5% or less of total energy) used by them. This was confirmed by Lindros and Jarvelainen[107]; this group also showed that such a chronic low carbohydrate diet reduces the glutathione peroxidase activity in the centrilobular zone of the liver which might exacerbate the lesions[108].

Low carbohydrate diets also increase the induction of the microsomal ethanol oxidizing system (MEOS)[109]. Thus, the chronic intragastric infusion of alcohol, when used in conjunction with an extremely low carbohydrate diet, reflects the effects of the carbohydrate deficiency and cannot be viewed as a model relevant to clinical alcoholic liver disease since alcoholics do not have a diet so severely deficient in carbohydrate. In fact, such a carbohydrate deficiency could not be achieved using commonly available food supplies.

Hepatic alcoholic injury in primates

In the aggregate of several studies[35,39,110,111], production of cirrhosis was observed in 14 of a total of 67 baboons fed ethanol for 5 years or more, with septal fibrosis developing in an additional 14 animals. No lesions developed in the corresponding pair-fed controls. The capacity of ethanol to produce fibrosis in well fed baboons was confirmed by Porto et al.[112,113]; these lesions were less severe than those produced before[15,110,111], but the amount of alcohol administered was also smaller and the duration of the study was shorter.

In man, epidemiological studies have clearly indicated a relationship between the development of various aspects of alcoholic liver injury and the amount of alcohol consumed, independent of nutritional factors. Indeed, the development of alcoholic liver disease correlated both with the magnitude and duration of alcohol consumption[114]. Pequignot et al.[115] estimated that the risk is increased 5 times with increased consumption between 80 and 160 g/day and 25 times if daily ethanol consumption exceeds 160 g.

A close correlation exists between per capita alcohol consumption and cirrhosis mortality[116–119]. During the First and Second World Wars in Europe and during the time of Prohibition in the United States, there was a clear decrease in mortality from cirrhosis[116], despite unchanged or even deteriorating nutritional conditions. High alcohol taxes were associated with decreased death rates from cirrhosis in England and Wales[120]. Similarly, the termination of alcohol rationing in Sweden in 1955 was followed by an increase in deaths attributable to cirrhosis[121] and economic growth in such countries as West Germany resulted in an increase of problem drinkers and cirrhosis mortality[122]. Thus, a variety of studies have clearly linked the incidence of cirrhosis and associated mortality with the amount and duration of alcohol consumption.

The most direct evidence of the hepatotoxicity of alcohol in man was obtained in judicious clinical experiments. In a series of controlled studies conducted under metabolic ward conditions, it was shown that individuals with a morphologically normal liver developed a fatty liver when given ethanol either in addition to a normal diet, or as an isocaloric substitution for carbohydrates in a variety of non-deficient diets. This was evident both by morphological examination[18,100] and by direct measurement of the lipid content of the liver biopsies[13,123,124]. Even with a high protein, vitamin-supplemented diet, there were significant increases in hepatic triglycerides[123]. Electron microscopic studies conducted in most of the above cited investigations as well as by Lane and Lieber[125] showed that, in addition to hepatic fat accumulation, alcohol also causes a striking injury to the organelles of the hepatocytes, especially the mitochondria and the endoplasmic reticulum.

Link of hepatotoxicity to the metabolism of ethanol

Many of the metabolic and toxic effects of alcohol in the liver have been linked to its metabolism in that organ. The hepatocyte contains three main pathways for ethanol metabolism, each located in a different subcellular compartment[126]: the alcohol dehydrogenase (ADH) pathway of the cytosol or soluble fraction of the cell, the microsomal ethanol oxidizing system located in the endoplasmic reticulum, and catalase located in the peroxisomes. Each of these pathways produces specific metabolic and toxic disturbances and all three result in the production of acetaldehyde, a highly toxic metabolite.

Metabolic disorders associated with alcohol oxidation by alcohol dehydrogenase

The oxidation of ethanol via the alcohol dehydrogenase pathway results in the production of acetaldehyde with loss of H which reduces NAD to NADH. The

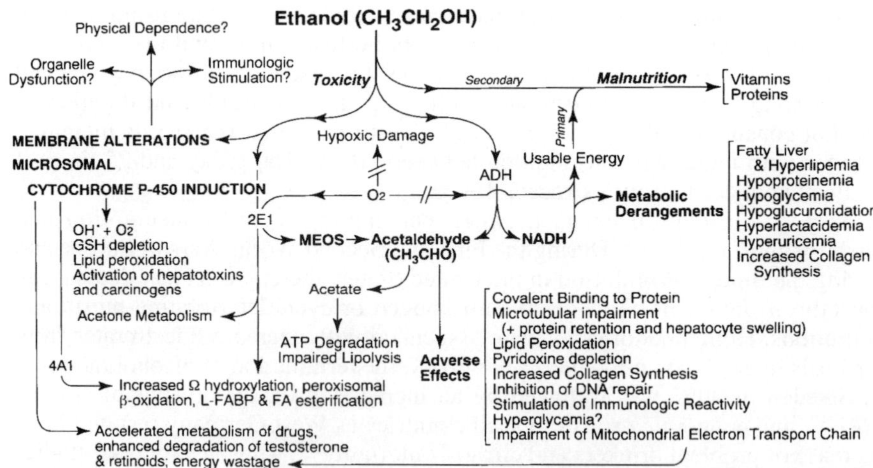

Figure 3. Hepatic, nutritional and metabolic abnormalities after ethanol abuse. Malnutrition, whether primary or secondary, can be differentiated from metabolic changes or direct toxicity, resulting partly from redox changes, or effects secondary to microsomal induction, including increased acetaldehyde production.

large amounts of reducing equivalents generated overwhelm the hepatocyte's ability to maintain redox homeostasis and a number of metabolic disorders ensue (Figure 3), including hyperlactacidaemia which contributes to the acidosis and also reduces the capacity of the kidney to excrete uric acid, leading to secondary hyperuricaemia. The latter is aggravated by the alcohol-induced ketosis and acetate-mediated enhanced ATP breakdown and purine generation[127]. Hyperuricaemia explains, at least in part, the common clinical observation that excessive consumption of alcoholic beverages frequently aggravates or precipitates gouty attacks.

Acute alcohol intoxication does occasionally cause severe hypoglycaemia, which can result in sudden death. As reviewed elsewhere[128], hypoglycaemia is due, in part, to the block by ethanol of hepatic gluconeogenesis, again as a consequence of the increased NADH/NAD ratio in subjects whose glycogen stores are already depleted by starvation or who have pre-existing abnormalities in carbohydrate metabolism. Under certain conditions, ethanol may accelerate rather than inhibit gluconeogenesis, and hyperglycaemia may also occur in association with alcoholism. Glucose intolerance may be due, at least in part, to decreased peripheral glucose utilization.

The increased NADH/NAD ratio also raises the concentration of α-glycerophosphate that favours hepatic triglyceride accumulation by trapping fatty acids. In addition, excess NADH may promote fatty acid synthesis[129,130]. Theoretically, enhanced lipogenesis can be considered a means for disposing of the excess hydrogen. Some hydrogen equivalents are transferred into mitochondria by various 'shuttle' mechanisms. The activity of the citric acid cycle is depressed, partly because of a slowing of the reactions of the cycle that require NAD; the mitochondria will use the hydrogen equivalents originating from ethanol, rather than those derived from the oxidation of fatty acids that normally serve as the main energy source of the liver. Indeed, the effects of ethanol were reproduced in vitro by an alternate NADH generating system (sorbitol-fructose) and were blocked by a H^+ acceptor (methylene blue)[129,131].

Decreased fatty acid oxidation results in the accumulation in the liver of dietary fat[124,132]. Theoretically, lipids that accumulate in the liver can originate from three main sources: dietary lipids (which reach the bloodstream as chylomicrons), adipose tissue lipids (which are transported to the liver as free fatty acids, FFA), and lipids synthesized in the liver itself[133]. These fatty acids of various sources can accumulate in the liver because of a large number of metabolic disturbances, primarily decreased lipid oxidation in the liver, enhanced hepatic lipogenesis, decreased hepatic release of lipoproteins, increased mobilization of peripheral fat, and enhanced hepatic uptake of circulating lipids. Depending on the experimental conditions, any of the three sources and the various mechanisms can be implicated. In addition to the functional changes that are a direct consequence of the metabolism of ethanol, chronic ethanol abuse results in more persistent changes in the mitochondria. The striking structural changes in the mitochondria are associated with corresponding functional abnormalities, including decreased capacity to oxidize fatty acids. Thus, decreased fatty acid oxidation, whether as a function of the reduced citric acid cycle activity (secondary to the altered redox potential) or as a consequence of permanent changes in mitochondrial structure, offers the most likely explanation for the deposition of fat in the liver, especially fat derived from the diet. In addition, with stressful amounts of ethanol and/or fasting conditions, some mobilization of fatty acids from adipose tissue may also contribute to the accumulation of lipids in the liver[132].

A characteristic feature of liver injury in the alcoholic is the predominance of steatosis and other lesions in the perivenular (also called centrilobular zone or zone 3) of the hepatic acinus. The mechanism for this zonal selectivity of the toxic effects has been postulated to involve a relative lack of oxygen supply, and propylthiouracil treatment has been proposed to attenuate this deficit.

The hypoxia hypothesis originated from the observation that liver slices from rats fed alcohol chronically consume more oxygen than those of controls[134]. It was then postulated that the enhanced consumption of oxygen would increase the gradient of oxygen tensions along the sinusoids to the extent of producing anoxic injury of perivenular hepatocytes[135]. Indeed both in human alcoholics[136] and in animals fed alcohol chronically[137,138], decreases in either hepatic venous oxygen saturation[136] or PO_2[137] and in tissue oxygen tensions[138] have been found during the withdrawal state. However, these changes in hepatic oxygenation found during the withdrawal state disappeared[137,139] or decreased[138] when alcohol was present in the blood. Acute ethanol administration increased splanchnic oxygen consumption in baboons, but the consequences of this effect on oxygenation in the perivenular zone were offset by increased blood flow resulting in unchanged hepatic venous oxygen tension[137]. Ethanol in fact induces an increase in portal hepatic blood flow[137,139–141]. In baboons fed alcohol chronically, defective O_2 utilization rather than lack of blood O_2 supply characterized liver injury produced by high concentration of ethanol[142]. The low oxygen tensions (normally prevailing in perivenular zones) exaggerate the redox shift produced by ethanol[137]. Indeed, ethanol increased the lactate/pyruvate ratio and decreased pyruvate more in hepatic venous blood than in total liver. In isolated rat hepatocytes, the ethanol-induced redox shift was markedly exaggerated by lowering the oxygen to a tension similar to that found in centrilobular zones. The process was also assessed in isolated perfused rat livers by varying the oxygen supply to produce the oxygen tensions prevailing in vivo along the sinusoid[143]. Hypoxia increased NADH which in turn inhibited the activity of NAD^+-dependent xanthine dehydrogenase, thereby favouring that of oxygen-dependent xanthine oxidase (XO)[144]. It has been postulated that, due to the acetate derived from ethanol, purine metabolites accumulate and could be metabolized via XO. This process may lead to the production of oxygen radicals which may mediate toxic effects towards liver cells, including peroxidation. Physiological substrates for XO, hypoxanthine and xanthine, as well as AMP, significantly increased in the liver after ethanol, together with an enhanced urinary output of allantoin (a final product of xanthine metabolism). Allopurinol pretreatment resulted in 90% inhibition of XO activity, and also significantly decreased ethanol induced lipid peroxidation[144]. Zonal distribution of some enzymes can influence the selective perivenular toxicity. Proliferation of the smooth endoplasmic reticulum after chronic ethanol consumption is maximal in the perivenular zone, with associated enzyme induction and related effects. Furthermore, by means of immunohistochemical techniques, human ADH has also been demonstrated mainly in hepatocytes around the terminal hepatic venule[145]. Thus, a presumably higher level of ethanol metabolism in the perivenular zone could contribute to the increased hepatotoxicity of ethanol in that area.

Adverse effects resulting from microsomal ethanol oxidation, its induction and interactions with other chemicals

That a cytochrome P-450 enzyme system can also metabolize ethanol was demonstrated in liver microsomes in vitro and found to be inducible by chronic alcohol feeding in vivo[146]; it was named the microsomal ethanol oxidizing system (MEOS)[146,147]. Its distinct nature was shown by isolation of a P-450-containing fraction from liver microsomes which, although devoid of any ADH or catalase activity, could still oxidize ethanol as well as higher aliphatic alcohols (e.g. butanol, which is not a substrate for catalase)[148,149]; and reconstitution of ethanol-oxidizing activity using NADPH-cytochrome P-450 reductase, phospholipids, and either partially-purified or highly-purified microsomal P-450 from untreated[150] or phenobarbital-treated[151] rats. That chronic ethanol consumption results in the induction of a unique P-450 was also shown by Ohnishi and Lieber[150] using a liver microsomal P-450 fraction isolated from ethanol-treated rats. An ethanol-inducible form of P-450, purified from rabbit liver microsomes[152], catalysed ethanol oxidation at rates much higher than other P-450 isozymes. The purified human protein (now called CYP2E1 or 2E1) was obtained in a catalytically active form, with a high turnover rate for ethanol and other specific substrates[153]. MEOS has a relatively high K_m for ethanol (8–10 mM compared to 0.2–2 mM for hepatic ADH) but, contrasting with hepatic ADH, which is not inducible in primates as well as most other animal species, a 4-fold induction of 2E1 was found in biopsies of recently drinking subjects, using the Western blot technique with specific antibodies against this 2E1[154], with a corresponding rise in mRNA[155].

Other cytochromes P-450 (1A2, 3A4) are also involved[156]. This induction contributes to the ethanol tolerance that develops in the alcoholic and spills over to other drugs that are microsomal substrates. The tolerance of the alcoholic to various psychoactive drugs has been generally attributed to central nervous system adaptation[157] but, in addition, metabolic adaptation must be considered, because the clearance rate of many drugs from the blood is enhanced in alcoholics[158]. Indeed, controlled studies have shown that chronic administration of pure ethanol with non-deficient diets either to rats or man (under metabolic ward conditions) results in a striking increase in the rate of blood clearance of ethanol[159], meprobamate, pentobarbital[158] and propranolol[160,161]. Similarly, increases were found in the metabolism of antipyrine[161], tolbutamide[162–164], warfarin[163], diazepam[165] and rifamycin[166].

In addition to the oxidation of ethanol, CYP2E1 also has an extraordinary capacity to activate many xenobiotics to highly toxic metabolites. These include industrial solvents such as bromobenzene[167] and vinylidene chloride[168]; as well as anaesthetics such as enflurane[169,170] and halothane[171]; commonly used medications, such as isoniazid and phenylbutazone[172]; illicit drugs (e.g., cocaine); and over-the-counter analgesics such as acetaminophen (paracetamol, N-acetyl-*p*-aminophenol) shown to be a good substrate for human CYP2E1[173]. The induction of 2E1 explains the increased vulnerability of the heavy drinker to the toxicity of these substances. Among alcoholic patients, hepatic injury associated with acetaminophen has been described following repetitive intake for headaches (including those associated with withdrawal symptoms), dental pain, or the pain of pancreatitis. Amounts well within the accepted tolerable rate (2.5–4 g) have been incriminated as the cause of hepatic injury in alcoholic patients[174,175]. It is likely that the enhanced hepatotoxicity of acetaminophen after chronic ethanol consumption is caused, at least in part, by an increased microsomal production of reactive metabolite(s) of acetaminophen. Consistent with this view is the observation that, in animals fed ethanol chronically, the potentiation of acetaminophen hepatotoxicity occurs after ethanol withdrawal[176] when production of the toxic metabolite may be at its peak, since at that time competition by ethanol for a common microsomal pathway has stopped. Thus, maximal vulnerability to the toxicity of acetaminophen occurs immediately after cessation of drinking, when there is also the greatest need for analgesia, because of the headaches and other symptoms associated with withdrawal. This also explains the synergistic effect between acetaminophen, ethanol and fasting[177], since all three deplete reduced glutathione (GSH), thereby contributing to the toxicity of each compound because GSH provides one of the cell's fundamental mechanisms for the scavenging of toxic free radicals.

There is increased evidence that ethanol toxicity is associated with an enhanced production of reactive oxygen intermediates at the microsomal level, especially through the intervention of the ethanol-inducible CYP2E1[178]. This induction is associated with proliferation of the endoplasmic reticulum, which is accompanied by increased oxidation of NADPH, with resulting H_2O_2 generation[179]. There is also increased superoxide radical production[180]. In addition, the CYP2E1 induction contributes to the well-known lipid peroxidation associated with alcoholic liver injury. Lipid peroxidation correlated with the amount of CYP2E1 in liver microsomal preparations, and it was inhibited by antibodies against CYP2E1 in control and ethanol-fed rats[181,182]. Indeed, 2E1 is rather 'leaky' and its operation results in a significant release of free radicals, including 1-hydroxyethyl-free radical intermediates[183,183], confirmed by detecting the hydroxyethyl radicals in vivo[185]. The presence of CYP2E1 was also shown in Kupffer cells[186]. In rats, ethanol treatment caused a sevenfold increase in CYP2E1 content of Kupffer cells which, in addition to endotoxin, may stimulate the Kupffer cells to release pro-inflammatory and fibrogenic cytokines.

Non-oxidative metabolism of ethanol and associated toxicity

The possible pathogenic role of a non-oxidative pathway of ethanol to form fatty acid ethyl esters was raised by Laposata and Lange[187] who found that in acutely intoxicated subjects, concentrations of fatty acid ethyl esters were significantly higher than in controls in pancreas, liver, heart, and adipose tissue. Since this non-oxidative ethanol metabolism occurs in humans in organs most commonly injured by alcohol abuse, and since some of these organs lack oxidative ethanol metabolism, Laposata and Lange[187] postulated that fatty acid ethyl esters may have a role in the production of alcohol-induced injury. This was corroborated by more recent evidence for experimental pancreatic damage[188], but further studies are needed to verify the possible role of this mechanism in the pathogenesis of alcohol-induced injury.

Toxic effects of acetaldehyde

Increased acetaldehyde and its adverse effects on antioxidant systems

Because of the inducibility of CYP2E1, chronic excessive alcohol consumption results in enhanced acetaldehyde production that, in turn, aggravates the oxidative stress directly as well as indirectly (by impairing defence systems against it).

Acetaldehyde, the product of ethanol oxidation, is highly toxic but is rapidly metabolized to acetate, mainly by a mitochondrial low K_m aldehyde dehydrogenase (ALDH). However, the activity of ALDH is significantly reduced by chronic ethanol consumption[189]. The decreased capacity of mitochondria of alcohol-fed subjects to oxidize acetaldehyde, associated with unaltered or even enhanced rates of ethanol oxidation (and therefore acetaldehyde generation because of MEOS induction), results in an imbalance between production and disposition of acetaldehyde. The latter causes the elevated acetaldehyde levels observed after chronic ethanol consumption in humans[190] and in baboons, with a tremendous increase of acetaldehyde in hepatic venous blood[142], reflecting high tissue levels.

The toxicity of acetaldehyde is due, in part, to its capacity to form protein adducts, resulting in antibody production, enzyme inactivation[191] and decreased DNA repair[192]. Indeed, acetaldehyde–protein adduct formation interferes with the activity of many key enzymes and repair systems, and thus becomes an important cause of direct toxicity at the tissue level, eventually resulting in cell necrosis. Minute concentrations of acetaldehyde (as low as 0.05 μmol/l) were found to impair the repair of alkylated nucleoproteins[192]. The toxicity is associated with a significant reduction in the capacity of the liver to utilize oxygen[142] and there is uncoupling of oxidation with phosphorylation in mitochondria damaged by chronic ethanol consumption[36]. By binding to the tubulin of the microtubules, acetaldehyde also seriously impairs the secretion of proteins from the liver into the plasma, with a corresponding hepatic retention[193]. The increases in lipid, protein, water[194], and electrolytes result in enlargement of the hepatocytes, the experimental counterpart of the ballooning of the hepatocyte seen in the alcoholic. Acetaldehyde adducts also promote collagen production.

Furthermore, acetaldehyde promotes glutathione (GSH) depletion, resulting in free radical-mediated toxicity, and lipid peroxidation. Indeed, in isolated perfused livers acetaldehyde was shown to cause lipid peroxidation[195,196]. In vitro, metabolism of acetaldehyde via xanthine oxidase or aldehyde oxidase may generate free radicals, but the concentration of acetaldehyde required is much too high for this mechanism to be of significance in vivo. However, another mechanism to promote lipid peroxidation is via GSH depletion. One of the three amino acids of this tripeptide is cysteine. Binding of acetaldehyde with cysteine and/or glutathione (GSH) may contribute to a depression of liver GSH[197]. Rats fed ethanol chronically have significantly increased rates of GSH turnover[198]. Acute ethanol administration inhibits GSH synthesis and produces an increased loss from the liver[199]. GSH is selectively depleted in the mitochondria[200] and many contribute to the striking alcohol-induced alterations of that organelle since GSH offers one of the mechanisms for the scavenging of toxic-free radicals, as shown in Figure 2.

Iron overload may play a contributory role, as chronic alcohol consumption results in an increased iron uptake by hepatocytes[201] and as iron exposure accentuates the changes of lipid peroxidation and in the glutathione status of the liver cell induced by acute ethanol intoxication[202].

Therapeutic use of GSH itself is complicated by the fact that its replenishment through supplementation is hampered by its lack of penetration into the hepatocytes, except for its ethyl derivative, which is not suitable for the treatment of alcoholic liver injury.

Cysteine is one of the three amino acids of GSH, and the ultimate precursor of cysteine is methionine (Figure 2). Compared to methionine, the administration of SAMe has the advantage of bypassing the deficit in SAMe synthesis (from methionine) referred to before (Figure 2).

Alterations in collagen metabolism; their prevention and treatment

Acetaldehyde stimulates collagen production in stellate cells[203], in part through inhibition of the feedback control of collagen synthesis by the propeptide because of corresponding adduct formation[204] (Figure 4). Furthermore, fibrosis is related to associated metabolic effects of ethanol. Indeed, the hepatic oxidation of ethanol to acetaldehyde in the alcohol dehydrogenase (ADH) pathway and the further oxidation of acetaldehyde to acetate reduce NAD to NADH, thereby producing striking redox changes that impact on collagen metabolism. Indeed, the rise in NADH shifts pyruvate to lactate which was found to stimulate collagen synthesis in cultured myofibroblasts[205]. This suggested that, in addition to the acetaldehyde and the aldehydic products of lipid peroxidation[206,207], ethanol-induced redox changes may play a role. This was confirmed by the

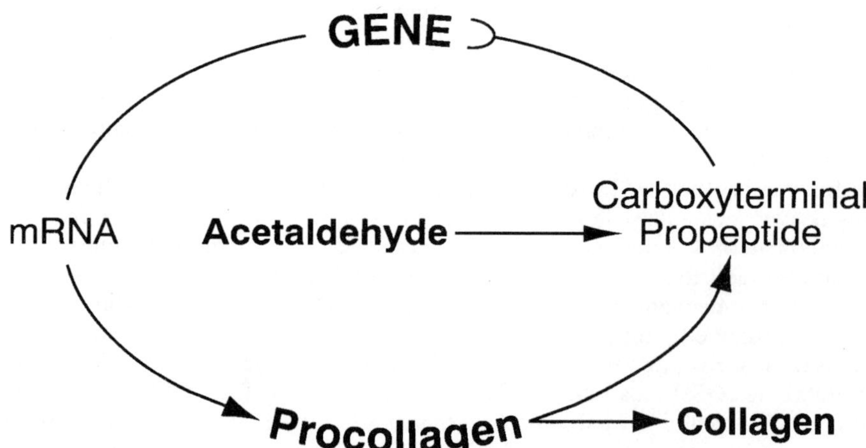

Figure 4. Feedback inhibition of collagen production and release from that control by acetaldehyde.

observation that methylene blue, a scavenger of reducing equivalents, totally inhibits the stimulatory effect of acetaldehyde on $\alpha 1$ (I) procollagen and fibronectin gene expression in stellate cells[208].

Individual susceptibility to the development of cirrhosis varies, and therefore recognition of those individuals prone to progress to cirrhosis at an early but still reversible stage is of practical importance. In that regard, recognition of perivenular fibrosis on liver biopsy is valuable. This lesion had been described in association with full-blown alcoholic hepatitis[209], but it can occur at the fatty liver stage in the absence of hepatitis[210]. Experimental data suggested that perivenular fibrosis is a common and early warning sign of impending cirrhosis if drinking continues[210], and similar conclusions were derived from clinical studies in alcoholics[211] and, interestingly, in diabetics[212].

The accumulation of hepatic collagen during the development of cirrhosis could theoretically be accomplished by increased synthesis, decreased degradation, or both. The role of increased collagen synthesis was suggested by increased activity of hepatic peptidylproline hydroxylase in rats and primates and increased incorporation of proline ^{14}C into hepatic collagen in rat liver slices[213]. Increased hepatic peptidylproline hydroxylase activity was also found in patients with alcoholic cirrhosis[214] and hepatitis[215]. In baboons given ethanol that developed significant fibrosis, molecular evaluation revealed that the ribonucleic acid (RNA) from these livers was more active in in vitro protein synthesis, and the type I procollagen mRNA content was significantly higher (per liver RNA) as determined by hybridization analysis[216]. Concerning the respective role of hepatocytes and stellate cells in the production of collagen in the liver, a consensus has been reached that stellate cells, which are activated after chronic alcohol consumption[77,217], appear to play the major role. Normal stellate cells, when isolated and cultured on plastic, undergo spontaneous transformation into transitional-like cells, thereby mimicking in vitro the condition that prevails in vivo after chronic alcohol consumption[203]. These cells in culture produce collagen[203]. When acetaldehyde, the active metabolite of ethanol, is added to these cells, they respond with a further increase in collagen accumulation[203], and enhanced synthesis with increased mRNA for collagen[208] because of release from feedback inhibition (Figure 4).

Collagen accumulation reflects not only enhanced synthesis, but it also results from an imbalance between collagen degradation and collagen production. Thus, cirrhosis might, in part, represent relative failure of collagen degradation to keep pace with synthesis. Interestingly, polyenylphosphatidylcholine (PPC) may affect this balance. Indeed, addition of PPC to transformed stellate cells was found to prevent the acetaldehyde-mediated increase in collagen accumulation, possibly by stimulation of collagenase activity[42]. If we can extrapolate from these in vitro data to the in vivo condition, these findings could explain, at least in part, why PPC attenuates the development of fibrosis, including cirrhosis after chronic alcohol administration in baboons and CCl_4 or heterologous albumin in rats[218]. This was also associated with a striking attenuation of the oxidative stress induced by alcohol in baboons[219], and CCl_4 in rats[220]. In vitro the capacity to stimulate collagenase activity was found to reside exclusively with dilinoleoylphosphatidylcholine, the major PC species present in the PPC extract[35].

Role of cytokines

As reviewed in detail elsewhere[221], it has been proposed that tumour necrosis factor, a mediator of endotoxic shock and sepsis, plays a role in alcoholic hepatitis, since cytokines cause metabolic disturbances that are similar to complications of alcoholic hepatitis.

Ethanol is known to affect several Kupffer cell functions which may also contribute to the development of alcoholic liver injury. Different mechanisms underlying these effects have been proposed, but their relative importance is still debated. A potent stimulant of Kupffer cell activation is the gut-derived endotoxin lipopolysaccharide[222–224].

Experimentally, acute administration of alcohol enhanced endotoxin hepatotoxicity when the dose of endotoxin was small, but the effect of alcohol was masked when larger doses of endotoxin were given[225]. Circulating tumour necrosis factor (TNF)-α, and interleukin-1 remained elevated for up to 6 months after the diagnosis of alcoholic hepatitis, whereas interleukin-6 normalized in parallel with clinical recovery[226]. Concentrations of all three cytokines correlated with biochemical parameters of liver injury. Sheron et al.[227] also found that the cytokine interleukin-6 is activated in severe alcoholic hepatitis and postulated that this may mediate hepatic or extrahepatic tissue damage. On the one hand, TNF appears to be a proximal mediator of multiple types of experimental injury and TNF activity is elevated in alcoholic liver disease, as are the levels of certain other cytokines. On the other hand, low physiological amounts of cytokines appear to be important for liver regeneration (and perhaps are beneficial to the organism as a whole).

An additional possible stimulator of Kupffer also is 2E1, shown recently to be increased after chronic alcohol consumption not only in hepatocytes but also in Kupffer cells[186]. In both acute and chronic liver diseases, Kupffer cells become activated to produce cytokines and reactive oxygen radicals[228–233], known mediators of hepatocellular injury. How and to what extent the induction of Kupffer cell CYP2E1 plays a role in these processes is now being investigated. The challenge is to acquire sufficient knowledge to conserve the positive growth enhancing effects of cytokines while attenuating their cytotoxic effects.

Role of immune factors and hepatitis viruses

Acetaldehyde adducts may serve as neoantigens, generating an immune response in mice[234] and in humans[235,236]. Niemela et al.[237] found antibodies against acetaldehyde in patients with alcoholic hepatitis, whereas Hoerner et al. detected them in most alcoholics[235], including some with simple fatty liver, early fibrosis, or both[236], and in even nonalcoholics with liver disease[236]. This immune reaction may contribute to the aggravation or perpetuation of liver injury. Alcoholism and viral hepatitis not infrequently occur in the same patients.

Most important is the association of alcoholic liver disease with hepatitis C: a quarter of all patients with alcoholic liver disease have also markers of HCV infection[238], with an even higher incidence in urban areas. We found that even in the absence of risk factors such as intravenous drug abuse, portal or lobular inflammation is strongly associated with the hepatitis C virus in alcoholics[239], · suggesting that alcohol may favour the acquisition, replication, or persistence of the virus. It was also clear that alcoholism is associated with hepatitis C but not hepatitis B in that population[240]. Alcohol consumption is clearly a risk factor for the progression of liver disease caused by HCV[241,242]. Furthermore, fibrosis correlates significantly with alcohol consumption, and even low alcohol intake increases viraemia and hepatic fibrosis[243]. Wiley et al.[244], who examined the effect of moderate alcohol intake on HCV infection, concluded that alcohol intake is an independent risk factor in the clinical and histological progression of HCV infection. Specifically, there was a 2- to 3- fold greater risk of liver cirrhosis and decompensated liver disease in the alcoholic, and the development of cirrhosis was faster in the alcohol group. Thus, HCV infection multiplies the alcohol-associated risk of cirrhosis[245] and alcohol and HCV together accelerate the development of hepatocellular carcinoma (HCC)[246]. In the latter group of patients, the incidence of HCC exceeded 50%.

Effect of gender and genetics

The average cirrhogenic doses as well as the threshold doses are lower in females than males: a daily intake of alcohol of 40–60 g in men but only 20 g in women resulted in a statistically significant increase in the incidence of cirrhosis in a well-nourished population[115,247]. There is also evidence that the progression to more severe liver injury is accelerated in women: Wilkinson et al.[248] found women to be more susceptible than men to the development of alcoholic cirrhosis, and other studies reported the incidence of chronic advanced liver disease to be higher among women than among men for a similar history of alcohol abuse[249–251]. Gender differences in ethanol metabolism, not only in the liver but also in the stomach[252,253], may be contributory. Thus, gender must be recognized as one of the factors that determines severity of alcoholic liver injury. Indeed, gender differences in ethanol distribution[254], bioavailability[252] and hepatic metabolism[255], with increased production of acetaldehyde[256], may contribute to women's vulnerability to alcohol consumption. In addition, gender differences in alcohol-induced derangements of hepatic lipid metabolism, affecting the disposition of potentially toxic fatty acids, have also been reported in experimental animals[257]. Furthermore, chronic alcohol administration increased ω-oxidation more effectively in male than in female rats[258], explaining the potentially deleterious accumulation of non-esterified fatty acids in the liver of the alcohol-fed females[257]. This was also associated with a much smaller ethanol-induced increase in cytosolic fatty acid binding protein (L-FABPc) and microsomal esterification in females than in males, whereas the inhibition of mitochondrial β-oxidation was similar in both genders. Related findings have been observed in humans[259] and explain, at least in part, the greater vulnerability of women to the development of alcoholic liver injury.

Although no group is immune to alcoholic cirrhosis, various segments of our society are affected differently. For instance, American Indians seem to be very prone to develop alcoholic cirrhosis. These differences are commonly attributed to cultural factors leading to alcoholism, although genetic influences favouring either alcoholism or cirrhosis or both have not been ruled out. Indeed, individual differences in rates of ethanol metabolism appear, in part, to be genetically controlled[260], and the role of heredity for the development of alcoholism in humans has been emphasized[261]. Its role in men is well established[262] and has now been shown to play a major role in the aetiology of alcoholism in women as well[263]. The dopamine D_2 gene has been incriminated[264,265], but this is disputed[266,267].

It is also suspected that genetic factors influence the severity of alcohol-induced liver disease[262]. It has been proven that the predisposition for many different diseases is significantly associated with specific histocompatibility antigens (as reviewed in refs 268 and 269). In patients with chronic alcoholic liver disease, the HLA-B8 was more prevalent in patients with alcoholic cirrhosis than in controls or in patients with fatty liver or minimal fibrosis[270]. Another difference was the absence of HLA-A28 in the cirrhotic patients[271]. The cirrhotics with HLA-B8 had been drinking for a shorter period of time than patients with comparable clinical and histological diseases but without HLA-B8[272]. These results supported the hypothesis that genetic factors may be implicated in alcohol-induced liver damage and particularly its progression to cirrhosis. These data, however, have not been confirmed[273–275]. Bell and Nordhagen[274] found an association with HLA-BW40 and Melendez et al.[276] with HLA-B13; but Scott et al.[273], Simon et al.[277], Shigeta et al.[278], and Gluud et al.[275] did not. These discrepancies in different populations of alcoholic patients with cirrhosis suggest that the HLA locus B is not implicated in alcoholic cirrhosis, but that it maintains a close association with nearby genes that are involved. Some results[279] also indicated different ADH3 allele frequencies in patients with alcohol-related end-organ damage compared to controls, suggesting that genetically determined differences in alcohol metabolism may, in part, explain differences in susceptibility to disease (possibly through enhanced generation of toxic metabolites), but this has been questioned[280].

Different polymorphic sites in the 5′-flanking region of the human CYP2E1 gene have been reported. Several restriction fragment length polymorphisms (RFLP) may affect transcriptional regulation or the functional activity of the expressed protein[281–286] and hence its pathogenic role. Two nucleotide exchanges are within restriction sites (*Pst*I and *Rsa*I) and were found to be in complete linkage disequilibrium. The *Rsa*I sites in the regulatory 5′-flanking region described in Japanese subjects were found to affect the rate of transcription when coupled to a reporter gene in an in vitro expression system[281,286]. Hayashi et al.[281] classified the genotypes as type A (homozygous normal alleles; *c1,c1*), type C (homozygous alleles with the nucleotide exchanges; *c2,c2*) and type B (heterozygous, having a normal and an altered allele; *c1,c2*). The rare mutant allele (termed the *c2* allele) that lacks the *Rsa*I restriction site is associated with higher transcriptional activity, protein levels and enzyme activity than the more common wild-type allele (*c1* allele)[281,286,287].

The frequency of the *Rsa*I-lacking *c2* allele varies in different populations[288]. The highest frequency has been observed in the Taiwanese (0.28) and Japanese (0.19–0.27), while in African-Americans, European-Americans and Scandinavians, the frequency is much lower, ranging between 0.01 and 0.05[288]. The *Rsa*I polymorphism has been investigated in the Japanese population by two groups; one showed a positive association of the *c2* allele with alcoholic liver disease[287], whereas the other reported an association between the *c1* (wild-type) allele and alcoholic liver disease[289]. A smaller study has also been performed in North American Caucasian men[290]; it did not show an association between alcoholic liver disease and *Rsa*l polymorphism, whereas others[290] found that the *c2* allele frequency in patients with alcoholic liver disease was significantly higher than in control subjects, suggesting that Caucasians carrying the *Rsa*l c2 allele of the *CYP2E1* gene may be at higher risk of developing ALD if they abuse alcohol. There was also no relationship between the *Rsa*l polymorphism and CYP2E1 activity[291] but this does not of course exclude the possibility of an effect of this polymorphism on inducibility of *CYP2E1*, as suggested by the observation that individuals who are heterozygote for the *Rsa*l mutation show reduced induction during exposure to alcohol[292].

A significant association of a particular restriction fragment length polymorphism (RFLP) haplotype of the COL1A2 locus and alcoholic cirrhosis has been reported[293], but questioned by others[294]. That susceptibility to alcoholic liver disease is, in part, genetically determined has been shown by twin studies[295] and, recently, a significant association was found between the occurrence of the null glutathione-S-transferase genotype and that of alcoholic liver cirrhosis[296].

Although these genetic markers are of great theoretical interest, from a practical point of view, there are no markers available as yet to easily identify individuals predisposed to the development of alcoholism. The same pertains to the early detection of individuals prone to develop alcoholic cirrhosis at an early stage prior to their development of full blown cirrhosis and their medical and social disintegration. Therefore, at the present time one must rely on empirical markers such as precirrhotic lesions (e.g. perivenular fibrosis, see above) to detect such individuals at an early stage, prior to their medical or social disintegration.

Acknowledgements

Original studies reviewed here were supported by NIH grants AA05934, AA11115, AA11160, AA07275 and the Department of Veterans Affairs. Skilful typing of the manuscript by Ms. D. Perez is gratefully acknowledged.

REFERENCES

1. Lieber CS. Herman Award Lecture, 1993: A personal perspective on alcohol, nutrition and the liver. Am J Clin Nutr. 1993;58:430–442.
2. Korsten MA, Lieber CS. Nutrition in pancreatic and liver disorders. In: Shils ME, Olson JA, Shike M, eds. Modern Nutrition in Health and Disease, 8th edn. Philadelphia, PA; Lea and Febiger, 1994:1066–1080.
3. Feinmann L, Lieber CS. Liver disorders: nutritional management, In: Sadler M, Caballero B, Strain S, eds. Encyclopedia of Human Nutrition. London, UK: Academic Press, 1988:1209–1226.
4. Perlow W, Baraona E, Lieber CS. Symptomatic intestinal disaccharidase deficiency in alcoholics. Gastroenterology. 1977;72:680–684.
5. Best CH, Hartroft WS, Lucas CC, Ridout JH. Liver damage produced by feeding alcohol or sugar and its prevention by choline. Br Med J. 1949;2:1001–1006.
6. Klatskin G, Krehl WA, Conn HO. The effect of alcohol on the choline requirement. I. Changes in the rat's liver following prolonged ingestion of alcohol. J Exp Med. 1954;100:605–614.
7. Thompson JA, Reitz RC. Studies of the acute and chronic effects of ethanol ingestion on choline oxidation. Ann NY Acad Sci. 1976;273:194–204.

8. Hoffbauer FW, Zaki PG. Choline deficiency in baboon and rat compared. Arch Pathol. 1965;79:364–369.

9. Volwiler W, Jones CM, Mallory TB. Criteria for the measurement of results of treatment in fatty cirrhosis. Gastroenterology. 1948;11:164–182.

10. Phillips GB, Davidson CS. Acute hepatic insufficiency of the chronic alcoholic. Arch Intern Med. 1954;94:585–603.

11. Post J, Benton JG, Breakstone R, Hoffman J. The effects of diet and choline on fatty infiltration of the human liver. Gastroenterology. 1952;20:403–410.

12. Olson RE. Modern nutrition in health and disease. In: Wohl MG, Goodhart RS, eds, Nutrition and Alcoholism, 3rd edn. Philadelphia: Lea and Febiger, 1964:779–795.

13. Rubin E, Lieber CS. Alcohol induced hepatic injury in nonalcoholic volunteers. N Engl J Med. 1968;278:869–876.

14. Chawla RK, Wolf DC, Kutner MH, Bonkovsky HL. Choline may be an essential nutrient in malnourished patients with cirrhosis. Gastroenterology. 1989;97:1514–1520.

15. Lieber CS, DeCarli LM. An experimental model of alcohol feeding and liver injury in the baboon. J Med Primatol. 1974;3:153–163.

16. Lieber CS, Leo MA, Mak KM, DeCarli LM, Sato S. Choline fails to prevent liver fibrosis in ethanol-fed baboons but causes toxicity. Hepatology. 1985;5:561–572.

17. Derr RF, Porta EA, Larkin EC, Rao GA. Is ethanol per se hepatotoxic? J Hepatol. 1990;10:381–386.

18. Lieber CS, Jones DP, DeCarli LM. Effects of prolonged ethanol intake: production of fatty liver despite adequate diets. J Clin Invest. 1965;44:1009–1021.

19. Lieber CS, Lasker JM, DeCarli LM, Saeli J, Wojtowicz T. Role of acetone, dietary fat and total energy intake in the induction of the hepatic microsomal ethanol oxidizing system. J Pharmacol Exp Ther. 1988;247:792–795.

20. Finkelstein JD, Martin JJ. Methionine metabolism in mammals. Adaptation to methionine excess. J Biol Chem. 1986;261:1582–1587.

21. Hardwick DF, Applegarth DA, Cockcroft DM, Ross PM, Cder RJ. Pathogenesis of methionine-induced toxicity. Metabolism. 1970;19:381–391.

22. Iob V, Coon WW, Sloan W. Free amino acids in liver, plasma and muscle of patients with cirrhosis of the liver. J. Surg Res. 1967;7:41–43.

23. Fischer JE, Yoshimura N, Aguirre A et al. Plasma amino acids in patients with hepatic encephalopathy. Am J Surg. 1974;127:40–47.

24. Iber FL, Rosen H, Stanley MA, Levenson SM, Chalmers TC. The plasma amino acids in patients with liver failure. J Lab Clin Med. 1957;50:417–425.

25. Montanari A, Simoni I, Vallisa D et al. Free amino acids in plasma and skeletal muscle of patients with liver cirrhosis. Hepatology. 1988;8:1034–1039.

26. Kinsell L, Harper HA, Barton HC, Michaels GD, Weiss HA. Rate of disappearance from plasma of intravenously administered methionine in patients with liver damage. Science. 1947;106:589–594.

27. Horowitz JH, Rypins EB, Henderson JM et al. Evidence for impairment of transsulfuration pathway in cirrhosis. Gastroenterology. 1981;81:668–675.

28. Duce AM, Ortiz P, Cabrero C, Mato JM. S-adenosyl-L-methionine synthetase and phospholipid methyltransferase are inhibited in human cirrhosis. Hepatology. 1988;8:65–68.

29. Finkelstein JD, Cello FP, Kyle WE. Ethanol-induced changes in methionine metabolism in rat liver. Biochem Biophys Res Commun. 1974;61:475–481.

30. Lieber CS, Casini A, DeCarli LM, Kim C, Lowe N, Sasaki R, Leo MA. S-adenosyl-L-methionine attenuates alcohol-induced liver injury in the baboon. Hepatology. 1990;11:165–172.

31. Hirata F, Axelrod J. Phospholipid methylation and biological signal transmission. Science. 1980;209:1082–1090.

32. Hirata F, Viveros OH, Diliberto EJ Jr, Axelrod J. Identification and properties of two methyltransferases in conversion of phosphatidylethanolamine to phosphatidylcholine. Proc Natl Acad Sci USA. 1978;75:1718–1721.

33. Yamada S, Mak KM, Lieber CS. Chronic ethanol consumption alters rat liver plasma membranes and potentiates release of alkaline phosphatase. Gastroenterology. 1985;88:1799–1806.

34. Mato JM, Cámara J, Fernández de Paz J. S-Adenosylmethionine in alcoholic liver cirrhosis: A randomized, placebo-controlled, double-blind, multicentre clinical trial. J Hepatol. 1999;30:1081–1089.

35. Lieber CS, Robins SJ, Li J, DeCarli LM, Mak KM, Fasulo JM, Leo MA. Phosphatidylcholine protects against fibrosis and cirrhosis in the baboon. Gastroenterology. 1994;106:152–159.
36. Arai M, Gordon ER, Lieber CS. Decreased cytochrome oxidase activity in hepatic mitochondria after chronic ethanol consumption and the possible role of decreased cytochrome aa_3 content and changes in phospholipids. Biochim Biophys Acta. 1984;797:320–327.
37. Navder KP, Baraona E, Lieber CS. Polyenylphosphatidylcholine attenuates alcohol-induced fatty liver and hyperlipemia in rats. J Nutr. 1997;127:1800–1806.
38. Lieber CS, Robins SJ, Leo MA. Hepatic phosphatidylethanolamine methyltransferase activity is decreased by ethanol and increased by phosphatidylcholine. Alcohol: Clin Exp Res. 1994;18:592–595.
39. Lieber CS, DeCarli LM, Mak KM, Kim C-I, Leo MA. Attenuation of alcohol-induced hepatic fibrosis by polyunsaturated lecithin. Hepatology. 1990;12:1390–1398.
40. Lekim D, Graf E. Tierexperimentelle Studien zur Pharmakokinetik der 'essentiellen' Phospholipide (EPL). Drug Res Arzneimittel-Forsch. 1976;26:1772–1782.
41. Poniachik J, Baraona E, Zhao J, Lieber CS. Dilinoleoylphosphatidylcholine decreases hepatic stellate cell activation. J Lab Clin Med. 1999;133:342–348.
42. Li J-J, Kim C-I, Leo MA, Mak KM, Rojkind M, Lieber CS. Polyunsaturated lecithin prevents acetaldehyde-mediated hepatic collagen accumulation by stimulating collagenase activity in cultured stellate cells. Hepatology. 1992;15:373–381.
43. Patek AJ, Haig C. The occurrence of abnormal dark adaptation and its relation to vitamin A metabolism in patients with cirrhosis of the liver. J Clin Invest. 1939;18:609–616.
44. Wald G. Molecular basis of visual excitation. Science. 1968;162:230–239.
45. Smith JC, Brown ED, White SC, Finkelson JD. Plasma vitamin A and zinc concentration in patients with alcoholic cirrhosis. Lancet. 1975;1:1251–1252.
46. McClain CJ, Van Thiel DH, Parker S, Badzin LK, Gilbert H. Alteration in zinc, vitamin A and retinol-binding protein in chronic alcoholics: A possible mechanism for night blindness and hypogonadism. Alcohol: Clin Exp Res. 1979;3:135–140.
47. Smith FR, Goodman DS. The effects of diseases of the liver, thyroid, and kidney on the transport of vitamin A in human plasma. J Clin Invest. 1971;50:2426–2436.
48. Smith JC, McDaniel EG, Fan FF, Halsted JA. Zinc. A trace element essential in vitamin A metabolism. Science. 1973;181:954–955.
49. Leo MA, Lieber CS. Hepatic vitamin A depletion in alcoholic liver injury. N Engl J Med. 1982;307:597–601.
50. Vahlquist A, Sjolund K, Norden A, Pererson PA, Stigmar G, Johansson B. Plasma vitamin A transport and visual dark adaptation in diseases of the intestine and liver. Scand J Clin Lab Invest. 1978;38:301–308.
51. Sato M, Lieber CS. Hepatic vitamin A depletion after chronic ethanol consumption in baboons and rats. J Nutr. 1981;111:2015–2023.
52. Leo MA, Lieber CS. Alcohol, vitamin A, and beta-carotene. Adverse interactions, including hepatotoxicity and carcinogenicity. Am J Clin Nutr. 1999;69:1071–1085.
53. Leo MA, Arai M, Sato M, Lieber CS. Exacerbation by ethanol of liver injury due to vitamin A deficiency and excess. In: Lieber CS, ed. Biological Approach to Alcoholism: Update. Research Monograph-11, DHHS Publication No. (ADM) 83–1261, Superintendent of Documents, Washington, DC: US Government Printing Office; 1983:195–233.
54. Leo MA, Sato M, Lieber CS. Effect of hepatic vitamin A depletion on the liver in humans and rats. Gastroenterology. 1983;84:562–572.
55. Green MH, Green JB, Berg T, Norum KR, Blomhoff R. Vitamin A metabolism in rat liver: a kinetic model. Am J Physiol. 1993;264:G509–G521.
56. Davis BH, Vucic A. The effect of retinol on Ito cell proliferation in vitro. Hepatology. 1988;8:788–793.
57. Davis BH, Kramer RJ, Davidson, NO. Retinoic acid modulates rat Ito cell proliferation, collagen, and transforming growth factor β production. J Clin Invest. 1990;86:2062–2070.
58. Friedman SL, Wei S, Blaner W. Retinol release by activated rat hepatic lipocytes: regulation by Kupffer cell-conditioned medium and PDGF. Am J Physiol. 1993;264:G947–G952.
59. Krupski M, Fine A, Berk JL, Goldstein RH. Retinoic acid-induced inhibitions of type I collagen gene expression by human lung fibroblasts. Biochim Biophys Acta. 1994;1219:335–341.
60. Wang X-D, Liu C, Chung J, Stickel F, Seitz HK, Russell RM. Chronic alcohol intake reduces retinoic acid concentration and enhances AP-1 (c-Jun and c-Fos) expression in rat liver. Hepatology. 1988;28:744-750.

61. Kvale G, Bielke F, Gart JJ. Dietary habits and lung cancer risk. Int J Cancer. 1983;31:397–405.
62. Pollack ES, Nomura AMY, Heilbrum L, Steimmermann GN, Green SB. Prospective study of alcohol consumption and cancer. N Engl J Med. 1984;310:617–621.
63. Russell RM, Boyer JL, Bagheri SA et al. Hepatic injury from chronic hypervitaminosis A resulting in portal hypertension and ascites. N Engl J Med. 1974;291:435–440.
64. Farrell GC, Bathal PS, Powell LW. Abnormal liver function in chronic hypervitaminosis A. Dig Dis Sci. 1977;22:724–728.
65. Jeghers H, Marraro H. Hypervitaminosis A: its broadening spectrum. Am J Clin Nutr. 1958;6:335–339.
66. Farris W, Erdman J. Protracted hypervitaminosis A following long term low-level intake. JAMA. 1982;247:1317–1318.
67. Herbert V. Toxicity of 25 000 IU vitamin A supplements in health food users. Am J Clin Nutr. 1982;36:185–186.
68. Minuk GY, Kelly JK, Hwang WS. Vitamin A hepatoxicity in multiple family members. Hepatology. 1988;8:272–275.
69. Geubel AP, DeGalocsy C, Alves N, Rahier J, Dive C. Liver damage caused by therapeutic vitamin A administration: estimate of dose related toxicity in 41 cases. Gastroenterology. 1991;100:1701–1709.
70. Oikarinen H, Oikarinen AI, Tan EML et al. Modulation of pro-collagen gene expression by retinoids. J Clin Invest. 1985;75:1545–1553.
71. Senoo H, Wale K. Suppression of experimental hepatic fibrosis by administration of vitamin A. Lab Invest. 1985;52:182–194.
72. Leo MA, Lieber CS. Hypervitaminosis A: a liver lover's lament. Hepatology. 1988;8:412–417.
73. Leo MA, Arai M, Sato M et al. Hepatotoxicity of vitamin A and ethanol in the rat. Gastroenterology. 1982;92:194–205.
74. Worner TM, Gordon G, Leo MA et al. Treatment with vitamin A of sexual dysfunction in male alcoholics. Am J Clin Nutr. 1988;48:1431–1435.
75. Leo MA, Lieber CS. Hepatic fibrosis after long term administration of ethanol and moderate vitamin A supplementation in the rat. Hepatology. 1983;3:1–11.
76. Chapman KMC, Prabhudesai M, Erdman JW. Vitamin A status of alcoholics upon admission and after two weeks of hospitalization. J Am Coll Nutr. 1993;12:77–83.
77. Mak KM, Leo MA, Lieber CS. Alcoholic liver injury in baboons: transformation of lipocytes to transitional cells. Gastroenterology. 1984;87:188–200.
78. Leo MA, Lieber CS. New pathway for retinol metabolism in liver microsomes. J Biol Chem. 1985;260:5228–5231.
79. Leo MA, Kim C, Lieber CS. NAD$^+$-dependent retinol dehydrogenase in liver microsomes. Arch Biochem Biophys. 1987;259:241–249.
80. Sato M, Lieber CS. Increased metabolism of retinoic acid after chronic ethanol consumption in rat liver microsomes. Arch Biochem Biophys. 1982;213:557–564.
81. Leo MA, Iida S, Lieber CS. Retinoic acid metabolism by a system reconstituted with cytochrome P-450. Arch Biochem Biophys. 1984;234:305–312.
82. Ahmed S, Leo MA, Lieber CS. Interactions between alcohol and beta-carotene in patients with alcoholic liver disease. Am J Clin Nutr. 1994;60:430–436.
83. Ward RJ, Peters TJ. The antioxidant status of patients with either alcohol-induced liver damage or myopathy. Alcohol Alcoholism. 1992;27:359–365.
84. Forman MR, Beecher GR, Lanza E et al. Effect of alcohol consumption on plasma carotenoid concentrations in premenopausal women: A controlled dietary study. Am J Clin Nutr. 1995;62:131–135.
85. Leo MA, Kim CI, Lowe N, Lieber CS. Interaction of ethanol with β-carotene: Delayed blood clearance and enhanced hepatotoxicity. Hepatology. 1992;15:883–891.
86. Leo MA, Rosman AS, Lieber CS. Differential depletion of carotenoids and tocopherol in liver disease. Hepatology. 1993;17:977–986.
87. Patek AJ, Toth IG, Saunders MG, Castro GAM, Engel JJ. Alcohol and dietary factors in cirrhosis. An epidemiological study of 304 alcohol patients. Arch Intern Med. 1975;135:1053–1057.
88. Leo MA, Aleynik S, Aleynik M, Lieber CS. B-carotene beadlets potentiate hepatotoxicity of alcohol. Am J Clin Nutr. 1997;66:1461–1469.

89. The α-Tocopherol, β-Carotene and Cancer Prevention Study Group. The effect of vitamin E and β-carotene on the incidence of lung cancer and other cancers in male smokers. N Engl J Med. 1994;330:1029–1035.

90. Omenn GS, Goodman GE, Thornquist MD et al. Effects of a combination of beta carotene and vitamin A on lung cancer and cardiovascular disease. N Engl J Med. 1996;334:1150–1155.

91. Leo MA, Lieber CS. Beta carotene, vitamin E, and lung cancer. N Engl J Med. 1994;331:612.

92. Garro AJ, Gordon BHJ, Lieber CS. Alcohol abuse. Carcinogenic effects and fetal alcohol syndrome. In: Lieber CS, ed., Medical and Nutritional Complications of Alcoholism: Mechanisms and Management. New York, Plenum Press, 1992:459.

93. Burton GW, Ingold KU. β-Carotene: an unusual type of lipid antioxidant. Science. 1984;224:569–573.

94. Albanese D, Heinonen OP, Taylor PR et al. α-Tocopherol and β-carotene supplements and lung cancer incidence in the Alpha-Tocopherol, Beta-Carotene Cancer Prevention Study: effect of base-line characteristics and the study compliance. J Natl Cancer Inst. 1996;88:1560–1571.

95. Omenn GS, Goodman GE, Thornquist MD et al. Risk factors for lung cancer and for intervention effects in CARET, the Beta-Carotene and Retinol Efficacy Trial. J Natl Cancer Inst. 1996;88:1550–1559.

96. Albanes D, Virtamo J, Taylor PR, Rautalahti M, Pietinen P, Heinonen OP. Effects of supplemental β-carotene, cigarette smoking, and alcohol consumption on serum carotenoids in the alpha tocopherol, beta-carotene cancer prevention study. Am J Clin Nutr. 1997;66:366–372.

97. Bjørneboe GEA, Bjørneboe A, Hagen BF, Morland J, Drevon CA. Reduced hepatic α-tocopherol content after long-term administration of ethanol to rats. Biochem Biophys Acta. 1987;918:236–241.

98. Kawase T, Kato S, Lieber CS. Lipid peroxidation and antioxidant defense systems in rat liver after chronic ethanol feeding. Hepatology. 1989;10:815–821.

99. von Herbay A, de Groot H, Hegi U, Stemmel W, Strohmeyer G, Sies H. Low vitamin E content in plasma of patients with alcoholic liver disease, hemochromatosis and Wilson's disease. J Hepatol. 1994;20:41–46.

100. Lieber CS, Jones DP, Mendelson J, DeCarli LM. Fatty liver, hyperlipemia and hyperuricemia produced by prolonged alcohol consumption, despite adequate dietary intake. Trans Assoc Am Phys. 1963;76:289–300.

101. Lieber CS, Lefevre A, Spritz N, Feinman L, DeCarli LM. Difference in hepatic metabolism of long- and medium-chain fatty acids: the role of fatty acid chain length in the production of the alcoholic fatty liver. J Clin Invest. 1967;46:1451–1460.

102. Lieber CS, DeCarli LM. Effects of mineral and vitamin supplementation on the alcohol induced fatty liver and microsomal induction. Alcohol: Clin Exp Res. 1989;13:142–143.

103. Tsukamoto H, French SW, Benson N, Delgado G, Rao GA, Larkin EC, Largman C. Severe and progressive steatosis and focal necrosis in rat liver induced by continuous intragastric infusion of ethanol and low fat diet. Hepatology. 1985;5:224–232.

104. Nanji AA, French SW. Dietary linoleic acid is required for development of experimentally induced alcoholic liver injury. Life Sci. 1989;44:223–227.

105. Nanji AA, Mendenhall CL, French SW. Beef fat prevents alcoholic liver disease in the rat. Alcohol: Clin Exp Res. 1989;13:15–19.

106. Badger TM, Korourian S, Hakkak R, Ronis MJJ, Shelnut SR, Ingelman-Sundberg M, Waldron J. Carbohydrate deficiency as a possible factor in ethanol-induced hepatic necrosis. Alcohol: Clin Exp Res. 1998;22:742–744.

107. Lindros K, Jarvelainen H. A new oral low-carbohydrate alcohol liquid diet producing liver lesions: a preliminary account. Alcohol Alcoholism. 1998;33:347–353.

108. Sippel H, Oinonen T, Lindros KO. Chronic low-carbohydrate ethanol diet: Further depletion of glutathione peroxidase activity in the centrilobular liver region. Alcohol: Clin Exp Res. 1998;22:171A.

109. Teschke R, Moreno F, Petrides AS. Hepatic microsomal ethanol oxidizing system (MEOS): respective roles of ethanol and carbohydrates for the enhanced activity after chronic alcohol consumption. Biochem Pharmacol. 1981;30:1745–1751.

110. Lieber CS, DeCarli LM, Rubin E. Sequential production of fatty liver, hepatitis and cirrhosis in subhuman primates fed ethanol with adequate diets. Proc Natl Acad Sci USA. 1975;72:437–441.

111. Popper H, Lieber CS. Histogenesis of alcoholic fibrosis and cirrhosis in the baboon. Am J Pathol. 1980;98;695–716.

112. Porto LC, Chevallier M, Crimaud J-A. Morphometry of terminal hepatic veins. 1. Comparative study in man and baboon. Virchows Arch. 1989;414:129–134.
113. Porto LC, Chevallier M, Crimaud J-A. Morphometry of terminal hepatic veins. 2. Follow up in chronically alcohol-fed baboons. Virchows Arch. 1989;414:299–307.
114. Lelbach WK. Cirrhosis in the alcoholic and its relation to the volume of alcohol abuse. Ann NY Acad Sci. 1975;252:85–105.
115. Pequignot G, Chabert C, Eydoux H, Corcowl MA. Increased risk of liver cirrhosis with intake of alcohol. Rev Alcoholism. 1974;20:191–202.
116. Jolliffe N, Jellinek EM. Vitamin deficiencies and liver cirrhosis in alcoholism. Part VII: Cirrhosis of the liver. QJ Stud Alcohol. 1941;2:544–583.
117. Schmidt W. Agreement, disagreement in experimental, clinical and epidemiological evidence on the etiology of alcoholic liver cirrhosis: a comment. In: Khanna JM, Israel Y, Kalant H, eds. Alcoholic Liver Pathology. Ontario: Addiction Research Foundation, 1975:19–30.
118. Lelbach WK. Epidemiology of alcoholic liver disease. In: Popper H, Schaffner, F, eds. Progress in Liver Disease. New York: Grune and Stratton, 1976:494–515.
119. Schmidt W. The epidemiology of cirrhosis of the liver: a statistical analysis of mortality data with special reference to Canada. In: Fischer MM, Rankin JG, eds. Alcohol and the Liver. New York: Plenum Press, 1977:1–26.
120. Stone WD, Islam NRK, Paton A. The natural history of cirrhosis. Q J Med. 1968;37:119–132.
121. Hällen J, Krook H. Follow-up studies on an unselected ten-year material of 360 patients with liver cirrhosis in one community. Acta Med Scand. 1963;173:479–493.
122. Martini GA, Bode CH. The epidemiology of cirrhosis of the liver. In: Engel A, Larsson T, eds. Alcoholic Cirrhosis and Other Toxic Hepatopathies. Stockholm: Nordiska Bokhandelinsforlog, 1970:315–335.
123. Lieber CS, Rubin E. Alcoholic fatty liver in man on a high-protein and low-fat diet. Am J Med. 1968;44:200–206.
124. Lieber CS, Spritz N. Effects of prolonged ethanol intake in man: role of dietary, adipose and endogenously synthesized fatty acids in the pathogenesis of the alcoholic fatty liver. J Clin Invest. 1966;45:1400–1411.
125. Lane BP, Lieber CS. Ultrastructural alterations in human hepatocytes following ingestion of ethanol with adequate diets. Am J Pathol. 1966;49:593–603.
126. Lieber CS, DeCarli LM. Hepatotoxicity of ethanol. J Hepatol. 1991;12:394–401.
127. Faller J, Fox IH. Evidence for increased urate production by activation of adenine nucleotide turnover. N Engl J Med. 1982;307:1598–1602.
128. Lieber CS (ed). Medical and Nutritional Complications of Alcoholism: Mechanisms and Management. New York: Plenum Medical Book Company, 1992.
129. Lieber CS, DeCarli LM, Schmid R. Effects of ethanol on fatty acid metabolism in liver slices. Biochem Biophys Res Commun. 1959;1:302–306.
130. Lieber CS, Pignon J-P. Ethanol and lipids. In: Fruchart JC, Shepherd J, eds. Human Plasma Lipoproteins: Chemistry, Physiology and Pathology. Berlin: Walter De Gruyter and Co., 1989:245–280.
131. Lieber CS, Schmid R. The effect of ethanol on fatty acid metabolism: Stimulation of hepatic fatty acid synthesis in vitro. J Clin Invest. 1961;40:394–399.
132. Lieber CS, Spritz N, DeCarli LM. Role of dietary, adipose and endogenously synthesized fatty acids in the pathogenesis of the alcoholic fatty liver. J Clin Invest. 1966;45:51–62.
133. Lieber CS, Savolainen M. Ethanol and lipids. Alcohol: Clin Exp Res. 1984;8:409–423.
134. Videla L, Israel Y. Factors that modify the metabolism of ethanol in rat liver and adaptive changes produced by its chronic administration. Biochem J. 1970;118:275–281.
135. Israel Y, Kalant H, Orrego H, Khanna JM, Videla L, Phillips JM. Experimental alcohol-induced hepatic necrosis: Suppression by prophylthiouracil. Proc Natl Acad Sci USA. 1975;72:1137–1141.
136. Kessler BJ, Lieber JB, Bronfin GJ, Sass M. The hepatic blood flow and splanchnic oxygen consumption in alcohol fatty liver. J Clin Invest. 1954;33:1338–1345.
137. Jauhonen P, Baraona E, Miyakawa H, Lieber CS. Mechanism for selective perivenular hepatotoxicity of ethanol. Alcohol: Clin Exp Res. 1982;6:350–357.
138. Sato N, Kamada T, Kawano S et al. Effect of acute and chronic ethanol consumption on hepatic tissue oxygen tension in rats. Pharmacology. 1983;18:443–447.
139. Shaw S, Heller E, Friedman H, Baraona E, Lieber CS. Increased hepatic oxygenation following ethanol administration in the baboon. Proc Soc Exp Biol Med. 1977;56:509–513.

140. Stein SW, Lieber CS, Leevy CM, Cherrick GR, Abelmann WH. The effect of ethanol upon systemic hepatic blood flow in man. Am J Clin Nutr. 1963;13:68–74.
141. Carmichael FJ, Saldivia V, Israel Y, McKaigney JP, Orrego H. Ethanol-induced increase in portal hepatic blood flow: interference by anesthetic agents. Hepatology. 1987;7:89–94.
142. Lieber CS, Baraona E, Hernández-Muñoz R et al. Impaired oxygen utilization: A new mechanism for the hepatotoxicity of ethanol in sub-human primates. J Clin Invest. 1989;83:1682–1690.
143. Jauhonen P, Baraona E, Lieber CS, Hassinen IE. Dependence of ethanol-induced redox shift on hepatic oxygen tensions prevailing in vivo. Alcohol. 1985;2:163–167.
144. Kato S, Kawase T, Alderman J, Lieber CS. Role of xanthine oxidase in ethanol-induced lipid peroxidation in rats. Gastroenterology. 1990;98:203–210.
145. Buhler R, Hess M, von Wartburg J-P. Immunohistochemical localization of human liver alcohol dehydrogenase in liver tissue, cultured fibroblasts and hela cells. Am J Pathol. 1982;108:89–99.
146. Lieber CS, DeCarli LM. Ethanol oxidation by hepatic microsomes: adaptive increase after ethanol feeding. Science. 1968;162:917–918.
147. Lieber CS, DeCarli LM. Hepatic microsomal ethanol oxidizing system: in vitro characteristics and adaptive properties in vivo. J Biol Chem. 1970;245:2505–2512.
148. Teschke R, Hasumura Y, Joly JG, Ishii H, Lieber CS. Microsomal ethanol-oxidizing system (MEOS): Purification and properties of a rat liver system free of catalase and alcohol dehydrogenase, Biochem Biophys Res Commun. 1972;49:1187–1193.
149. Teschke R, Hasumura Y, Lieber CS. Hepatic microsomal alcohol oxidizing system: Solubilization, isolation and characterization. Arch Biochem Biophys. 1974;163:404–415.
150. Ohnishi K, Lieber CS. Reconstitution of the microsomal ethanol-oxidizing system: qualitative and quantitative changes of cytochrome P-450 after chronic ethanol consumption. J Biol Chem. 1977;252:7124–7131.
151. Miwa GT, Levin W, Thomas PE, Lu AYH. The direct oxidation of ethanol by catalase- and alcohol dehydrogenase-free reconstituted system containing cytochrome P-450. Arch Biochem Biophys. 1978;187:464–475.
152. Koop DR, Morgan ET, Tarr GE, Coon MJ. Purification and characterization of a unique isozyme of cytochrome P-450 from liver microsomes of ethanol-treated rabbits. J Biol Chem. 1982;257:8472–8480.
153. Lasker JM, Raucy J, Kubota S, Bloswick BP, Black M, Lieber CS. Purification and characterization of human liver cytochrome P-450-ALC. Biochem Biophys Res Commun. 1987;148:232-238.
154. Tsutsumi M, Lasker JM, Shimizu M, Rosman AS, Lieber CS. The intralobular distribution of ethanol-inducible P450IIE1 in rat and human liver. Hepatology. 1989;10:437–446.
155. Takahashi T, Lasker JM, Rosman AS, Lieber CS. Induction of cytochrome P-4502E1 in the human liver by ethanol is caused by a corresponding increase in encoding messenger RNA. Hepatology. 1993;17:236–245.
156. Salmela KS, Kessova IG, Tsyrlov IB, Lieber CS. Respective roles of human cytochrome P4502E1, 1A2, and 3A4 in the hepatic microsomal ethanol oxidizing system. Alcohol: Clin Exp Res. 1998;22:2125–2132.
157. Kalant H, Khanna JM, Marshman J. Effect of chronic intake of ethanol on pentobarbital metabolism. J Pharmacol. 1970;175:318–324.
158. Misra PS, Lefévre A, Ishii H, Rubin E, Lieber CS. Increase of ethanol meprobamate and pentobarbital metabolism after chronic ethanol administration in man and in rats. Am J Med. 1971;51:346–351.
159. Salaspuro MP, Lieber CS. Non-uniformity of blood ethanol elimination: its exaggeration after chronic consumption. Ann Clin Res. 1978;10:294–297.
160. Pritchard JF, Schneck DW. Effects of ethanol and phenobarbital on the metabolism of propranolol by 9000 g rat liver supernatant. Biochem Pharmacol. 1977;26:2453–2454.
161. Sotaniemi EA, Anttila M, Rautio A, Stengard J, Saukko P, Jarvensivu P. Propranolol and sotalol metabolism after a drinking party. Clin Pharmacol Ther. 1981;29:705–710.
162. Carulli N, Manenti F, Gallo M, Salvioli GF. Alcohol-drugs interaction in man: Alcohol and tolbutamide. Eur J Clin Invest. 1971;1:421–424.
163. Kater RMH, Roggin G, Tobon F, Zieve P, Iber FL. Increased rate of clearance of drugs from the circulation of alcoholics. Am J Med Sci. 1969;258:35–39.
164. Kater RMH, Tobon F, Iber FL. Increased rate of tolbutamide metabolism in alcoholic patients. JAMA. 1969;207:363–365.

165. Sellman R, Kanto J, Raijola E, Pekkarinen A. Human and animal study on elimination from plasma and metabolism of diazepam after chronic alcohol intake. Acta Pharmacol Toxicol. 1975;36:33–38.
166. Grassi GG, Grassi C. Ethanol-antibiotic interactions at hepatic level. Int J Clin Pharmacol. 1975;11:216–225.
167. Hetu C, Dumont A, Joly JG. Effect of chronic ethanol administration on bromobenzene liver toxicity in the rat. Toxicol Appl Pharmacol. 1983;67:166–167.
168. Siegers C-P, Heidbuchel K, Younes M. Influence of alcohol, dithiocarb and (+)-catechin on the hepatotoxicity and metabolism of vinylidene chloride in rats. J Appl Toxicol. 1983;3:90–95.
169. Kharasch ED, Thummel KE. Identification of cytochrome P4502E1 as the predominant enzyme catalyzing human liver microsomal defluorination of sevoflurane, isoflurane, and methoxyflurane. Anesthesiology. 1993;79:795–807.
170. Tsutsumi R, Leo MA, Kim CI, Tsutsumi M, Lasker J, Lowe N, Lieber CS. Interaction of ethanol with enflurane metabolism and toxicity: Role of P450IIE1. Alcohol: Clin Exp Res. 1990;14:174–179.
171. Takagi T, Ishii H, Takahashi H et al. Potentiation of halothane hepatotoxicity by chronic ethanol administration in rat. An animal model of halothane hepatitis. Pharmacol Biochem Behav. 1983;18:461–465.
172. Beskid M, Bialek J, Dzieniszewski J, Sadowski J, Tlalka J. Effect of combined phenylbutazone and ethanol administration on rat liver. Exp Pathol. 1980;18:487–491.
173. Raucy JL, Lasker JM, Lieber CS, Black M. Acetaminophen activation by human liver cytochromes P450IIE1 and P4501A2. Arch Biochem Biophys. 1989;271:270–283.
174. Black M. Acetaminophen hepatotoxicity. Annu Rev Med. 1984;35:577–593.
175. Seeff LB, Cucherini BA, Zimmerman HJ, Alder E, Benjamin SB. Acetaminophen hepatotoxicity in alcoholics: A therapeutic misadventure (clinical review). Ann Intern Med. 1986;104:399–404.
176. Sato C, Matsuda Y, Lieber CS. Increased hepatotoxicity of acetaminophen after chronic ethanol consumption in the rat. Gastroenterology. 1981;80:140–148.
177. Whitecomb DC, Block GD. Association of acetaminophen hepatotoxicity with fasting and ethanol use. JAMA. 1994;272:1845–1850.
178. Nordmann R, Ribiére C, Rouach H. Implication of free radical mechanisms in ethanol-induced cellular injury. Free Radical Biol Med. 1992;12:219–240.
179. Lieber CS, DeCarli LM. Reduced nicotinamide-adenine dinucleotide phosphate oxidase: Activity enhanced by ethanol consumption. Science. 1970;170:78–80.
180. Dai Y, Rashba-Step J, Cederbaum AI. Stable expression of human cytochrome P4502E1 in HepG2 cells: characterization of catalytic activities and production of reactive oxygen intermediates. Biochemistry. 1993;32:6928–6937.
181. Ekstrom G, Ingelman-Sundberg M. Rat liver microsomal NADPH-supported oxidase activity and lipid peroxidation dependent on ethanol-inducible cytochrome P-450 (P-450IIE1). Biochem Pharmacol. 1989;38:1313–1319.
182. Castillo T, Koop DR, Kamimura S, Triadafilopoulos G, Tsukamoto H. Role of cytochrome P-450 2E1 in ethanol-, carbon tetrachloride- and iron-dependent microsomal lipid peroxidation. Hepatology. 1992;16:992–996.
183. Albano E, Tomasi A, Goria-Gatti L, Poli G, Vannini B, Dianzani MU. Free radical metabolism of alcohols in rat liver microsomes. Free Rad Res Commun. 1987;3:243.
184. Reinke L, Lai EK, DuBose CM, McCay PB, Janzen EG. Reactive free radical generation in vivo in heart and liver of ethanol-fed rats: Correlation with radical formation in vitro. Proc Natl Acad Sci USA. 1987;84:8223–8227.
185. Reinke LA, Kotake Y, McCay PB, Janzen EG. Spin trapping studies of hepatic free radicals formed following the acute administration of ethanol to rats: in vivo detection of l-hydroxyethyl radicals with PBN. Free Rad Biol Med. 1991;11:31–39.
186. Koivisto T, Mishin VM, Mak KM, Cohen PA, Lieber CS. Induction of cytochrome P-4502E1 by ethanol in rat Kupffer cells. Alcohol: Clin Exp Res. 1996;20:207–212.
187. Laposata EA, Lange LG. Presence of nonoxidative ethanol metabolism in human organs commonly damaged by ethanol abuse. Science. 1986;231:497–499.
188. Werner J, Laposata M, Fernandez-Del Castillo C et al. Pancreatic injury in rats induced by fatty acid ethyl ester, a nonoxidative metabolite of alcohol. Gastroenterology. 1997;113: 286–294.

189. Hasumura Y, Teschke R, Lieber CS. Hepatic microsomal ethanol oxidizing system (MEOS): Dissociation from reduced nicotinamide adenine dinucleotide phosphate-oxidase and possible role of form 1 of cytochrome P-450. J Pharmacol Exp Ther. 1975;194:469–474.

190. Di Padova C, Worner TM, Julkunen RJK, Lieber CS. Effects of fasting and chronic alcohol consumption on the first pass metabolism of ethanol. Gastroenterology. 1987;92:1169–1173.

191. Dicker E, Cederbaum AI. Increased oxygen radical-dependent inactivation of metabolic enzymes by liver microsomes after chronic ethanol consumption. FASEB J. 1988;2:2901–2906.

192. Espina N, Lima V, Lieber CS, Garro AJ. In vitro and in vivo inhibitory effect of ethanol and acetaldehyde on O^6methylguanine transferase. Carcinogenesis. 1988;9:761–766.

193. Baraona E, Leo MA, Borowsky SA, Lieber CS. Pathogenesis of alcohol-induced accumulation of protein in the liver. J Clin Invest. 1977;60:546–554.

194. Wondergem R, Davis J. Ethanol increases hepatocyte water volume. Alcohol: Clin Exp Res. 1994;18:1230–1236.

195. Müller A, Sies H. Role of alcohol dehydrogenase activity and of acetaldehyde in ethanol-induced ethane and pentane production by isolated perfused rat liver. Biochem J. 1982;206:153–156.

196. Müller A, Sies H. Inhibition of ethanol- and aldehyde-induced release of ethane from isolated perfused rat liver by Pargyline and Disulfiram. Pharmacol Biochem Behav. 1983;18:429–432.

197. Shaw S, Rubin KP, Lieber CS. Depressed hepatic glutathione and increased diene conjugates in alcoholic liver disease: evidence of lipid peroxidation. Dig Dis Sci. 1983;28:585–589.

198. Morton S, Mitchell MC. Effects of chronic ethanol feeding on glutathione turnover in the rat. Biochem Pharmacol. 1985;34:1559–1563.

199. Speisky H, MacDonald A, Giles G, Orrego H, Israel Y. Increased loss and decreased synthesis of hepatic glutathione after acute ethanol administration. Biochem J. 1985;225:565.

200. Hirano T, Kaplowitz N, Tsukamoto H, Kamimura S, Fernandez-Checa JC. Hepatic mitochondrial glutathione depletion and progression of experimental alcoholic liver disease in rats. Hepatology. 1992;6:1423–1427.

201. Zhang H, Loney LA, Potter BJ. Effect of chronic alcohol feeding on hepatic iron status and ferritin uptake by rat hepatocytes. Alcohol: Clin Exp Res. 1993;17:394–400.

202. Valenzuela A, Fernandez V, Videla LA. Hepatic and biliary levels of glutathione and lipid peroxides following iron overload in the rat: Effect of simultaneous ethanol administration. Toxicol Appl Pharmacol. 1983;70:87–95.

203. Moshage H, Casini A, Lieber CS. Acetaldehyde stimulates collagen production in cultured rat liver fat-storing cells but not in hepatocytes. Hepatology. 1990;12:511–518.

204. Ma X, Svegliati-Baroni G, Poniachik J, Baraona E, Lieber CS. Collagen synthesis by liver stellate cells is released from its normal feedback regulation by acetaldehyde-induced modification of the carboxyl-terminal propeptide of procollagen. Alcohol: Clin Exp Res. 1997;21:1204–1211.

205. Savolainen E-R, Leo MA, Timple R, Lieber CS. Acetaldehyde and lactate stimulate collagen synthesis of cultured baboon liver myofibroblasts. Gastroenterology. 1984;87:777–787.

206. Geesin JC, Hendricks LJ, Falkenstein PA, Gordon JS, Berg RA. Regulation of collagen synthesis by ascorbic acid: Characterization of the role of ascorbate stimulated lipid peroxidation. Arch Biochem Biophys. 1991;290:127–132.

207. Tsukamoto H. Oxidative stress, antioxidants, and alcoholic liver fibrogenesis. Alcohol. 1993;10:465–467.

208. Casini A, Cunningham M, Rojkind M, Lieber CS. Acetaldehyde increases procollagen type I and fibronectin gene transcription in cultured rat fat-storing cells through a protein synthesis-dependent mechanism. Hepatology. 1991;13:758–765.

209. Edmondson HA, Peters RL, Frankel HH, Borowsky S. The early stage of liver injury in the alcoholic. Medicine. 1967;46:119–129.

210. Van Waes L, Lieber CS. Early perivenular sclerosis in alcoholic fatty liver: an index of progressive liver injury. Gastroenterology. 1977;73:646–650.

211. Worner TM, Lieber CS. Perivenular fibrosis as precursor lesion of cirrhosis. JAMA. 1985;254:627–630.

212. Falchuk KR, Fiske S, Federman C, Trey C. Pericentral hepatic fibrosis and intracellular hyaline in diabetes mellitus. Gastroenterology. 1980;78:535–541.

213. Feinman L, Lieber CS. Hepatic collagen metabolism: effect of alcohol consumption in rats and baboons. Science. 1972;176:795.

214. Patrick RS. Alcohol as a stimulus to hepatic fibrogenesis. J Alcoholism. 1973;8:13–27.
215. Mezey E, Potter JJ, Iber FL, Maddrey WC. Hepatic collagen proline hydroxylase activity in alcoholic hepatitis: effect of d-penicillamine. J Lab Clin Med. 1979;93:92–100.
216. Zern MA, Leo MA, Giambrone MA, Lieber CS. Increased type I procollagen mRNA levels and in vitro protein synthesis in the baboon model of chronic alcoholic liver disease. Gastroenterology. 1985;89:1123–1131.
217. Mak KI, Lieber CS. Lipocytes and transitional cells in alcoholic liver disease: a morphometric study. Hepatology. 1988;8:1027–1033.
218. Ma X, Zhao J, Lieber CS. Polyenylphosphatidylcholine attenuates non-alcoholic hepatic fibrosis and accelerates its regression. J Hepatol. 1996;24:604–613.
219. Lieber CS, Leo MA, Aleynik SI, Aleynik MK, DeCarli LM. Polyenylphosphatidyl-choline decreases alcohol-induced oxidative stress in the baboon. Alcohol: Clin Exp Res. 1997;21:375–379.
220. Aleynik S, Leo MA, Ma X, Aleynik MK, Lieber CS. Polyenylphosphatidylcholine prevents carbon tetrachloride induced lipid peroxidation while it attenuates liver fibrosis. J Hepatol. 1997;26:554–561.
221. McClain C, Hill D, Schmidt J, Diehl AM. Cytokines and alcoholic liver disease. Semin Liver Dis. 1993;13:170–182.
222. Nolan JP. Intestinal endotoxins as mediators of hepatic injury – An idea whose time has come again. Hepatology. 1989;10:887–891.
223. Nolan JP, Camara DS. Intestinal endotoxins as co-factors in liver injury. Immunol Invest. 1989;18:325–337.
224. Adachi Y, Moore LE, Bradford BU, Gao W, Thurman RG. Antibiotics prevent liver injury in rats following long term exposure to ethanol. Gastroenterology. 1995;108:218–224.
225. Shibayama Y, Asaka S, Nakata K. Endotoxin hepatotoxicity augmented by ethanol. Exp Mol Pathol. 1991;55:196–301.
226. Khoruts A, Stahnke L, McClain CJ, Logan G, Allen JI. Circulating tumor necrosis factor, interleukin-1 and interleukin-6 concentrations in chronic alcoholic patients. Hepatology. 1991;13:267–276.
227. Sheron N, Bird G, Goka J, Alexander G, Williams R. Elevated plasma interleukin-6 and increased severity and mortality in alcoholic hepatitis. Clin Exp Immunol. 1991;84:449–453.
228. Decker K. Biologically active products of stimulated liver macrophages (Kupffer Cells) J Biochem. 1990;192:245–261.
229. Matsuoka M, Tsukamoto H. Stimulation of hepatic lipocyte collagen production by Kupffer cell-derived transforming growth factor beta: implication for a pathogenetic role in alcoholic liver fibrogenesis. Hepatology. 1990;11:599–605.
230. Kamimura S, Tsukamoto H. Cytokine gene expression by Kupffer cells in experimental alcoholic liver disease. Hepatology. 1995;22:1304–1309.
231. Bautista AP. The role of Kupffer cells and reactive oxygen species in hepatic injury during acute and chronic alcohol intoxication. Alcohol: Clin Exp Res. 1998;22:255S–259S.
232. Batey R, Cao Q, Madsen G, Pang G, Russell A, Clancy R. Decreased tumor necrosis factor-α and interleukin-1α production from intrahepatic mononuclear cells in chronic ethanol consumption and up regulation by endotoxin. Alcohol: Clin Exp Res. 1998;22:150–156.
233. Tsukamoto H. Molecular mechanism of induced hepatic macrophage cytokine gene expression in experimental alcoholic liver injury. Alcohol: Clin Exp Res. 1998;22:253S–254S.
234. Israel Y, Hurwitz E, Niëmelä O, Arnon R. Monoclonal and polyclonal antibodies against acetaldehyde-containing epitopes in acetaldehyde-protein adducts. Proc Natl Acad Sci USA. 1986;83:7923–7927.
235. Hoerner M, Behrens UJ, Worner T, Lieber CS. Humoral immune response to acetaldehyde adducts in alcoholic patients. Res Commun Chem Pathol Pharmacol. 1986;54:3–12.
236. Hoerner M, Behrens UJ, Worner TM et al. The role of alcoholism and liver disease in the appearance of serum antibodies against acetaldehyde adducts. Hepatology. 1988;8:569–574.
237. Niemela O, Klajner F, Orrego H, Vidins E, Blendis L, Israel Y. Antibodies against acetaldehyde-modified protein epitopes in human alcoholics. Hepatology. 1987;7:1210–1214.
238. Koff RS, Dienstag JL. Extrahepatic manifestations of hepatitis C and the association with alcoholic liver disease. Semin Liver Dis. 1995;15:101–109.

239. Rosman AS, Paronetto F, Galvin K, Williams RJ, Lieber CS. Hepatitis C virus antibody in alcoholic patients. Association with the presence of portal and/or lobular hepatitis. Arch Intern Med. 1993;153:965–969.
240. Rosman AS, Waraich A, Galvin K, Casiano J, Paronetto F, Lieber CS. Alcoholism is associated with hepatitis C but not hepatitis B in an urban population. Am J Gastroenterol. 1996;91:498–505.
241. Schiff ER. Hepatitis C and alcohol. Hepatology. 1997;26:39S–42S.
242. Ostapowicz G, Watson KJR, Locarnini SA, Desmond PV. Role of alcohol in the progression of liver disease caused by hepatitis C virus infection. Hepatology. 1998;27:1730–1735.
243. Pessione F, Degos F, Marcellin P et al. Effect of alcohol consumption on serum hepatitis C virus RNA and histological lesions in chronic hepatitis C. Hepatology. 1998;27:1717–1722.
244. Wiley TE, McCarthy M, Breidi L, McCarthy M, Layden TJ. Impact of alcohol on the histological and clinical progression of hepatitis C infection. Hepatology. 1998;28:805–809.
245. Corrao G, Arico S. Independent and combined action of hepatitis C virus infection and alcohol consumption on the risk of symptomatic liver cirrhosis. Hepatology. 1998;27:914–919.
246. Tsutsumi M, Ishizaki M, Takada A. Relative risk for the development of hepatocellular carcinoma in alcoholic patients with cirrhosis: A multiple logistic-regression coefficient analysis. Alcohol: Clin Exp Res. 1996;20:758–762.
247. Pequignot G, Tuyns AJ, Berta JL. Ascitic cirrhosis in relation to alcohol consumption. Int J Epidemiol. 1978;7:113–120.
248. Wilkinson P, Santamaria JN, Rankin JG. Epidemiology of alcoholic cirrhosis. Aust Ann Med. 1969;18:222–226.
249. Morgan MY, Sherlock S. Sex-related differences among 100 patients with alcoholic liver disease. Br Med J. 1977;1:939–941.
250. Maier KP, Haag SG, Peskar BM, Gerok WA. Verlaufsformen alkoholischer Lebererkrankungen. Klini Wochenschr. 1979;57:311–317.
251. Nakamura S, Takezawa Y, Sato T, Kera K, Maeda T. Alcoholic liver disease in women. Tohoku J Exp Med. 1979;129:351–355.
252. Frezza M, Di Padova C, Pozzato G, Terpin M, Baraona E, Lieber CS. High blood alcohol levels in women: role of decreased gastric alcohol dehydrogenase activity and first pass metabolism. N Engl J Med. 1990;322:95–99.
253. Lieber CS. Women and alcohol: Gender differences in alcohol metabolism and susceptibility. In: Wilsnack RW, Wilsnack SC, eds. Gender and Alcohol. Rutgers Center for Alcohol Studies, Piscataway, NJ. 1997;3:77–89.
254. Jones BM, Jones MK. Male and female intoxication levels for three alcohol doses or do women really get higher than men? Alcohol Technical Report. 1976;5:544–583.
255. Mishra L, Sharma S, Potter JJ, Mezey E. More rapid elimination of alcohol in women as compared to their male siblings. Alcohol: Clin Exp Res. 1989;13:752–754.
256. Eriksson CJP, Fukunaga T, Sarkola T, Linholm H, Ahola L. Estrogen-related acetaldehyde elevation in women during alcohol intoxication. Alcohol: Clin Exp Res. 1996;20:1192–1195.
257. Shevchuk O, Baraona E, Ma XL, Pignon JP, Lieber CS. Gender differences in the response of hepatic fatty acids and cytosolic fatty acid-binding capacity to alcohol consumption in rats. Proc Soc Exp Biol Med. 1991;198:584–590.
258. Ma XL, Baraona E, Lieber CS. Alcohol consumption enhances fatty acid ω oxidation, with a greater increase in male than in female rats. Hepatology. 1993;18:1247–1253.
259. Ma X, Baraona E, Goozner BG, Lieber CS. Gender differences in medium chain dicarboxylic aciduria in alcoholics. Am J Med. 1999;106:70–75.
260. Vesell ES, Page JG, Passananti GT. Genetic and environmental factors affecting ethanol metabolism in man. Clin Pharmacol Ther. 1971;12:192–201.
261. Goodwin DW. Is alcoholism hereditary? Arch Gen Psychiatry. 1971;25:545–549.
262. Lumeng L, Crabb DW. Genetic aspects and risk factors in alcoholism and alcoholic liver disease. Gastroenterology. 1994;107:572–578.
263. Kendler KS, Heath AC, Neale MC, Kessler RC, Eaves LJ. A population-based twin study of alcoholism in women. JAMA. 1992;268:1877–1882.
264. Blum K, Noble EP, Sheridan PJ et al. Allelic association of human dopamine D2 receptor gene in alcoholism. JAMA. 1990;263:2055–2060.
265. Higuchi S, Muramatsu T, Murayama M, Hayashida M. Association of structural polymorphism of the dopamine D2 receptor gene and alcoholism. Biochem Biophys Res Commun. 1994;204:1199–1205.

266. Bolos AM, Dean M, Lucas-Derse S, Rasonsburg M, Brown GL, Goldman D. Population and pedigree studies reveal a lack of association between the dopamine D2 receptor gene and alcoholism. JAMA. 1990;264:356–360.
267. Gejman PV, Ram A, Gelernter J et al. No structural mutation in the dopamine D_2 receptor gene in alcoholism or schizophrenia. Analysis using denaturing gradient gel electrophoresis. JAMA. 1994;271:204–208.
268. McDevitt HO, Bodmer WF. Histocompatibility antigens, immune responsiveness and susceptibility to disease. Am J Med. 1972;52:1–8.
269. Bell H, Nordhagen R. HLA antigens in alcoholics, with special reference to alcoholic cirrhosis. Scand J Gastroenterol. 1980;15:453–456.
270. Bailey RJ, Krasner N, Eddleston ALW et al. Histocompatibility antigens, autoantibodies, and immunoglobulins in alcoholic liver disease. Br Med J. 1976;2:727–729.
271. Morgan MY, Ross MGR, Ng CM, Adams DM, Thomas HC, Sherlock S. HLA-B8-immunoglobulins, and antibody responses in alcohol-related liver disease. J Clin Pathol. 1980;3:488–492.
272. Saunders JB, Wodak AD, Haines A et al. Accelerated development of alcoholic cirrhosis in patients with HLA-B8. Lancet. 1982;1:1381–1384.
273. Scott BB, Rajah SM, Losowsky MD. Histocompatibility antigens in chronic liver disease. Gastroenterology. 1977;72:122–125.
274. Bell H, Nordhagen R. Association between HLA-BW40 and alcoholic liver disease with cirrhosis. Br Med J. 1978;1:822.
275. Gluud C, Aldershvile J, Dietrichson O et al. Human leucocyte antigens in patients with alcoholic liver cirrhosis. Scand J Gastroenterol. 1980;15:337–341.
276. Melendez M, Vargas-Tank L, Fuentes C et al. Distribution of HLA histocompatibility antigens. ABO blood groups and RH antigens in alcoholic liver disease. Gut. 1979;20:288–290.
277. Simon M, Bourel M, Genetet B, Fauchet R, Edan G, Brissot P. Idiopathic hemochromatosis and iron overload in alcoholic liver disease: Differentiation by HLA phenotype. Gastroenterology. 1977;73:655–658.
278. Shigeta Y, Ishii H, Takagi S et al. HLA antigens as immunogenetic markers of alcoholism and alcoholic liver disease. Pharmacology. 1980;13:89–94.
279. Day CP, Bashir R, James O et al. Investigation of the role of polymorphisms at the alcohol and aldehyde dehydrogenase loci in genetic predisposition to alcohol-related end-organ damage. Hepatology. 1991;14:798–801.
280. Poupon RE, Napalas B, Coutelle C, Fleury B, Couzigou P, Higueret D, the French Group for Research on Alcohol and Liver. Polymorphism of the alcohol dehydrogenase, alcohol and aldehyde dehydrogenase activities: implications in alcoholic cirrhosis in white patients. Hepatology. 1992;15:1017–1022.
281. Hayashi S, Watanabe J, Kaname K. Genetic polymorphism in the 5'-flanking region change transcriptional regulation of the human cytochrome P450IIE1 gene. J Biochem. 1991;110:559–565.
282. Persson I, Johansson I, Bergling H et al. Genetic polymorphism of cytochrome P4502E1 in a Swedish population: relationship to incidence of lung cancer. FEBS Lett. 1993;319:207–211.
283. Uematsu F, Kikuchi H, Motomiya M et al. Association between restriction fragment length polymorphism of the human cytochrome P450IIE1 gene and susceptibility to lung cancer. Jpn J Cancer Res. 1991;82:254–256.
284. Uematsu F, Ikawa S, Kikuchi H et al. Restriction fragment length polymorphism of the human CYP2E1 (cytochrome P450IIE1) gene and susceptibility to lung cancer: possible relevance to low smoking exposure. Pharmacogenetics. 1994;4:58–63.
285. Hirvonen A, Husgafvel-Pursiainen K, Anttila S, Karjalainen A, Vainio H. The human CYP2E1 gene and lung cancer: Dra1 and Rsa1 restriction fragment length polymorphisms in a Finnish study population. Carcinogenesis. 1993;14:85–88.
286. Watanabe J, Hayashi S, Kawajiri K. Different regulations and expression of the human CYP2E1 gene due to the Rsa1 polymorphism in the 5' flanking region. J Biochem. 1994;116:321–326.
287. Tsutsumi M, Takada A, Wang JS. Genetic polymorphism of cytochrome P4502E1 related to the development of alcoholic liver disease. Gastroenterology. 1994;107:1430–1435.
288. Stephens EA, Taylor JA, Kaplan N et al. Ethnic variation in the CYP2E1 gene: polymorphism analysis of 695 African-Americans, European-Americans and Taiwanese. Pharmacogenetics. 1994;4:185–192.

289. Maezawa Y, Yamauchi M, Toda G. Association between restriction fragment length polymorphism of the human cytochrome P450IIE1 gene and susceptibility to alcoholic liver cirrhosis. Am J Gastroenterol. 1994;89:561–565.
290. Pirmohamed M, Kitteringham NR, Quest LJ et al. Genetic polymorphism of cytochrome P4502E1 and risk of alcoholic liver disease in Caucasians. Pharmacogenetics. 1995;5:351–357.
291. Powell H, Kitteringham NR, Pirmohamed M, Smith DA, Park BK. Expression of cytochrome P4502E1 in human liver: assessment by MRNA, genotype and phenotype. Pharmacogenetics. 1998;8:411–421.
292. Lucas D, Menez C, Girre C et al. Cytochrome P450 2E1 genotype and chlorzoxazone metabolism in healthy and alcoholic Caucasian subjects. Pharmacogenetics. 1995;5:298–304.
293. Weiner FR, Eskreis D, Compton KV, Orrego H, Zern MA. Haplotype analysis of type I collagen gene and its association with alcoholic cirrhosis in man. Mol Aspects Med. 1988;10:159–168.
294. Bashir R, Day CP, James OFW, Ogilvie DJ, Sykes B, Bassendine MF. No evidence for involvement of type I collagen structural genes in 'genetic predisposition' to alcoholic cirrhosis. J Hepatol. 1992;16:316–319.
295. Hrubec Z, Omenn GS. Evidence of genetic predisposition to alcoholic cirrhosis and psychosis: Twin concordances for alcoholism and its biological end points by zygosity among male veterans. Alcohol: Clin Exp Res. 1981;5:207–215.
296. Savolainen VT, Pajarinen J, Perola M, Pentillä A, Karhunen PJ. Glutathione-S-transferase GST M1 'null' genotype and the risk of alcoholic liver disease. Alcohol: Clin Exp Res. 1996;20:1340–1345.
297. Lieber CS. Alcohol, liver and nutrition. J Am Col Nutr. 1991;10:602–632.
298. Lieber CS. Hepatic and other medical disorders of alcoholism: From pathogenesis to treatment. J Stud Alcohol 1998;59:9–25.

15
Clinical aspects of alcoholic liver disease

R. WILLIAMS

The clinical presentation of alcoholic liver disease varies widely and the most commonly used classification is based upon histological criteria. Fatty liver is present in at least 90% of chronic alcohol misusers, but is almost invariably asymptomatic and this review will therefore concentrate on the more severe forms of damage. Alcoholic hepatitis is an intermediate stage, and is characterized histologically by hepatocellular necrosis, an acute inflammatory infiltrate and the presence of an eosinophilic material – Mallory's hyaline. Some patients with this lesion may be totally asymptomatic, but more commonly they present with illness ranging from hepatomegaly and jaundice to an acute, life-threatening syndrome with encephalopathy, hepatorenal failure, coagulopathy, fever, and gastrointestinal bleeding. A proportion of patients presenting with acute alcoholic hepatitis (up to 50% in some series) have underlying cirrhosis already. Cirrhosis may also arise without a clinically apparent stage of hepatitis.

End-stage cirrhosis manifests clinically with the consequences of hepatocellular failure and portal hypertension, particularly variceal bleeding, ascites, oedema, encephalopathy and general debility. A small proportion of patients with long-standing cirrhosis develop hepatocellular carcinoma.

Well-conducted studies from the Toronto group in the 1980s demonstrated the importance of alcoholic hepatitis in the progression of alcoholic liver damage and in determining the final prognosis. As shown in Table 1, if there is evidence of hepatitis histologically on examination of liver biopsy, whether or not the

Table 1. Effects of excess alcohol

Fatty liver ↓	Present in > 90% patients, usually asymptomatic
Alcoholic hepatitis ↓	Variable presentation. Hepatomegaly and mild jaundice → acute liver failure
Cirrhosis ± chronic alcoholic hepatitis	Compensation or decompensated with portal hypertension, encephalopathy, infections, HCC

Table 2. Prognosis of alcoholic liver disease in the presence and absence of hepatitis and cirrhosis (data from ref. 1)

% mortality	Non-cirrhotics		Cirrhotics	
	No hepatitis	Hepatitis	No hepatitis	Hepatitis
1 year	6.9	5.3	7.1	26.5
5 years	24.1	36.8	31.0	46.9

patient has already developed cirrhosis, the prognosis at 5 years is significantly worse. The data in Table 2 also make clear the very poor prognosis of patients with alcoholic cirrhosis and hepatitis[1]. Less than 50% of such patients live 5 years, a survival worse than many forms of cancer. However, with abstinence, patients with alcoholic liver disease even at the stage of cirrhosis, provided this has not decompensated, have survival rates which are very little different from normal.

Although I have indicated the sequence of changes from fatty change of little consequence clinically through to acute alcoholic hepatitis and then cirrhosis as occurring sequentially, cirrhosis can also develop insidiously without clinical or biochemical signs becoming apparent. Indeed it has been suggested that only about 60% of patients with cirrhosis have signs or symptoms of liver disease: the remaining 40% are discovered fortuitously during routine testing or at autopsy[2].

CO-FACTORS OF HEPATITIS B AND C INFECTION: INTERACTION IN LIVER DAMAGE

Not surprisingly, an excessive alcohol intake often exacerbates other liver diseases. The condition in which this has been best demonstrated, and is of major contemporary interest, is chronic hepatitis from HCV infection. In this condition, the rate of progression and development of severe fibrosis is greatly enhanced in those who consume alcohol in excess, as compared to those who drink mildly or not at all. Indeed, alcoholic excess is a major factor in the development of cirrhosis from HCV infection. In such cases the histological changes are of hepatitis C-related liver disease and not those of alcoholic hepatitis and cirrhosis. However, there is also evidence that hepatitis B or C infection may lead to a worsening of alcoholic liver disease. In Japan, patients with alcoholic liver disease who on liver biopsy had, as well as the changes characteristic of that aetiology, features of an active chronic hepatitis type lesion with interface hepatitis which were more likely to be infected with hepatitis B or C virus. These patients also did less well with abstinence than those in whom hepatitis B and C infection (and the associated histological changes) were absent. Different combinations of lesions in association with alcoholic liver disease are most likely to be seen in Mediterranean countries, particularly Italy, where viral hepatitis infection is common and where the population has a relatively high alcohol intake. Recent data showing the coincidence of these infections with alcoholic cirrhosis in a large multicentre series are given in Table 3. It is

Table 3. Associations with both hepatitis virus infection and alcohol in an Italian multicentre study on 1829 cases with cirrhosis (% cases) (data from ref. 26)

	Alone	+ HCV	+ HBV/HDV	+ Alcohol
HCV	47.7	–	3.2	21.2
HBV/HDV	7.4	3.2	–	3.0
Alcohol	8.7	21.2	3.0	–

apparent that patients considered to have primarily alcoholic cirrhosis frequently have chronic infection with hepatitis C, and to a lesser extent with hepatitis B, virus. Chronic HBV carriers in Italy who misuse alcohol have been shown to have a more rapid progression of HBV-related liver damage[3] and a study from Spain suggests that the presence of HCV antibody is associated with a more severe histology[4]. In this country, although there is some increase in prevalence of hepatitis B markers in both alcohol misusers and patients with alcoholic liver disease, HBV does not appear to be a major exacerbating factor for alcoholic liver disease.

Recognition of non-alcoholic steatohepatitis (NASH)

Existence of a non-alcoholic form of steatohepatitis with liver lesions identical to those due to alcohol, ranging from fatty liver through necroinflammatory features with fibrosis to cirrhosis and occasionally acute liver failure, has been recognized since the term was first used by Ludwig and colleagues at the Mayo Clinic in 1980[5]. In such cases the tendency is to doubt the truth of the alcohol history obtained and indeed this is the reason for my wanting to draw attention to this condition. Such patients are usually diagnosed, as with alcoholic liver disease, following the incidental finding of abnormal liver function tests on routine screening or insurance examination. Currently, there is considerable interest in the concept that NASH represents an acquired metabolic disorder as shown by associated features of hyperlipidaemia, obesity and diabetes, with one study also reporting mild iron overload in association with heterozygosity for the C282Y mutant of the haemochromatosis gene[6]. Although at one time obesity was thought to be the most important aetiological factor, the frequency of obesity in one recent series was 39% and the previously described female preponderance was less, with 53% of cases occurring in males[7]. Most interestingly, in relation to the similarity of the histological spectrum in liver lesions to alcoholic liver disease, the cases are described where NASH has recurred over a short period of time (1–3 years) following successful orthotopic liver transplantation.

TREATMENT MEASURES

The cornerstones of therapy in alcoholic hepatitis are abstinence, adequate diet, correction of vitamin deficiencies and management of complications. In addition several therapeutic approaches have been studied in order to reduce short-term mortality and stop progression to cirrhosis (Table 4).

Table 4. Treatment measures

Spectrum of illness – Stable asymptomatic cirrhosis to acute fulminating alcoholic hepatitis

1. Abstinence

2. Directed to complications – portal hypertension, encephalopathy, ascites, malnutrition.

3. Given to reverse or prevent progress of histological abnormalities – steroid therapy, insulin and glucagon, propylthiouracil, colchicine

4. Liver transplantation

Several trials have shown that corticosteroids appear to reduce short-term mortality in the subgroup of patients with acute alcoholic hepatitis who have prolongation of prothrombin time, increased levels of bilirubin and hepatic encephalopathy[8,9]. There is no evidence that corticosteroid therapy, even though it is associated with more frequent and rapid recovery, can prevent progression to cirrhosis. Infusions of insulin and glucagons have been used in an attempt to stimulate liver regeneration. The results are conflicting and the resulting insulin-induced hypoglycaemia can be dangerous[10,11]. There is also a question as to whether these stimulants of regeneration can be taken up and used by injured hepatocytes.

Propylthiouracil (PTU) has also been given with the rationale of reducing hypermetabolism and protecting the vulnerable zone III of the hepatic lobule from hypoxic injury. Again, there are conflicting results as to short-term benefits and whether PTU improves mortality. In a 2-year controlled clinical trial of 310 patients with alcoholic liver disease there was a 48% reduction in the cumulative mortality rate from 0.25 (placebo group) to 0.13 (PTU group; $p < 0.05$), with the most pronounced therapeutic benefit found in patients with alcohol hepatitis[1,12].

Anabolic-androgenic steroids have been studied with overall poor results[13]. In addition, long-term therapy could be a factor in the development of hepato-cellular carcinoma[14].

Use of orthotopic liver transplantation

The use of orthotopic liver transplantation in end-stage alcoholic liver disease has become increasingly accepted over the past 10 years. The most common clinical indications are ascites and oedema resistant to conventional therapy, repeated episodes of variceal bleeding, recurrent encephalopathy and small (< 4 cm) hepatocellular carcinomas detected by ultrasound screening. The pre-transplant assessment includes careful screening for other alcohol-related end-organ damage, particularly cardiomyopathy, pancreatic and CNS disease, as well as consideration of the psychosocial background. Few patients with acute alcoholic hepatitis have been transplanted because of the severity of the multi-organ failure and the difficulties at the time of assessing alcohol abuse apart from priority considerations in obtaining a donor organ.

Series from the major centres have shown that survival rates after organ liver transplantation are in the medium term compatible with the results obtained for end-stage cirrhosis of other aetiologies[14–17]. However, this form of treatment is never likely to be available for more than a small proportion of patients with end-stage alcoholic liver disease because of concerns regarding relapse of alcohol misuse, poor rehabilitation and failure to comply with immuno-suppressive treatment or to attend regularly for follow-up. With the increasing donor organ shortage, transplant centres are paying even greater attention to patient selection and the complex ethical issues involved[18,19].

In the UK the number of transplants performed for alcoholic liver disease increased from 31 cases (6.1% of the total number of liver transplants) in 1992 to 92 (14.1%) in 1996 (UKTSSA, personal communication). These low figures are attributable in part to the relatively low prevalence of chronic liver disease in the UK: in 1989 the age-standardized mortality rates from cirrhosis in Britain were 4.4/100 000 men and 3.1/100 000 women compared with figures in the USA of 12.5/100 000 and 5.5/100 00, respectively[20]. It seems, however, that only a small proportion of the patients with alcoholic cirrhosis who might benefit from liver transplantation are currently being referred. In England and Wales in 1994, almost 2000 patients aged < 65 years were reported to die of chronic liver disease, of which approximately two-thirds were caused by alcohol[21]. Based on the results of one survey, up to 10% of these alcoholic patients may be eligible for liver transplantation each year[22].

Information on the effects of a return to alcohol consumption after otherwise successful liver transplantation on long-term graft and patient survival is relatively limited. In a series of 60 patients transplanted at King's College Hospital with a diagnosis of end-stage alcoholic liver disease as one of the indications for transplantation[23], (Pereira and Williams, personal communication), five patients developed recurrent cirrhosis and/or graft failure due to continued drinking within 5 years. Two of these patients died of recurrent alcoholic hepatitis and graft failure within 2 years (Table 5). In 47 of those 60 patients, alcohol was considered the sole causative factor whereas 13 (22%) had at least one other aetiological agent identified as contributing to the cirrhosis, including chronic hepatitis B or C in 12. In nine of the 60 patients (15%) the development of HCC was the indication for liver transplantation and two others were found to have incidental HCC in the explanted grafts.

Table 5. Five cases with severe graft damage from alcohol ingestion in a series of 60 cases transplanted for alcoholic liver disease (data from ref. 23 and Pereira and Williams, personal communication)

Patient	Abstinent pre-transplantation	Effect on graft	Outcome
1	18 months	Cirrhosis at 4 years	Now abstinent
2	No	Severe alcoholic hepatitis at 9 months	Now abstinent
3	11 months	Cirrhosis at 5 years	Now abstinent
4	5 months	Severe alcoholic hepatitis at 10 months	Died of liver failure
5	6 months	Severe alcoholic hepatitis at 2 years	Died of liver failure

Although insistence on a period of abstinence of at least 6 months pre-transplant does not guarantee that the patient will not return to some drinking post-transplant, or even drink excessively again, it does provide a period of time during which the effect of abstinence on the liver disease can be determined. Even patients with decompensated liver cirrhosis can improve dramatically once they are no longer drinking and they may no longer need a transplant. In our experience, a period of abstinence prior to transplantation is insufficient to guarantee future sobriety. A study carried out in collaboration with the Department of Psychiatry showed that only one of 20 patients was totally abstinent at 2 years post-transplant, despite a mean abstinent period before transplantation of 26 months[24]. However, on average they drank less than before transplantation and had levels of physical and psychiatric morbidity similar to those of patients receiving transplants for non-alcoholic liver disease.

The data of Poynard et al.[25] should be kept in mind when selecting patients for transplant. The results of this large multicentre study carried out in France are summarized in Table 6. The 5-year survival of patients after transplantation was found to be significantly better than for matched control patients or for control data where the patients' own findings were assessed by a prognostic score, only in those with the most severe liver disease, namely Child-Pugh Grade C (score 11+). In those with less severe categories of disease, namely Child-Pugh Grades B and A, there was no improvement in 5-year survival for those transplanted compared with the controls.

CONCLUSION

There is a wide spectrum of histological liver lesions in association with alcohol excess and considerable variation in the clinical picture resulting. Additional infection with the hepatitis viruses, particularly HCV, may be important in certain population groups. Many cases of alcoholic liver damage do not reach clinical recognition for reasons including the constitutional susceptibility of the patient to the damaging effects of alcohol, the pattern of drinking or other coincidental dietary and environmental factors. Except in the most severe instances of alcoholic hepatitis presenting with acute liver failure, patients with alcoholic cirrhosis can show marked improvement with abstinence. In those cases where manifestations of severe liver decompensation continue in the absence of other

Table 6. Transplantation for alcoholic cirrhosis – 5 year survival (data from ref. 25)

	Transplanted	Controls	
		Matched	Simulated
Total series (169 patients)	66	52	52
Pugh 11+	58	31	32
Pugh 6–11	67	57	56
Pugh 5.6	78	75	73

serious organ damage, then liver transplantation can give an excellent improvement in survival and quality of life, with only a low risk to the graft from recidivism post-transplant. Nevertheless, the number of cases currently being transplanted in the UK remains small and it is likely that there is a considerable under-referral of suitable cases to transplant centres.

REFERENCES

1. Orrego H, Blake JE, Blendis LM et al. Long term treatment of alcoholic liver disease with propylthiouracil. N Engl J Med. 1987;317:1421–1427.
2. Dufour MC, Stinson FS, Caces MF. Trends in cirrhosis morbidity and mortality: United States, 1979–1988. Semin Liver Dis. 1993;13:109–125.
3. Villa E, Barchi T, Grisendi A et al. Susceptibility of chronic symptomless HBsAg carriers to ethanol-induced hepatic damage. Lancet. 1982;ii:1243–1244.
4. Pares A, Barrera JM, Caballeria J et al. Hepatitis C virus antibodies in chronic alcoholic liver patients: association with severity of liver injury. Hepatology. 1990;12:1295–1299.
5. Ludwig J, Viggiano TR, McGill DB, Ott BJ. Non-alcoholic steatohepatitis. Mayo Clinic experiences with a hitherto unnamed disease. Mayo Clin Proc. 1980;55:434–438.
6. James OFW, Day CP. Non-alcoholic steatohepatitis (NASH): a disease of emerging identity and importance. J Hepatol. 1998;29:495–501.
7. Bacon BR, Farahvash MJ, Janney CG, Neuschwander-Tetri BA. Nonalcoholic steatohepatitis: an expanded clinical entity. Gastroenterology. 1994;107:1103–1109.
8. Carithers RL, Herlong HF, Diehl AM et al. Methylprednisolone therapy in patients with severe alcoholic hepatitis: a randomized multicentre trial. Ann Intern Med. 1989;110:685–690.
9. Reynolds TB, Benhamou JP, Blake J, Nacarato R, Orrego H. Treatment of acute alcoholic hepatitis. Gastroenterol Int. 1989;2:208–216.
10. Feher J, Cornides A, Romany A et al. A prospective multi-center study of insulin and glucagon infusion therapy in acute alcoholic hepatitis. J Hepatol. 1987;5:224–231.
11. Bird G, Lau JYN, Koskinas J, Wicks C, Williams R. Insulin and glucagon infusion in acute hepatitis: a prospective randomized controlled trial. Hepatology. 1991;14:1097–1101.
12. Israel Y, Walfish PG, Orrego H et al. Thyroid hormones in alcoholic liver disease: effect of treatment with 6-n-propylthioracil. Gastroenterology. 1979;76:116–122.
13. Copenhagen Study Group. Testosterone treatment of men with alcoholic cirrhosis: a double blind study. Hepatology. 1986;6:807–813.
14. Maddrey WC. Is therapy with testosterone or anabolic-androgenic steroids useful in the treatment of alcoholic liver disease? Hepatology. 1986;6:1033–1035.
15. Knechtle SJ, Fleming MF, Barry KL et al. Liver transplantation for alcoholic liver disease. Surgery. 1992;112:694–701.
16. Lucey MR, Merion RM, Henley KS et al. Selection for and outcome of liver transplantation in alcoholic liver disease. Gastroenterology. 1992;102:1736–1741.
17. Berlakovich GA, Steininger R, Herbst F, Barlan M, Mittlbock M, Muhlbacker F. Efficacy of liver transplantation for alcoholic cirrhosis with respect to recidivism and compliance. Transplantation. 1994;58:560–565.
18. Neuberger J. An ethical code for everybody in health care. Patients should help to shape such a code. Br Med J. 1998;316:1459.
19. Pereira SP, Williams R. Limits to liver transplantation in the UK. Gut. 1998;42:883–885.
20. La Vecchia C, Levi F, Lucchini F, Franceschi S, Negri E. Worldwide patterns and trends in mortality from liver cirrhosis, 1955 to 1990. Ann Epidemiol. 1994;4:480–486.
21. OPCS (Office of Population Censuses and Surveys). Deaths in 1994 by cause, and by area of residence: Provisional numbers. OPCS Monitor DH2 95/1, London, 1995.
22. Davies MH, Langman MJ, Elias E, Neuberger JM. Liver disease in a district hospital remote from a transplant centre: a study of admissions and deaths. Gut. 1992;33:1397–1399.
23. Pereira SP, Williams R. Liver transplantation for alcoholic liver disease at King's College Hospital: Survival and quality of life. Liver Transplant Surg. 1997;3:245–250.
24. Howard L, Fahy T, Wong P, Sherman D, Gane E, Williams R. Psychiatric outcome in alcoholic liver transplant patients. Q J Med. 1994;87:731–736.

25. Poynard T, Naveau S, Doffoel M et al. Evaluation of liver transplantation in alcoholic cirrhosis by comparison with matched and simulated controls' 5 year survival. Hepatology. 1996;24(Suppl):184A.
26. De Bac C, Stroffolini T, Gaeta GB, Taliani G, Giusti G. Pathogenic factors in cirrhosis with and without hepatocellular carcinoma: a multicenter Italian study. Hepatology. 1994;20:1225–1230.

Section VI
Bile acid therapy

16
Ursodeoxycholic acid in the treatment of alcoholic liver disease*

J.N. PLEVRIS, P.C. HAYES and I.A.D. BOUCHIER

INTRODUCTION

Oral bile salts have been used for many years in the treatment of gallstone disease. Ursodeoxycholic acid (UDCA) has largely replaced chenodeoxycholic acid because of its safety and efficacy. In 1987, Poupon et al.[1] suggested that UDCA may be of value in the treatment of primary biliary cirrhosis (PBC), improving liver function tests and perhaps slowing progression of disease.

Since then, several groups have reported that UDCA may be beneficial in PBC[2-4]. Although precisely how it works remains largely unknown, the initial reassuring results in the treatment of PBC have led to the use of UDCA in other cholestatic liver disorders, namely primary sclerosing cholangitis (PSC)[5,6]. Treatment of chronic active hepatitis has shown similar promising results[7,8] and there are also reports that UDCA has been used with apparent benefit in congenital cholestatic diseases such as biliary atresia[9,10] and cystic fibrosis associated with cholestasis and malabsorption[11].

Although the use of UDCA in these disorders is still limited to clinical trials, one of its main attractions is that this form of therapy is safe, well tolerated and virtually free from side effects.

There are no reports so far on the use of UDCA in the treatment of alcoholic liver disease. Because most studies on UDCA have been in patients with cholestatic disorders and have demonstrated a fall in biochemical markers of cholestasis, namely bilirubin and alkaline phosphatase, we have decided to investigate its effect in alcoholic liver disease.

METHOD

Twelve patients (11 males, one female) mean age 56 ± 5 years with biopsy-proven alcoholic cirrhosis were included in this study. All patients had

*This chapter was first published in European Journal of Gastroenterology and Hepatology 1991;3:653–656 and is reproduced here by permission of Lippincott Williams and Wilkins.

biochemical evidence of impaired liver function with bilirubin > 25 μmol/l and or serum alkaline phosphatase > 150 IU/l at entry to the study. All patients admitted active drinking except one; there was, however, biochemical evidence of continuing alcohol abuse.

Seven patients were Pugh A, three were Pugh B and two were Pugh C grade of liver disease[12].

Patients were randomized in a single-blind cross-over fashion to receive UDCA (15 mg/kg) or placebo for 4 weeks after a 4-week observation period. A thorough medical history and clinical examination was performed at the beginning of the observation period, and blood tests including full blood count prothrombin time, liver function tests, urea and electrolytes and alcohol levels were taken. Patients were asked not to change their usual drinking habits throughout the study period and they attended the outpatients clinic at biweekly intervals for repeat of the blood tests, to check for compliance to treatment by counting the tablets and to report any adverse effects.

Patients were studied for 12 weeks (4 weeks observation period, 4 weeks on UDCA or placebo and 4 weeks vice versa).

The effect of UDCA on liver function tests was assessed by applying the Wilcoxon's rank sum test. Paired Student's t-test was used to assess changes in the liver function tests during the observation period. Variation in the blood alcohol levels during the study was assessed by using one-way analysis of variance. All results were expressed as mean (s.e.m.). The study has been approved by the local ethical committee.

RESULTS

Eleven patients completed the study. Six received the treatment in the order: placebo, UDCA, and five: UDCA, placebo. One patient was withdrawn from the

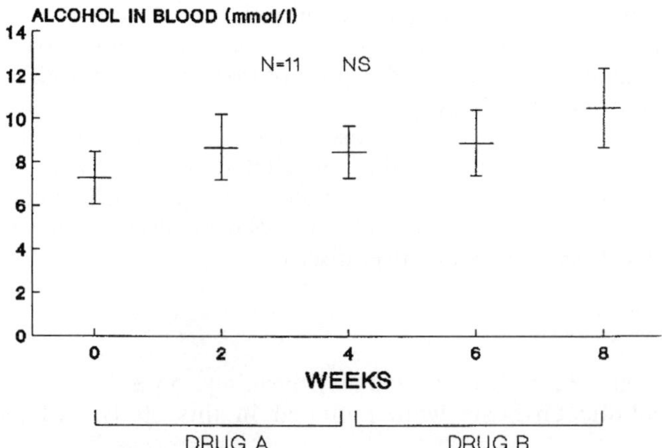

Figure 1. Mean blood alcohol levels during treatment with Drug A [ursodeoxycholic acid (UDCA) or placebo] and Drug B (vice versa) (NS, no significant changes).

study because of development of diarrhoea; he was on placebo treatment. None of the other patients who completed the study developed any side-effects during the trial period. All patients had their blood alcohol levels checked at every hospital visit and there was no significant variation in the mean alcohol levels between these visits throughout the study, alcohol usually being detected in most patients (Fig. 1).

Treatment with UDCA for 4 weeks resulted in a significant decrease of gamma-glutamyl transpeptidase (γ GT) ($p < 0.01$), total bilirubin ($p < 0.01$) (Fig. 2a,c), and alanine aminotransferase levels (ALT) ($p < 0.05$) (Fig. 3) compared with placebo treatment. There was no significant difference in serum alkaline phosphatase (Fig. 2b), prothrombin time, urea or electrolytes between UDCA and placebo treatment. The improvement in the liver biochemistry was apparent from the 2nd week of treatment with UDCA. UDCA had no adverse effect on full blood count or platelets.

There was a small but significant decrease of mean total albumin levels at the end of UDCA treatment compared with placebo ($p < 0.05$).

None of the patients changed Pugh class at the end of UDCA or placebo treatment.

DISCUSSION

In this study, we have demonstrated that UDCA induces a significant improvement in biochemical liver function as measured by the conventional liver function tests, in patients with alcoholic liver disease. This improvement was apparent from the first 2 weeks of treatment, and withdrawal of UDCA resulted in deterioration of liver function to the pre-treatment levels. The improvement in liver function was most pronounced in those with more active disease. None of the patients changed their drinking patterns and all but one (11 out of 12) continued drinking throughout the trial period.

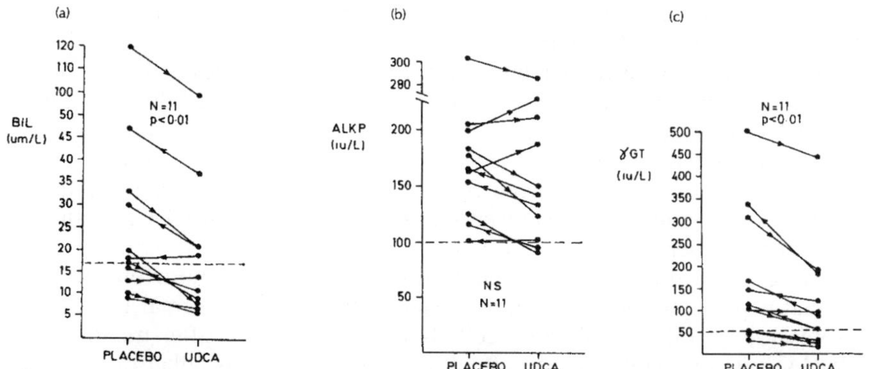

Figure 2. (a) BIL, bilirubin; (b) ALKP, alkaline phosphatase; (c) GGT, gamma-glutamyl transpeptidase; levels after treatment with ursodeoxycholic acid (UDCA) and placebo. Arrows indicate the order of treatment and dotted lines indicate the upper level of normal values.

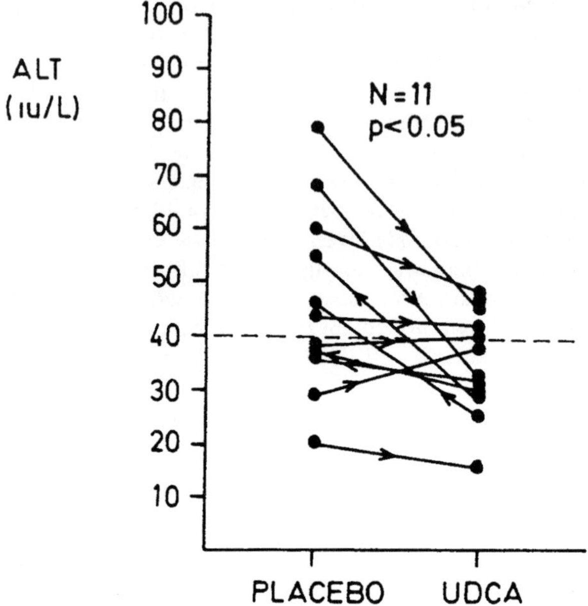

Figure 3. Changes in alanine aminotransferase (ALT) levels after treatment with ursodeoxycholic acid (UDCA) and placebo. (Arrows indicate the order of treatment and dotted line indicates the upper level of normal value for ALT.)

The mechanism whereby UDCA may produce beneficial effects on the liver function remains unclear. It has been hypothesized that UDCA treatment increases the hydrophilic properties of the bile salt pool and replaces the more hydrophobic bile salts which are hepatotoxic and can cause liver damage in prolonged hepatic cholestasis[2,3,7,13]. More recent studies have shown that UDCA stimulates transport of organic ions such as bilirubin level[14]. UDCA is also capable of reversing the adverse effect of the cholestatic factor (lymphokine) on bile flow and bile acid secretion[15].

Our study is of particular interest not only because elevated bilirubin and γGT levels, but the transaminase levels were also decreased during treatment with UDCA, which suggests a protective role of UDCA on hepatocytes in vivo. This is supported by recent evidence that UDCA may exert a protective effect against hepatic necrosis induced by endotoxin in vitro[15]. Recently published work from Calmus et al.[16] showed that the treatment with UDCA resulted in reduction of aberrant class I HLA antigen on hepatocytes, which, it has been suggested, is a direct effect of cholestasis. In addition, improvements in abnormal hepatocyte membrane fluidity and reduction in abnormal HLA class II expression on biliary epithelial cells have been reported after treatment with UDCA[17]. It is possible that the effect on antigen display is either due to altered composition of bile or improvement of cholestasis; such an immunomodulatory effect may play a role in reducing autoimmune liver damage in alcoholic liver disease.

Although in the majority of studies UDCA has been shown to produce a significant improvement in the liver function tests, namely bilirubin, alkaline phosphatase and γGT in patients with PBC, some long-term studies[18] suggest that this effect may not be sustained and is not always matched by histological improvement. The pathophysiology of PBC, however, is quite different from that of alcohol-associated liver disease as it mainly affects the biliary ducts. The improvement in the liver function tests, in particular ALT levels, in patients with alcoholic liver disease may reflect a hepatoprotective effect of UDCA against alcohol-associated liver damage. Although histological data is not available in this trial, measurement of ALT activity in hepatic disorders with direct hepatotoxicity has been shown to be an accurate and widely used biochemical parameter to monitor disease activity in clinical practice. Improvement in this biochemical analyte in patients with alcoholic liver disease justifies further long-term trials, including histological data to assess the effect of UDCA in alcohol associated liver damage.

We conclude that UDCA improves biochemical tests in a number of cholestatic disorders[19] and may also have a beneficial effect on disease activity in alcoholic liver disease, as measured by transaminase levels. We believe that longer term trials of UDCA in alcoholic liver disease, irrespective of whether or not cholestasis is present, should be undertaken and should include histological monitoring of disease activity.

Acknowledgement

We would like to thank Dr R.A. Elton, Department of Medical Statistics, University of Edinburgh for his statistical advice on the analysis of data.

REFERENCES

1. Poupon R, Poupon RE, Calmus Y, Chretien Y, Ballet F, Darnis F: Is ursodeoxycholic acid an effective treatment for primary biliary cirrhosis? Lancet. 1987;i:834–836.
2. Chretien Y, Poupon R, Gherardt MF, Chazouilleres O, Labbe D, Myara A, et al.: Bile acid glycine and taurine conjugates in serum of patient with primary biliary: effect of ursodeoxycholic acid treatment. Gut. 1989;30:1110–1115.
3. Batta AK, Salen G, Arora R, Shefer S, Tint GS, Abroon J, et al.: Effect of ursodeoxycholic acid on bile acid metabolism in primary biliary cirrhosis. Hepatology. 1989;10:414–419.
4. Bateson MC, Ross PE, Diffey BL: Ursodeoxycholic acid in primary biliary cirrhosis. Lancet. 1989;i:898–899.
5. Chazouilleres O, Poupon R, Capron JP, Metman EH, Dhumeaux D, Amouretti M et al.: Ursodeoxycholic acid for primary sclerosing cholangitis. J Hepatol. 1990;11:16–21.
6. O'Brien C, Senior JR, Batta AK, Arora R, Tint GS, Salen G: Ursodeoxycholic acid treatment produces marked clinical and biochemical amelioration of primary sclerosing cholangitis. Gastroenterology. 1989;10:A640 (abstract).
7. Podda M, Ghezzi C, Battezzati PM, Crosignani A, Zuin M, Roda Eskreis D et al.: Effects of ursodeoxycholic acid and taurine on serum liver enzymes and bile acids in chronic hepatitis. Gastroenterology. 1990;98:1044–1050.
8. Bellentani S, Tabarroni G, Barchi T, Ferretti I, Fratti N, Villa E et al.: Effect of ursodeoxycholic acid treatment on alanine aminotransferase and gamma-glutamyl transpeptidase levels in patients with hypertransaminasaemia. J Hepatol. 1989;8:7–12.
9. Ullrich D, Rating D, Schroter W, Hanefeld F, Bircher J: Treatment with ursodeoxycholic acid renders children with biliary atresia suitable for liver transplantation. Lancet. 1987;ii:1324.

10. Nittono H, Tokita A, Hayashi M, Nakatsu N, Obinata K, Wanatabe T, et al.: Ursodeoxycholic acid in biliary atresia. Lancet. 1988;i:528.
11. Cotting J, Lentze M, Reichen J: Amelioration of cholestasis and nutritional state in patients with cystic fibrosis treated with ursodeoxycholic acid. J Hepatol. 1989;9:S21 (abstract).
12. Pugh RNH, Murray Lyon IM, Dawson JL, Pietroni MC, Williams R: Transection of the oesophagus for bleeding oesophageal varices. Br J Surg. 1973;60:646–649.
13. Scholmerich J, Becher MS, Schmidt K, Schubert R, Kremer B, Feldhaus S et al.: Influence of hydroxylation and conjugation of bile salts on their membrane damaging properties. Studies on isolated hepatocytes and lipid membrane vesicles. Hepatology. 1984;4:661–666.
14. Kitani K: Strategies for the Treatment of Hepatobiliary Diseases edited by Paumgarter et al. Boston: Kluwer Academic Publishers. 1990:43–56.
15. Mizogushi Y, Kodama C, Skagami Y, Seki S, Kobayashi K, Yamamoto S et al.: Effects of bile acids on liver cell injury by cultured supernatants of activated liver adherent cells. Gastroenterol Jpn. 1989;24:25–30.
16. Calmus Y, Gane P, Rouger P, Poupon R: Hepatic expression of class I and class II major histocompatibility complex molecules in primary biliary cirrhosis; effect of ursodeoxycholic acid. Hepatology. 1990;11:12–15.
17. Bateson MC: New directions in primary biliary cirrhosis. BMJ. 1990;301:1290–1291.
18. Hadziyannis SJ, Hadziyannis ES, Makris A: A randomized controlled trial of ursodeoxycholic acid (UDCA) in primary biliary cirrhosis (PBC). Hepatology. 1989;10:580 (abstract).
19. James OFW: Ursodeoxycholic acid treatment for cholestatic liver disease. J Hepatol. 1990;11:5–8.

17
Fibrosis markers and ursodeoxycholic acid

J.M.C. STENNER, R.P. JAZRAWI, H.A. AHMED, A. VERMA and
T.C. NORTHFIELD

INTRODUCTION

Fibrosis

Hepatic fibrosis is the abnormal accumulation of connective tissue in the extra-cellular matrix (ECM) of the liver. This can result from a number of insults, of which alcohol is but one. Fibrosis is the term used to represent the total amount

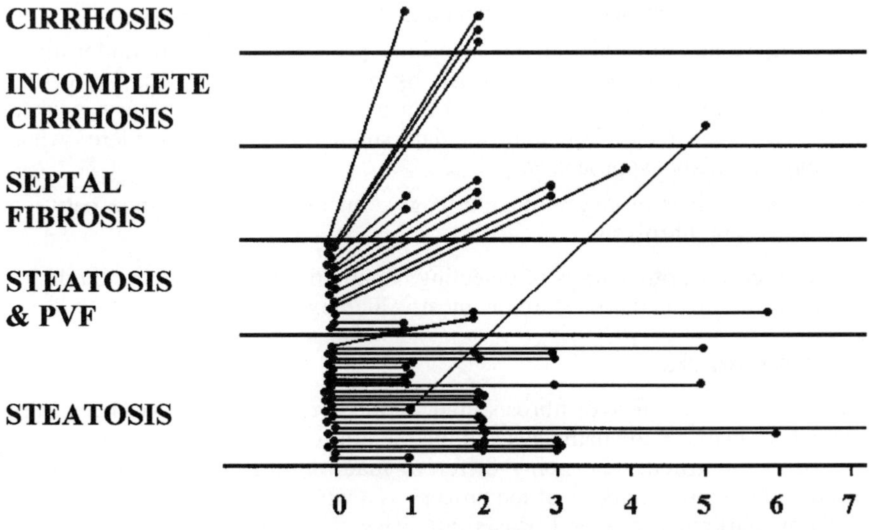

Figure 1. Progression of fibrosis in alcoholics followed up to 8 years after initial liver biopsy. From Worner et al.[1]

of connective tissue present within the liver at a given time. In reality this is a dynamic process of new connective tissue formation (fibrogenesis) and removal (fibrolysis), fibrosis being the net balance between these two active processes.

The clinical significance of fibrosis is easy to appreciate in the end-stage scenario of cirrhosis, where mortality and morbidity are apparent. However, even small amounts of fibrosis are significant. Worner et al.[1] showed how the presence of perivenular fibrosis significantly increased the risk of disease progression in alcoholic liver disease (Figure 1). Marbet[2] showed the same, but interestingly also reported that after a period of reduced alcohol intake, six out of eight patients with severe fibrosis on an initial biopsy showed marked reduction on a second biopsy, thus supporting the concept that fibrosis is a dynamic and reversible process. Therefore, there is great clinical importance in being able to accurately diagnose fibrosis, especially at an early stage. Equally, it is important to be able to decide whether, in the context of fibrosis, there is disease progression (fibrogenesis) or regression (fibrolysis).

DIAGNOSIS OF HEPATIC FIBROSIS

The current gold standard for diagnosis of fibrosis is by histological examination of a liver biopsy. This procedure is not without its problems:

Invasive: although the complication rate is remarkably low at < 0.1%[3], it must be remembered that this is in a selected group, and that there are some situations where a biopsy is rarely attempted (e.g. marked coagulopathy).

Unpleasant: despite reassurance, many patients find this procedure painful and unpleasant and are consequently reluctant to have repeat biopsies.

Sampling error: this is the most serious problem in that it undermines the whole validity of assessing fibrosis by biopsy. In one series, five of the 14 patients with cirrhosis would have been missed on the first biopsy if taken alone[4]. The inaccuracy of the gold standard should always be considered when assessing alternative approaches.

'Snapshot': a liver biopsy is unable to give an idea of the balance between fibrogenesis and fibrolysis.

For these reasons, other ways of detecting hepatic fibrosis have been sought, of which serum fibrosis markers are the most valuable.

Fibrosis markers

Although the exact cause of fibrosis in alcoholic liver disease has not been fully established, many of the pathways and interactions of fibrogenesis and fibrolysis have been identified. The many different macromolecules involved can be considered potential markers of the process as a whole.

Serum markers for liver fibrosis comprise the above markers for which biochemical assays are available. The ideal marker should be specific to liver fibrosis, reflect the degree of fibrosis and be independent of liver function. The natural history should be known and a reliable and accurate assay available. There is currently no such marker. Those that are in use are shown in Table 1.

Table 1. Serum assays for fibrosis

	Fibrogenesis	Fibrolysis	'Liver Specific'
PICP	+	−	(+) bone
PIIINP	+	+ (acute)	+
PIVCP	− (?)	+	+ (fibrosis)
PIVNP	− (?)	+	+ (fibrosis)
Hyaluronic Acid	+ (?)	+ (?)	+ (fibrosis)
Laminin	+ (?)	+ (?)	+ (fibrosis)
Collagen VI	−	+ (portal)	(+)
Undulin	−	−	+
Tenascin	+ (lobular)	−	+ (?)
TIMP-1	+	−	+ (?)
Collagenase 1	−	+	+ (?)

PICP, C terminal propeptide of procollagen I: PIINP, N-terminal propeptide of procollagen III:
PIVCP, C terminal propeptide of procollagen IV (NC1-fragment): PIVNP, N terminal propeptide of
procollagen IV (7-S collagen): TIMP-1, tissue inhibitor of metalloproteinases 1
Taken from Schuppan D. Falk Workshop 1995.

They have been listed according to whether they predominantly reflect fibrogenesis or fibrolysis. As a group they can be considered as being safe, repeatable, giving values reflecting whole liver fibrosis and differentiating between fibrogenesis and fibrolysis. However, there are also general limitations, since fibrosis occurs elsewhere in the body and this can affect the interpretation. However, other sources of fibrosis are usually easy to detect clinically.

Several assays are available for some markers, especially procollagen III N-terminal peptide (PIIIP). In this case, they measure slightly different antigenic parts of the target molecule and result in different absolute values. Furthermore, the different antigens are produced in differing amounts during fibrogenesis and fibrolysis, to add to the complexity of interpretation. This means it is very difficult to compare trials using different assays for the same fibrosis marker. For each method inter-assay and intra-assay variations are usually in the region of 5–10% and there is no established reference range.

FIBROSIS MARKERS AND ALCOHOLIC LIVER DISEASE

There is good correlation between the degree of histological fibrosis and fibrosis markers (Figure 2). Most of this work has been done using PIIIP and hyaluronic acid. The highest marker values in any of these series are always in those patients with alcoholic hepatitis, especially when associated with cirrhosis[5–8]. Unfortunately, the general conclusion must be that fibrosis markers lack the ability to differentiate accurately between steatosis and fibrosis, a major clinical and prognostic factor[9]. The overlap in absolute values between the histological stages limits the use of single measurements. However, serial measurements

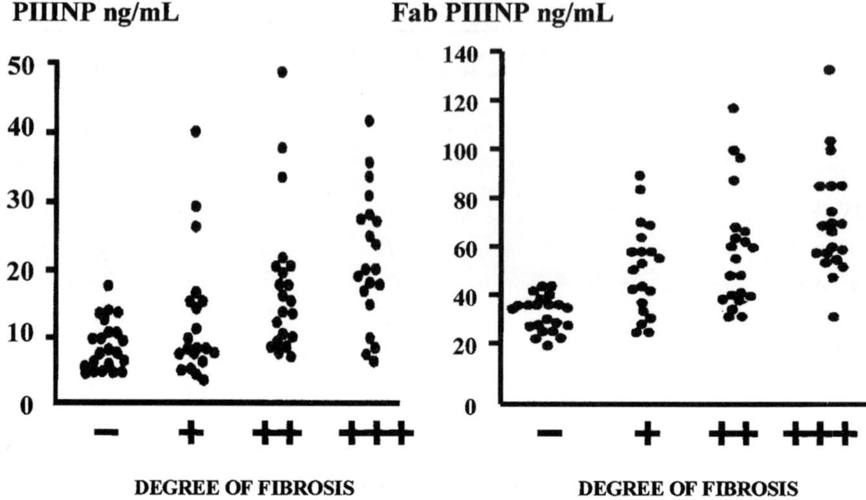

Figure 2. Correlation of PIIIP with histological staging of fibrosis in alcoholic liver disease. Taken from Sato et al.[9]

seem to have far more clinical use, as changes in fibrosis markers reflect changes in disease state; and that abstinence results in a fall in marker values[10]. This relationship between fibrosis markers and clinical condition has been best shown in treatment of hepatitis C with interferon. It has been shown that only those patients who are 'cured' have a persistent normalization of the fibrosis markers and a corresponding regression of fibrosis on histological staging[11–14]. Furthermore, in patients with psoriasis treated with methotrexate a persistently low PIIIP value strongly predicts the lack of hepatic fibrosis, and vice versa[15].

FIBROSIS MARKERS AND BILE ACID THERAPY

UDCA has been shown to be effective in a number of cholestatic liver conditions, and it is accepted that alcoholic liver disease has cholestatic features. Despite this, there is only one published trial on bile acid therapy in alcoholic liver disease, and this showed a biochemical improvement in the treatment group over a 1-month period[16]. We have completed a 6-month, double blind, placebo controlled trial using UDCA in alcoholic liver disease, with fibrosis markers as our outcome measure. The trial has been in patients with biopsy confirmed alcoholic liver disease.

The published literature on fibrosis markers and bile acid therapy is therefore limited to UDCA in PBC. As with alcoholic liver disease, there is a reasonable correlation between the stage of PBC and fibrosis markers[17,18], although not all authors agree on this[19]. There is work to support the use of fibrosis markers as prognostic variables in the Mayo Clinic model, especially when patients are receiving UDCA[20,21].

In the bile duct ligated rat model the absolute amount of fibrosis was reduced in the rats on UDCA therapy, supporting the idea that UDCA has an anti-fibrotic effect[22]. This has also been shown in humans with PBC. The work by Oesterling et al.[23] is interesting, as they not only showed a slight fall in PIIIP level, an indication of decreased fibrogenesis, but also a rise in collagen VI, an indication of fibrolysis, the clinically desirable pattern. The study by Beukers et al.[24] showed no relationship between fibrosis markers and histological disease progression, but it is difficult to interpret the data without the absolute values. There certainly appears to be a trend in that patients who progressed had higher fibrosis marker values, and almost all had a high value at some point in the trial. Equally, in the apparently negative report by Poupon[25] there was no convincing change in clinical condition, and hence the lack of change in fibrosis markers may have represented the true situation[26]. In another similar study there was certainly a strong trend to a reduction in PIIIP levels in the treatment group (16% decrease vs 6% increase)[27].

CONCLUSIONS

The assessment of hepatic fibrosis is of major clinical importance, not only for diagnosis but also for follow up. Fibrosis markers currently cannot replace a liver biopsy as initial assessment since it has been consistently shown that absolute values, except at very high levels, are not accurate predictors of hepatic fibrosis stage. Equally, it is unrealistic to expect the majority of patients to accept multiple liver biopsies, so that fibrosis markers could replace subsequent biopsies. Fibrosis markers can be done repeatedly and safely. Therefore, fibrosis markers are well suited to monitor the effect of treatment, especially if a selection of markers is used which reflects different parts of the fibrosis process.

REFERENCES

1. Worner TM, Lieber CS. Perivenular fibrosis as precursor lesion of cirrhosis. JAMA 1985;254:627–630.
2. Marbet UA, Bianchi L, Meury U, Stalder GA. Long-term histological evaluation of the natural history and prognostic factors of alcoholic liver disease. J Hepatol. 1987;4:364–372.
3. Piccinino F, Sagnelli E, Pasquale G, Giusti G. Complications following percutaneous liver biopsy. A multicentre retrospective study on 68,276 biopsies. J Hepatol. 1986;2:165–173.
4. Maharaj B, Maharaj RJ, Leary WP et al. Sampling variability and its influence on the diagnostic yield of percutaneous needle biopsy of the liver. Lancet. 1986;523–525.
5. Niemela O, Risteli L, Sotaniemi EA, Risteli J. Aminoterminal propeptide of type III procollagen in serum in alcoholic liver disease. Gastroenterology. 1983;85:254–259.
6. Torres-Salinas M, Pares A, Caballeria J et al. Serum procollagen type III peptide as a marker of hepatic fibrogenesis in alcoholic hepatitis. Gastroenterology. 1986;90:1241–1246.
7. Bell H, Raknerud N, Orjasaeter H, Haug E. Serum procollagen III peptide in alcoholic and other chronic liver diseases. Scand Gastroenterol. 1989;24:1217–1222.
8. Annoni G, Colombo M, Cantaluppi MC, Khlat B, Lampertico P, Rojkind M. Serum type III procollagen peptide and laminin (Lam-P1) detect alcoholic hepatitis in chronic alcohol abusers. Hepatology. 1989;9:693–697.
9. Sato S, Nouchi T, Worner TM, Lieber CS. Liver fibrosis in alcoholics. Detection by Fab radioimmunoassay of serum procollagen III peptides. JAMA. 1986;256:1471–1473.
10. Niemela O, Risteli J, Blake JE, Risteli L, Compton KV, Orrego H. Markers of fibrogenesis and basement membrane formation in alcoholic liver disease. Relation to severity, presence of hepatitis, and alcohol intake [see comments]. Gastroenterology. 1990;98:1612–1619.

11. Capra F, Casaril M, Gabrielli GB et al. alpha-Interferon in the treatment of chronic viral hepatitis: effects on fibrogenesis serum markers [see comments]. J Hepatol. 1993;18:112–118.
12. Suou T, Hosho K, Kishimoto Y, Horie Y, Kawasaki H. Long-term decrease in serum N-terminal propeptide of type III procollagen in patients with chronic hepatitis C treated with interferon alfa. Hepatology. 1995;22:426–431.
13. Gallorini A, Plebani M, Pontisso P et al. Serum markers of hepatic fibrogenesis in chronic hepatitis type C treated with alfa-2A interferon. Liver. 1994;14:257–264.
14. Guechot J, Loria A, Serfaty L, Giral P, Giboudeau J, Poupon R. Serum hyaluronan as a marker of liver fibrosis in chronic viral hepatitis C: effect of alpha-interferon therapy. J Hepatol. 1995;22:22–26.
15. Boffa MJ, Smith A, Chalmers RJ et al. Serum type III procollagen aminopeptide for assessing liver damage in methotrexate-treated psoriatic patients. Br J Dermatol. 1996;135:538–544.
16. Pleuris JN, Hayes PC, Bouchier IAD. Ursodeoxycholic acid in the treatment of alcoholic liver disease. Eur J Gastroenterol Hepatol. 1991;3:653–656. (reprinted as Chapter 16 of this volume).
17. Nyberg A, Lindqvist U, Engstrom-Laurent A. Serum hyaluronan and aminoterminal propeptide of type III procollagen in primary biliary cirrhosis: relation to clinical symptoms, liver histopathology and outcome. J Intern. Med. 1992;231:485–491.
18. Eriksson S, Zettervall O. The N-terminal propeptide of collagen type III in serum as a prognostic indicator in primary biliary cirrhosis. J Hepatol. 1986;2:370–378.
19. van Zanten RA, van Leeuwen RE, Beukers R, Wilson JH. Procollagen III peptide levels in alcoholic liver disease and primary biliary cirrhosis. Netherlands J Med. 1988;32:278–284.
20. Poupon RE, Balkau B, Guechot J, Heintzmann F. Predictive factors in ursodeoxycholic acid-treated patients with primary biliary cirrhosis: role of serum markers of connective tissue. Hepatology. 1994;19:635–640.
21. Babbs C, Smith A, Hunt LP, Rowan BP, Haboubi NY, Warnes TW. Type III procollagen peptide: a marker of disease activity and prognosis in primary biliary cirrhosis. Lancet. 1988;1:1021–1024.
22. Poo JL, Feldmann G, Erlinger S et al. Ursodeoxycholic acid limits liver histologic alterations and portal hypertension induced by bile duct ligation in the rat. Gastroenterology. 1992;102:1752–1759.
23. Oesterling C, Aksu T, Somasundaram R. Serum markers of collagen synthesis and breakdown suggest an antifibrotic effect of ursodeoxycholic acid in patients with PBC stage I–IV. Gut. 1995;37(Suppl 2): A121.
24. Beukers R, van Zanten RA, Schalm SW. Serial determination of type III procollagen amino propeptide serum levels in patients with histologically progressive and non-progressive primary biliary cirrhosis. J Hepatol. 1992;14:22–29.
25. Poupon RE, Huet PM, Poupon R, Bonnand AM, Nhieu JT, Zafrani ES. A randomized trial comparing colchicine and ursodeoxycholic acid combination to ursodeoxycholic acid in primary biliary cirrhosis. UDCA-PBC Study Group. Hepatology. 1996;24:1098–1103.
26. Floreani A, Zappala F, Mazzetto M, Naccarato R, Plebani M, Chiaramonte M. Different response to ursodeoxycholic acid (UDCA) in primary biliary cirrhosis according to severity of disease. Dig Dis Sci. 1994;39:9–14.
27. Vuoristo M, Farkkila M, Karvonen AL et al. A placebo-controlled trial of primary biliary cirrhosis treatment with colchicine and ursodeoxycholic acid. Gastroenterology. 1995;108: 1470–1478.

18
Ursodeoxycholic acid for treatment of chronic hepatitis C: an 'interferon sparing' effect

A. LANZINI, M.G. PIGOZZI, L. DISTEFANO, A. REGGIANI,
G.P. LORINI, R. SORBARA, M.G. DE TAVONATTI, L. BETTINI,
G. MONTANI, O. BAISINI, F. LANZAROTTO, D. QUATROCCHI,
A. COMINOTTI and M. FAVRET

INTRODUCTION

Infection with hepatitis C virus (HCV) affects an estimated 250 000 individuals worldwide, and is a major cause of chronic liver disease. The disease may progress to liver cirrhosis and ultimately to hepatocellular carcinoma, indicating the need for effective treatment of this condition. Interferon-α (IFN) is the only drug licensed for treatment of chronic hepatitis C in western countries. This drug has both immunomodulating and antiviral properties. The former includes the stimulation of cytotoxic T cells and TNF-α release, and the latter the induction of at least 12 proteins with antiviral properties[1]. It is the antiviral effect of IFN, rather than its immunostimulatory effect, which is regarded as its main mechanism of action, involving a direct inhibitory effect on hepatitis C virus replication[2].

Clinical studies have shown treatment with IFN alone to have a low response rate and a high recurrence rate after treatment[3,4]. IFN is particularly ineffective in patients with long-lasting HCV infection and in those with advanced liver disease, i.e. in those patients who most need effective treatment. Better treatment is clearly needed.

Alternative approaches for treatment of chronic hepatitis C include combining IFN treatment with antiviral (ribavirin, amantadine), antiinflammatory (NSAIDs) or immunomodulator (thymosin-α-1) drugs, or with ursodeoxycholic acid (UDCA). UDCA was amongst the first drugs to be used as an adjuvant to IFN treatment, and the combination of IFN + UDCA has been particularly attractive to clinical researchers because of the 'hepatoprotective effect' of UDCA, well documented in a variety of chronic liver diseases, and because of the safety of long-term administration of this drug.

UDCA FOR TREATMENT OF CHRONIC HEPATITIS C

The rationale for using UDCA in chronic hepatitis C is that this bile acid has both cytoprotective and immunomodulatory effects. Evidence for the cytoprotective effect comes from both experimental and clinical studies. Studies in vitro clearly indicate that this bile acid may protect isolated hepatocytes against the cytotoxic effect of damaging substances such as hydrophobic bile acids[5,6]. This hepatoprotective effect may involve not only protection against the membrane damaging effects of hydrophobic bile acids, but also modulation of apoptosis induced by toxic bile acids[7,8]. Evidence for an immune modulating effect of UDCA comes from the treatment of patients with primary biliary cirrhosis (PBC), in whom it reduces aberrant HLA class-I expression on the hepatocyte and of HLA class-II expression on biliary epithelium[9,10], and from in vitro studies of cultured mononuclear cells, in which it reduces the secretion of cytokines[11]. These immune modulating effects, together with the stabilization of mitochondrial membranes, are currently regarded as the main mechanisms underlying the beneficial effect of UDCA in the treatment of PBC[12–14].

The efficacy of UDCA in treating cholestatic liver diseases is particularly important because subclinical cholestasis is frequent in chronic hepatitis C: this form of hepatitis is often characterized histologically by damaged bile ductules and cholestasis, and biochemically by increased serum γ-glutamyl transpeptidase (GGT) in the absence of alcohol or drug abuse. Cholestasis may in turn reduce the efficacy of IFN treatment, as indicated by an in vitro study in which incubation of human mononuclear cells with cholestatic bile acids reduced the capacity of IFN to stimulate them to produce the antiviral protein $2',5'$-oligoadenylate synthetase[15]. Our report[16] that patients with chronic nonA-nonB hepatitis with pretreatment GGT above the normal range were resistant to IFN treatment also supports this theory.

Clinical confirmation of the potential efficacy of UDCA and of its taurine-conjugate (t-UDCA) in the treatment of chronic hepatitis C has been reported by several authors[17–20]. Chronic administration of UDCA or t-UDCA has been reported to cause a significant reduction in serum transminases, but the effect is transitory, and hypertransaminasaemia recurs in the majority of patients after treatment is stopped. UDCA administration has no effect on viral clearance in chronic hepatitis C[21]. These findings indicate that UDCA alone is of limited value for treating chronic hepatitis C, but may provide the rationale for combining UDCA with antiviral treatment. Many studies have compared the efficacy of UDCA + IFN with IFN alone[22–27] in the treatment of chronic hepatitis C. Virtually all studies have reported that a combination of IFN with UDCA is better than IFN alone in some respects. Three studies[22–24] have reported that the combination delays the relapse of hypertransaminasaemia after stopping treatment, and one study[25] has reported that it reduces the frequency of relapse, in comparison with IFN monotherapy. One study[26] has reported more rapid normalization of transminases with UDCA + IFN than with IFN alone. Another study in 108 patients[27], however, found no difference in biochemical response between UDCA + IFN and IFN alone, although both regimes were better than UDCA alone.

Only two of these studies have compared the effect of IFN with that of IFN + UDCA on liver histology, and their results conflict. Angelico et al.[23] compared the effect of IFN 6 MU tiw plus UDCA 10 mg/kg/day given for 6 months and that of the same dose of IFN alone in a total of 40 patients, and reported that relapse of hypertransaminasaemia occurred significantly later after combination treatment (7 months) than after IFN alone (2 months). Liver histology showed a similar improvement in lobular necrosis with both regimens, but portal inflammation improved only with UDCA + IFN. Boucher et al.[22] studied 80 patients using the same trial design and regimens, and reported a significantly higher relapse rate 6 months after stopping IFN alone (59%) than after combination therapy (27%), but no differences in either the histological or the virological response between the two regimens.

THE 'INTERFERON SPARING' EFFECT OF t-UDCA

This discrepancy between the two trials led us to undertake a randomized trial comparing the effect of IFN alone with that of IFN + UDCA in the treatment of chronic hepatitis C. We chose t-UDCA rather than UDCA because treatment with the latter has been reported to cause significant increase of the cytotoxic bile acid lithocholic acid in patients with PBC, an effect that has not been observed with equimolar t-UDCA.

We carried out a multicentre study in 106 patients with biopsy-proven chronic hepatitis C and an increased serum ALT for more than 6 months. The end-points were serum biochemistry, viraemia and liver histology. Patients with evidence of liver cirrhosis at histology and those with a history of drug or ethanol abuse were excluded from the study. None of the patients was HIV or HBsAg positive at enrolment, and all patients were screened and found to be negative for organ and non-organ specific antibodies.

The study was performed three phases:

Phase 1 (0–6 months): patients were allocated to IFN-α lymphoblastoid (3MU/m^2/three times a week) either alone or with t-UDCA 10 mg/kg/day.

Phase 2 (7–12 months): patients whose ALT was < 1.5 the upper limit of normal (uln) at the end of phase 1 had their dose of IFN tapered down to the minimum required to maintain ALT < 1.5 uln (minimum 1.5 MU three times a week) while maintaining full dose t-UDCA for those patients randomized to combination treatment.

Phase 3 (18 months): control liver biopsy was carried out in all patients 6 months after stopping IFN, while maintaining full dose t-UDCA for those patients randomized to combination treatment.

There was no difference in pre-treatment male/female ratio, age, BMI, ALT and GGT levels in the 51 patients randomized to IFN alone the 55 randomized to combination therapy. In both groups HCV genotype 1b was present in 50% of the patients. The histological score for fibrosis[28] before treatment was, however, significantly higher in patients randomized to the IFN + t-UDCA combination (Table 1).

The results are summarized in Table 1. The proportion of patients with normal ALT at the end of phase 1 was similar for IFN alone (33/51) and for t-UDCA + IFN (35/55, NS) and at the end of phase 2 (25/51 vs 31/55 respect-

Table 1. Biochemical, virological and histological response to IFN alone compared with that of IFN + t-UDCA combination treatment

Parameters	IFN	IFN + t-UDCA	p
On treatment responders	33/51	35/55	NS
End of treatment responders	25/51	31/55	NS
Sustained responders	21/51	24/55	NS
Negative viraemia end of phase 3*	11/26	12/28	NS
Phase 1: cumulative IFN dose (MU)	381	373	NS
Phase 2: cumulative IFN dose (MU)	180 ± 12	142 ± 4	< 0.006
Phase 2: no. patients reducing IFN dose > 50%	26/38	38/41	< 0.001
Necro-inflammatory score:			
basal	6.9 ± 0.4	6.9 ± 0.4	NS
after treatment	4.4 ± 0.5	4.7 ± 0.5	NS
Fibrosis score:			
basal	1.2 ± 0.1	1.6 ± 0.1	< 0.05
after treatment	1.2 ± 0.1	1.7 ± 0.1	< 0.05

*Viraemia results available in a sub-group of patients only.

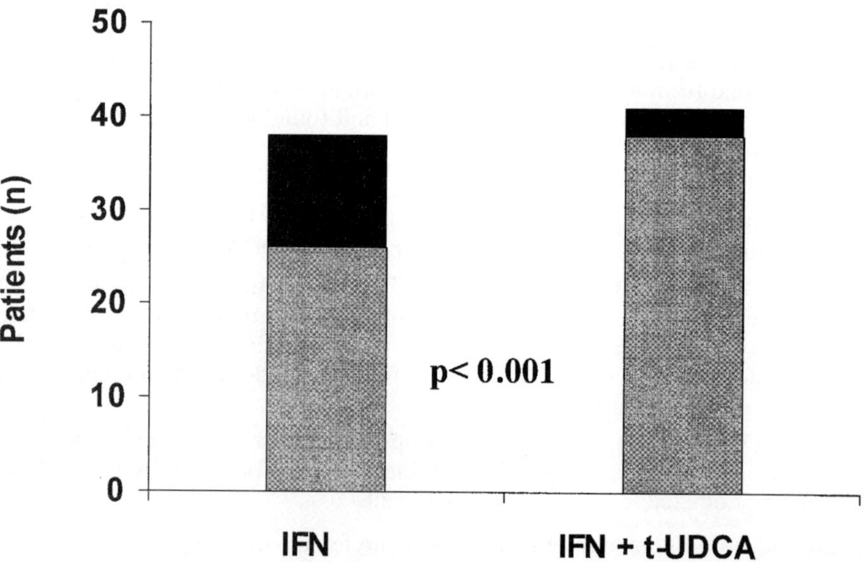

Figure 1. The 'interferon sparing' effect of t-UDCA. Number of patients reducing cumulative IFN dose by > 50% (grey) during IFN dose tapering (phase 2 of the study) shown as a proportion of total number of patients (black)

ively, NS) after 12 months treatment (on-treatment response). Sustained biochemical response at the end of phase 3, 6 months after stopping treatment, was also similar (21/51 vs 24/55, NS) and a similar proportion of patients were HCV-RNA negative (11/26 vs 12/28 respectively, NS).

Although biochemical and virological response rates did not differ between the two regimens, the dose of IFN needed to maintain response in phase 2 was lower with combination therapy than with IFN alone (mean cumulative IFN dose 142 ± 4 MU with IFN + UDCA, 180 ± 12 MU with IFN alone, $p < 0.006$). We have called this the 'interferon sparing' effect of t-UDCA[29]. This concept is further illustrated by the finding that that during phase 2 only 26 of the 38 patients treated with IFN alone who were suitable for tapering could reduce their IFN dose to less than 50% of the dose administered during phase 1, compared with 38/41 patients treated with INF + t-UDCA ($p < 0.001$, Figure 1).

The necro-inflammatory score decreased from 6.9 ± 0.4 to 4.4 ± 0.5 ($p < 0.01$) in patients treated with IFN alone and from 6.9 ± 0.4 to 4.7 ± 0.5 ($p < 0.01$) in those treated with IFN + t-UDCA, but the size of the effect was similar for both regimens. Fibrosis score remained unchanged with both regimens (Table 1).

We have also examined whether pre-treatment characteristics affected histological outcome, using a stepwise analysis. We found no effect of age, sex, pre-treatment serum ALT levels and BMI in predicting response to treatment. By contrast serum GGT was the most powerful predictor of lack of histological response to treatment.

OVERVIEW

The balance of evidence suggests that the combination of UDCA or t-UDCA with IFN has little effect in improving the response of chronic hepatitis C to IFN. Adjuvant t-UDCA does, however, allow remission to be maintained with a lower cumulative dose of IFN after initial full-dose therapy. This interferon sparing effect of t-UDCA may be important, particularly in conditions where patients cannot tolerate high-dose IFN because of unwanted effects.

REFERENCES

1. Dianzani F, Baron S. The interferons: a biological system with therapeutic potentials in viral infections. In: Dianzani F and Valtuena JP, editors. Lymphoblastoid Alpha-Interferon. London: Current Medical Literature Ltd. 1995;7–17.
2. Shindo M, Arai K, Tang MN et al. Hepatitis C virus RNA as a predictor of a long-term response to interferon-alpha therapy. Ann Intern Med. 1995;122:586–591.
3. Poynard T, Leroy V, Cohard M et al. Meta-analysis of interferon randomized trials in the treatment of viral hepatitis C: effects of dose and duration. Hepatology. 1996;24:778–789.
4. Poynard T, Beossa P, Chevallier M et al. A comparison of three interferon alfa-2b regimens for long term treatment of chronic non-A non-B hepatitis. N Engl J Med. 1995;332:1347–1462.
5. Heuman DM, Mills AS, McCall J et al. Conjugates of ursodeoxycholate protect against cytotoxicity of more hydrophobic bile salts. Hepatology. 1991;14:920–926.
6. Galle PR, Theilmann L, Raedsch R et al. Ursodeoxycholate reduces hepatotoxicity of bile salts in primary human hepatocytes. Hepatology. 1990;12:486–491.
7. Rodrigues CM, Fan G, Ma X et al. A novel role for ursodeoxycholic acid in inhibiting apoptosis by modulating mitochondrial membrane perturbation. J Clin Invest. 1998;101:2790–2799.
8. Benz C, Angermuller S, Tox U et al. Effect of tauroursodeoxycholic acid on bile acid induced apoptosis and cytolysis in rat hepatocytes. J Hepatol. 1998;28:99–106.
9. Spengler U, Pape GR, Hofmann RM et al. Differential expression of MHC Class II subregion products of bile duct epithelial cells and hepatocytes in patients with primary biliary cirrhosis. Hepatology. 1998;8:459–462.

10. Calmus Y, Gane P, Riuger P et al. Hepatic expression of class I and class II major histocompatibility complex molecules in primary biliary cirrhosis: effect of ursodeoxycholic acid. Hepatology. 1990;11:12–15.
11. Yoshikawa M, Tsujii T, Matsumura K et al. Immunomodulatory effects of ursodeoxycholic acid on immune responses. Hepatology. 1992;16:358–364.
12. Poupon RE, Balkau B, Eschwege P, Poupon R. The UDCA-PBC Study Group: a multicenter, controlled trial of ursodiol for treatment of primary biliary cirrhosis. N Engl J Med. 1991;324:1548–1554.
13. Heathcote EJ, Cauch-Dudek K, Walter V et al. The Canadian multicenter double-blind randomised controlled trial of ursodeoxycholic acid on primary biliary cirrhosis. Hepatology. 1994;19:1149–1156.
14. Lindor KD, Therneau TM, Jorgensen RA et al. Effect of ursodeoxycholic acid on survival in patients with primary biliary cirrhosis. Gastroenterology. 1996;110:1515–1518.
15. Podevin P, Calmus Y, Bonnefis MT et al. Effect of cholestasis and bile acids on interferon induced 2′,5′-adenylate synthetase and NK cell activities. Gastroenterology. 1995;108:1192–1198.
16. Battezzati PM, Podda M, Bruno S et al. Factors predicting early response to treatment with recombinant interferon alpha-2a in chronic non-A, non-B hepatitis. Preliminary report of a long-term trial. Ital J Gastroenterol. 1992;24:481–484.
17. Podda M, Ghezzi C, Battezzati PM. Effect of ursodeoxycholic acid and taurine on serum liver enzymes and bile acids in chronic hepatitis. Gastroenterology. 1990;90:1044–1050.
18. Crosignani A, Battezzati PM, Setchell KDR et al. Effect of ursodeoxycholic acid on serum liver enzymes and bile acid metabolism in chronic active hepatitis. A dose-response study. Hepatology. 1991;13:339–344.
19. Bellentani S, Podda M, Tiribelli C et al. Ursodiol in the long term treatment of chronic hepatitis: a double blind multicenter clinical trial. J Hepatol. 1993;19:459–464.
20. Simko V, Michael S, Prego. Ursodeoxycholic therapy in chronic liver disease: a meta-analysis in primary biliary cirrhosis and in chronic hepatitis. Am J Gastroenterol. 1994;89:92–98.
21. Mohler CM, Seipp S, Tox U et al. Effect of ursodeoxycholic acid on HCV replication in subtyped chronic hepatitis. Dig Dis Sci. 1996;41:1266–1267.
22. Boucher E, Jouanolle H, Ruffault A et al. Interferon and ursodeoxycholic acid combined therapy in the treatment of chronic viral C hepatitis: results from a controlled randomised trial in 80 patients. Hepatology. 1995;21:322–327.
23. Angelico M, Gandin C, Pescarmona E et al. Recombinant interferon-alpha and ursodeoxycholic acid versus interferon-alpha alone in the treatment of chronic hepatitis C: a randomised clinical trial with long-term follow-up. Am J Gastoenterol. 1995;90:263–269.
24. Tanaka K, Kondo M, Sakaguchi T et al. Efficacy of ursodeoxycholic acid in combination with interferon-alpha in treating chronic hepatitis C: results of a long-term follow-up trial. J Gastroenterol Hepatol. 1996;11:1155–1160.
25. Kiso S, Kawata S, Tamura S et al. Efficacy of combination therapy of interferon-alpha with ursodeoxycholic acid in chronic hepatitis C: a randomised controlled clinical trial. J Gastroenterol. 1997;32:56–62.
26. Clerici C, Distrutti E, Gentili G et al. Interferon plus ursodeoxycholic acid versus interferon in the treatment of chronic C viral hepatitis. Minerva Med. 1997;88:219–225.
27. Senturk H, Ozden U, Yucel B et al. Long-term efficacy of interferon-alpha and ursodeoxycholic acid in treatment of chronic type C hepatitis. Dig Dis Sci. 1997;42:1438–1444.
28. Knodell RG, Ishak KG et al. Formulation and application of a numerical scoring system for assessing histological activity in asymptomatic chronic active hepatitis. Hepatology. 1981;1:431–435.
29. Pigozzi MG, Sorbara R, Reggiani A et al. Interferon (IFN) sparing effect of adjuvant tauro-ursodeoxycholic acid (T-UDCA) therapy for treatment of chronic hepatitis C. Results of liver histology. Gut. 1997;40:A16.

Section VII
Cholesterol gallstone disease

19
Pathogenesis of cholesterol gallstone disease: role of the liver

M.C. CAREY and B. PAIGEN

INTRODUCTION

In general, cholesterol gallstone disease results from hepatic hypersecretion of cholesterol into bile[1]. The pathophysiological mechanisms of altered secretion of other biliary lipids are somewhat different in the normal weight and obese subjects. In normal weight subjects, bile salt pool size is reduced, but the recycling frequency is increased in compensation[2], hence bile salt and phosphatidylcholine secretion rates are normal or only slightly decreased[1,2]. There is strong evidence that these changes in the homeostasis of cholesterol solubilizing lipids are secondary to gallbladder dysmotility[3], apparently a consequence of cholesterol absorbed by the gallbladder from supersaturated bile[1]. It has been demonstrated that excess molecular cholesterol in the sarcolemmae of the gallbladder's smooth muscle cells[4] decreases plasma membrane fluidity[4] and causes signal transduction decoupling[5,6]. This results in both contractile[4,6] and relaxation[7] dysfunction of the gallbladder in response to cholecystokinin and vasoactive intestinal polypeptide, respectively. In contrast, in obese individuals with cholesterol gallstones, the secretion rates of all three biliary lipids are increased[8,9] but cholesterol hypersecretion is out of proportion to the others, resulting in abnormally high cholesterol supersaturation of bile[2]. On the basis of racial, family pedigree and twin studies, susceptibility to cholesterol gallstones in humans appears to have an important genetic basis[10] but the genomic or functional underpinnings have not yet been documented, although inroads on quantifying the genetic epidemiology are being made[11,12]. When fed a lithogenic diet, some strains of laboratory monkeys, hamsters, and mice are susceptible and others resistant to cholesterol gallstone formation[13].

In recent work, we have confined our focus to inbred mice and in 1995 discovered the first gallstone (*Lith1*) gene[14]. In subsequent years, a number of other cholesterol gallstone (*Lith*) genes[10,15] were discovered by our group. We employed a powerful genetic technique, namely quantitative trait locus (QTL) analysis, developed over the last decade[16] to define the chromosomal regions containing each gene. QTL analysis correlates genotype via microsatellite markers covering the entire genome with the phenotype of the disease, in our case gallstone weight[14]. As determined by high LOD ('log of the odds ratio') scores, we identified *Lith* genes on mouse chromosomes 2[14], 19[17,18], 17[19] and X[20], which were officially named and numbered *Lith1, Lith2, Lith3* and *Lith4*, respectively. Another group, also using the QTL method, obtained evidence for additional gallstone genes on mouse chromosomes 5, 7, and 11[21,22]. *Lith1* determines cholesterol gallstone formation in congenic mice[23] wherein, by selective breeding, the QTL region of the susceptible C57L strain is introgressed into the resistant AKR strain (AK.L *Lith1ˢ*). It is clear, therefore, that *Lith1* is a major cholesterol gallstone-determining gene. Employing phenotypic, genetic, and molecular analysis, we have now determined[24] that the bile salt export pump (*Bsep*)[25], previously known as sister to P-glycoprotein[26], is a highly promising candidate gene for *Lith1*[40]. Surprisingly *Bsep*, which is expressed solely on the canalicular membrane of the hepatocyte, appears to be up-regulated and its function overexpressed in C57L mice. Here we will summarize our findings and speculate on how overexpression of *Bsep* may enhance susceptibility to cholesterol gallstone disease[20].

FUNCTIONALITY STUDIES: HEPATIC PHENOTYPES OF *Lith1*

We characterized several hepatic phenotypes in gallstone-susceptible (C57L) and resistant (AKR) mice:

(i) HDL using blood levels to infer hepatic uptake of cholesterol since HDL is likely to be a principal plasma source of biliary cholesterol[27,28] and regulated, in part, by activity of the scavenger receptor B1 (*Srb1*)[29,30];

(ii) de novo hepatic cholesterol synthesis rates by measuring 3-hydroxy-3-methylglutaryl (HMG)-CoA reductase activity[2];

(iii) hepatic cholesterol catabolism to bile salts utilizing activities of cholesterol 7α-hydroxylase (C7H) and sterol 27-hydroxylase (S27H), key regulatory enzymes in bile salt synthetic pathways[2];

(iv) synthesis of cholesteryl esters by activity of acyl CoA:cholesterol acyl-transferase (ACAT)[2,31];

(v) cytosolic transport of de novo synthesized cholesterol via hepatic expression of sterol carrier protein 2 (*Scp2*)[32];

(vi) activities of canalicular export pumps, i.e., the bile salt export pump (*Bsep*) and the lecithin transmembrane translocator (multiple drug resistance protein 2, *Mdr2*), as inferred from their mRNA and protein expression levels and secretion rates of their major lipid substrates into bile[5,23,24].

Mice were fed a lithogenic diet containing 1% cholesterol, 15% dairy fat, and 0.5% cholic acid[14]. Dairy fat is not essential for induction of cholesterol gall-stones, but is important for rapid atherogenesis in the same strains[33]. After absorption and taurine conjugation by the liver, dietary cholic acid is essential for cholesterol gallstone formation because it aids cholesterol absorption from the intestine, facilitates biliary cholesterol hypersecretion, and promotes a solid phase transition in gallbladder bile, allowing cholesterol monohydrate crystals to form[34].

To assess the contribution of HDL cholesterol to biliary cholesterol secretion, we measured plasma HDL cholesterol levels at days 0 and 28, and found a 37% lowering in C57L mice with no appreciable change in AKR mice[14]. This is consistent with up-regulation of *Srb1*, the HDL docking receptor on the sinusoidal membrane of hepatocytes in susceptible mice[35]. Activities of HMG-CoA reductase, ACAT, C7H, and S27H were similar between susceptible and resistant strains of mice in the basal state, but at day 28 of lithogenic diet feeding, the gallstone-susceptible mice displayed significantly higher HMG-CoA reductase activities and lower C7H and S27H activities[31]. As expected for a dietary challenge with cholesterol, ACAT activities were increased markedly in both strains of mice[31]. Therefore, the activities of the regulatory enzymes in hepatic lipid metabolism may be responsible for augmenting the hepatocyte's pool of free and esterified cholesterol[31]. The resistance of HMG-CoA reductase to downregulation in C57L mice was observed in both males[31] and females[14] and was unanticipated in view of the high cholesterol content of the lithogenic diet[33]. The very low levels of C7H and S27H activities in gallstone-susceptible mice were probably related to marked increases in deoxycholate (a highly hydrophobic bile salt) levels in C57L (but not AKR) mice[36] and hence an intrahepatic downregulatory effect on transcription of C7H and S27H enzymes.

With respect to *Scp2*, believed to be involved in cytosolic transport of newly synthesized cholesterol to the plasma membrane[37], both its mRNA and protein levels were increased in the gallstone-susceptible (C57L) but not in gallstone-resistant (AKR) mice[32]. Moreover, the levels of *Scp2* expression became increased immediately following institution of the lithogenic diet and continued to increase substantially before microscopic crystals and gallstones appeared[32].

We measured biliary lipid secretion rates in hepatic bile over the first hour following construction of an acute biliary fistula. This procedure, although interrupting the enterohepatic circulation of bile salts[2], does not appreciably perturb physiological biliary lipid secretion rates because of the short collection period. Prior to institution of the lithogenic diet, we found that biliary lipids were pumped into bile at higher rates in gallstone-susceptible mice than in gallstone-resistant mice[38]. With both strains ingesting the lithogenic diet for 4 weeks, cholesterol and phospholipid secretion rates increased significantly, but bile salt secretion rates did not change[24,38]. Within a few days to weeks of lithogenic diet feeding in C57L mice, the cholesterol saturation indices (CSI) showed marked and sustained increases[36], indicating absolute and relative hypersecretion of cholesterol (mean CSI at 28 days = 1.8). However, an elevation in CSI was not observed initially in AKR mice, and at 28 days cholesterol supersaturation was moderate (mean CSI = 1.2). As inferred from the cholesterol/phospholipid, cholesterol/bile salt, and phospholipid/bile salt ratios in bile, it is likely that lecithin vesicles secreted from the hepatocyte's canalicular membrane[39] of C57L mice are, or subsequently become, appreciably ($\approx 30\%$) more enriched in cholesterol than in control mice[15,24].

Mice with susceptible *Lith1* alleles displayed approximately six-fold higher levels of *Bsep* mRNA and protein[15,24] than did mice with the normal *Lith1* alleles. No changes in *Bsep* expression were observed with lithogenic diet feeding as reflected in the constant biliary bile salt secretion rates. Nonetheless, an increase in *Mdr2* expression occurred on the lithogenic diet, which was most marked in C57L mice[15,24] and consistent with higher biliary phospholipid secretion rates in the gallstone-susceptible strain[38].

GENOMIC STUDIES: GENOTYPES OF *Lith1*

Phenotypic characterization of the gallstone-susceptible and -resistant mice and the susceptible AKR.L *Lith1* congenics suggested several candidate genes for *Lith1*[10,15]. These included the HDL docking receptor *Srb1*, HMG-CoA reductase, the rate-limiting enzyme in cholesterogenesis, C7H, and S27H enzymes controlling the first steps in bile salt synthesis, *Scp2*, the cytosolic sterol carrier protein, the hepatic P-glycoprotein *Mdr2*, and *Bsep*, the bile salt export pump. All of the genes encoding these functions, with the exception of *Bsep*, had been shown earlier to map to other chromosomes[10] and not chromosome 2, where *Lith1* is located[14]. Therefore, their differential expression and activities presumably represent secondary feedback and/or regulatory events. The chromosomal map position of *Bsep* in the mouse was unknown at the time we first communicated these studies[10]. When mapped genetically by linkage to micro-satellite markers in backcrosses of inbred mice, *Bsep* localized to proximal chromosome 2[10,15,24,40]. With further refinements of the chromosomal region for *Lith1*, first by QTL mapping and then by genotyping and progeny testing of large numbers of backcrossed mice, we found that both *Lith1* and *Spgp* were non-recombinant with the micro-satellite marker *D2Mit56*[24,40]. This strongly suggests that the gene encoding the canalicular monovalent bile salt transporter is a strong candidate gene for *Lith1*, the first cholesterol gallstone gene[24].

CONVERGENCE OF MOUSE PHENOTYPE AND GENOTYPE

How can we explain pathophysiologically why a primary up-regulation of the canalicular bile salt transporter determines cholesterol gallstone formation in the mouse? This question appears paradoxical since it contradicts time-honoured paradigms based on the interrelationships between the biliary lipid secretion rates in humans as well as laboratory animals[2,41]. These inter-relationships state that bile salt secretion rate into bile is a linear function of itself, i.e. bile salt return to the liver, and that lecithin as well as cholesterol secretion rates have different rectangular parabolic relationships to bile salt secretion, plateauing at distinctly different secretion rates[2,41]. It follows, then, that at high rates of bile salt secretion, smaller CSI values result from decreases in the molar ratios of cholesterol and lecithin to bile salts and therefore, bile becomes highly unsaturated with cholesterol[42]. Since these concepts are believed to hold true in both lithogenic and normal humans as well as laboratory animals[2,41], it follows that the high constitutive expression of *Bsep* in gallstone-susceptible C57L mice could not, by itself, account for the observed hypersecretion of biliary cholesterol. What was found in our experiments was that the bile salt secretion rate was constant in both basal and lithogenic states[24]. However, the secretion rates of lecithin and cholesterol increased, and proportionally more cholesterol was secreted in gallstone-susceptible mice than in gallstone-resistant mice[10,15,24]. In gallstone-susceptible mice[31], increased hepatic cholesterol uptake from HDL[14], augmented intracellular cholesterol transport[32], as well as increased de novo synthesis of cholesterol all occurred[14,31]. In other studies employing dual-isotope methodology, we found that cholesterol absorption from the intestine was also increased in C57L compared with AKR mice[43]. Therefore, the hepatocytes of gallstone-susceptible mice probably receive a continuous supply of cholesterol molecules in abundance. In particular, the canalicular plasma membrane would be enriched in cholesterol, making the molecules freely available for biliary hyper-secretion in the setting of *Bsep* over-expression and heightened bile salt (and phosphatidylcholine) secretion rates[38,39].

This scenario is reminiscent of hepatic cholesterol metabolism in obese cholesterol gallstone patients who are typified by cholesterol hypersecretion in the setting of elevated bile salt and phospholipid secretion rates as well as up-regulated de novo hepatic cholesterol synthesis[8,9,44]. It is clear that in gallstone-susceptible mice, as well as cholesterol gallstone patients, much more work will be required at molecular biological, genetic, and biophysical levels for a complete understanding of the role of the liver in the pathogenesis of cholesterol gallstone disease[45].

Acknowledgements

The authors' laboratories are supported by grants DK36588, DK52911, DK34854 (MCC), and DK51568 (B.P.) from the National Institutes of Health (U.S. Public Health Service). The discoveries, insights, and concepts summarized here represent mostly work-in-progress from the authors' laboratories carried out by Drs Frank Lammert, David Q-H Wang, David E. Cohen, Patsy M. Nishina, Guylaine Bouchard, Michael Fuchs, and David R. Beier, as well as the authors' research assistants Mark Hunt, Heather M. Nelson, Bhupinder Khanuja, and research manager Monika Leonard.

REFERENCES

1. LaMont JT, Carey MC. Cholesterol gallstone formation. 2. Pathobiology and pathomechanics. Prog Liver Dis. 1992;10:165–191.
2. Carey MC, Duane WC. Enterohepatic circulation. In: Arias IM, Boyer JL, Fausto N, Jakoby WB, Schachter D, Shafritz DA, eds. The Liver: Biology and Pathobiology, 3rd edn. New York: Raven Press, 1994;719–767.
3. Jazrawi RP, Pazzi P, Petroni ML et al. Postprandial gallbladder motor function: Refilling and turnover of bile in health and cholelithiasis. Gastroenterology. 1995;109:582–591.
4. Chen Q, Amaral J, Biancani P, Behar J. Excess membrane cholesterol alters human gallbladder muscle contractility and membrane fluidity. Gastroenterology. 1999;116:678–685.
5. Yu P, Chen Q, Hartnett KM, Amaral J, Biancani P, Behar J. Direct G-protein activation reverses impaired CCK signaling in human gallbladders with cholesterol stones. Am J Physiol. 1995;269:G659–G665.
6. Yu P, Chen Q, Biancani P, Behar J. Membrane cholesterol alters gallbladder muscle contractility in prairie dogs. Am J Physiol. 1996;271:G56–G61.
7. Chen Q, Amaral J, Oh S, Biancani P, Behar J. Gallbladder relaxation in patients with pigment and cholesterol stones. Gastroenterology. 1997;113:930–937.
8. Bennion LJ, Grundy SM. Effects of obesity and caloric intake on biliary lipid metabolism in men. J Clin Invest. 1975;56:966–1011.

9. Shaffer EA, Small DM. Biliary lipid secretion in cholesterol gallstone disease. The effect of cholecystectomy and obesity. J Clin Invest. 1977;59:828–840.

10. Paigen B, Carey MC. Gallstones. In: King RA, Rotter JI, Motulsky AC, eds. Genetic Basis of Common Diseases. 2nd edn. London: Oxford University Press, 1999. (In Press)

11. Miquel JF, Covarrubias C, Villaroel L et al. Genetic epidemiology of cholesterol cholelithiasis among Chilean Hispanics, Amerindians, and Maoris. Gastroenterology. 1998;115:937–946.

12. Duggirala R, Mitchell BD, Blangero J, Stern MP. Genetic determinants of variations in gallbladder disease in the Mexican-American population. Genet Epidemiol. 1999;16:191–204.

13. Liepa GU, Gorman MA, Duffy AM. The use of animals in studying the effects of diet on gallstone formation. In: Breynen AC, West CE, eds. Use of Animal Models for Research in Human Nutrition. Basel: Karger, 1988;6:149–173.

14. Khanuja B, Cheah YC, Hunt M et al. *Lith1*, a major gene affecting cholesterol gallstone formation among inbred strains of mice. Proc Natl Acad Sci USA. 1995;92:7729–7733.

15. Lammert F, Wang DQH, Cohen DE, Paigen B, Carey MC. Functional and genetic studies of biliary cholesterol secretion in inbred mice: Evidence for a primary role of sister to P-glycoprotein, the canalicular bile salt export pump, in cholesterol gallstone pathogenesis. In: Paumgartner G, Stiehl A, Gerok W, Keppler D, Leuschner U, eds. Bile Acids and Cholestasis. Dordrecht. Kluwer, 1999:224–228.

16. Lander ES, Botstein D. Mapping Mendelian factors underlying quantitative traits using RFLP linkage maps. Genetics. 1989;121:185–199.

17. Lammert F, Cohen DE, Paigen B, Carey MC, Beier DR. The gene encoding the multispecific organic anion transporter (*Cmoat*) of the hepatocyte canalicular membrane maps to mouse Chromosome 19. Mammal Genome. 1998;9:87–88.

18. Bouchard G, Chao HC, Lammert F, Wang DQH, Carey MC, Paigen B. *Cmoat* is a candidate for *Lith2*, a cholesterol gallstone gene found on chromosome 19 in inbred mice. Hepatology. 1998;28:502A.

19. Lammert F, Nelson HM, Wang DQH, Carey MC, Paigen B. Quantitative trait locus (QTL) mapping identifies a new murine gallstone gene on chromosome 17. Hepatology. 1997;26:401A.

20. Lammert F, Wang DQH, Nelson HM, Bouchard G, Carey MC, Paigen B. Quantitative trait loci mapping in mice identifies X-chromosome-linked cholesterol gallstone genes. Hepatology. 1998;28:502A.

21. Machleder D, Ivandic B, Welch C, Castellani L, Reue K, Lusis AJ. Complex genetic control of HDL levels in mice in response to an antherogenic diet. Coordinate regulation of HDL levels and bile acid metabolism. J Clin Invest. 1997;99:1406–1419.

22. Bahar RJ, Allayee H, Davis RC et al. A locus on mouse chromosome seven influences gallstone formation on a high-fat diet. Gastroenterology. 1997;112:A1219.

23. Wang DQH, Lammert F, Paigen B, Carey MC. The major gallstone gene (*Lith1*) is responsible for biliary cholesterol (Ch) hypersecretion and Ch gallstone formation in congenic mice (AK.L-*Lith1*ˢ). Gastroenterology. 1998;114:A1361.

24. Lammert F, Wang DQH, Cohen DE et al. The sister gene of P-glycoprotein as candidate for the first gallstone gene *Lith1*. Overexpression of the hepatocyte's canalicular bile salt export pump induces cholesterol cholelithiasis in inbred mice. 1999. (Submitted)

25. Gerloff T, Stieger B, Hagenbuch B et al. The sister of P-glycoprotein represents the canalicular bile salt export pump of mammalian liver. J Biol Chem. 1998;273:10046–10050.

26. Childs S, Yeh RL, Georges E, Ling V. Identification of a sister gene to P-glycoprotein. Cancer Res. 1995;55:2029–2034.

27. Robins SJ, Fasulo JM. High density lipoproteins, but not other lipoproteins provide a vehicle for sterol transport to bile. J Clin Invest. 1997;99:380–384.

28. Robins SJ, Fasulo JM. Delineation of a novel hepatic route for the selective transfer of unesterified sterols from high-density lipoproteins to bile: Studies using the perfused rat liver. Hepatology. 1999;29:1541–1584.

29. Acton S, Rigotti A, Landschultz KT, Hobbs HH, Krieger M. Identification of scavenger receptor SR-BI as a high-density lipoprotein receptor. Science. 1997;271:518–520.

30. Landschultz KT, Pathak RK, Rigotti A, Krieger M, Hobbs HH. Regulation of scavenger receptor class B, type I, a high-density lipoprotein receptor, in liver and steroidogenic tissues of the rat. J Clin Invest. 1996;98:984–995.

31. Lammert F, Wang DQH, Paigen B, Carey MC. *Lith* genes modify hepatic activities of the major lipid regulatory enzymes during cholesterol gallstone formation in inbred mice. Gastoenterology. 1997;112:A1312.

32. Fuchs M, Lammert F, Wang DQH, Paigen B, Carey MC, Cohen DE. Sterol carrier protein 2 participates in hypersecretion of biliary cholesterol during cholesterol gallstone formation in genetically gallstone-susceptible mice. Biochem J. 1998;336:33–37.
33. Nishina PM, Wang J, Toyofuku W, Kuypers FA, Ishida BY, Paigen B. Atherosclerosis and plasma and liver lipids in nine inbred strains of mice. Lipids. 1993;28:599–605.
34. Wang DQH, Lammert F, Cohen DE, Paigen B, Carey MC. Cholic acid aids absorption, biliary secretion, and phase transitions of cholesterol in murine cholelithogenesis. Am J Physiol. 1999;276:G751–G760.
35. Fuchs M, Steimann G, Müller O, Schalla C, Bartsch P, Stange EF. Hepatic overexpression of class B scavenger receptor (SR-BI) during cholesterol (Ch) gallstone formation in inbred mice. Hepatology. 1998;28:502A.
36. Wang DQH, Paigen B, Carey MC. Phenotypic characterization of *Lith* genes that determine susceptibility to cholesterol cholelithiosis in inbred mice. Physical chemistry of gallbladder bile. J Lipid Res. 1997;38:1395–1411.
37. Puglielli L, Rigotti A, Amigo L et al. Modulation of intrahepatic cholesterol trafficking. Evidence by in vivo antisense treatment for the involvement of sterol carrier protein 2 in newly-synthesized cholesterol transport into rat bile. Biochem J. 1996;317:681–687.
38. Wang DQH, Lammert F, Paigen B, Carey MC. *Lith* genes induce biliary cholesterol hyper-secretion as a prelude to cholesterol gallstone formation in inbred mice. Gastroenterology. 1997;112:A1411.
39. Crawford JM, Möckel GM, Crawford AR et al. Imaging biliary lipid secretion in the rat: ultra-structural evidence for vesiculation of the hepatocyte canalicular membrane. J Lipid Res. 1995;36:2147–2163.
40. Lammert F, Beier DR, Wang DQH, Carey MC, Paigen B, Cohen DE. Genetic mapping establishes Sister P-glycoprotein (*Spgp*) as candidate for the major gallstone gene (*Lith1*). Hepatology. 1997;26:358A.
41. Mazer NA, Carey MC. Mathematical model of biliary lipid secretion: A quantitative analysis of physiological and biochemical data from man and other species. J Lipid Res. 1984;25:932–953.
42. Carey MC. Critical tables for calculating the cholesterol saturation of native bile. J Lipid Res. 1978;19:945–955.
43. Wang DQH, Paigen B, Carey MC. Genetic variations in cholesterol (Ch) absorption efficiency are associated with Ch gallstone formation in inbred mice. Hepatology. 1998;28:163A.
44. Roda E, Mazzella G, Roda A et al. Effect of chenodeoxycholic acid and ursodeoxycholic acid administration on biliary lipid secretion in normal weight and obese gallstone patients. In: Paumgartner G, Stiehl A, Gerok W, eds. Bile Acids and Lipids. Lancaster: MTP, 1981;189–193.
45. Apstein MD, Carey MC. Pathogenesis of cholesterol gallstones: A parsimonious hypothesis. Eur J Clin Invest. 1996;26:343–352.

20
Pathogenesis of gallstones: events in bile

T. GILAT, G. SOMJEN and F. KONIKOFF

This brief overview will deal with the major lithogenic factors operating in bile after its secretion from the liver. It is now clear that the proportions of the three major biliary lipids, as expressed in the cholesterol saturation index (CSI), do not in themselves account for the majority of gallstones. In fact, only one out of 4–5 people with supersaturated bile develops gallstones. Clearly, additional factors must operate. Despite three decades of intensive research, not all factors have been identified yet. Of the known factors, we frequently ignore their relative importance, their interactions and often their mechanism of action.

GALLBLADDER STASIS

Stasis of bile in the gallbladder is well proven to be a lithogenic factor preceding and inducing gallstone formation. This has been shown repeatedly in experimental animals[1] and in humans[2] with gallstones. It is also important in gallstone recurrence[3] and in gallstone formation in various clinical situations such as parenteral alimentation[4] and octreotide therapy[5]. It has also been shown in humans that concentration of bile in the gallbladder shortens the nucleation time in a concentration-dependent manner[6]. What is the mechanism of this effect? It is certainly not supersaturation with cholesterol, as the opposite occurs: concentration of bile in the gallbladder decreases the CSI in a time-dependent manner[7]. This is because the concentration of bile decreases the amount of inter-micellar bile salts and increases the number of micelles, and because cholesterol and phospholipids are absorbed much more than the bile salts by the gallbladder mucosa. Nor is it the effect of stasis itself: crystallography has shown that motion accelerates crystallization, and cholesterol crystals form more slowly under conditions of hypomotility. Konikoff et al.[8] have shown in model biles that motion accelerated the formation of cholesterol crystals in a dose dependent manner. We are, therefore, left with a problem: stasis in the gallbladder is definitely lithogenic, but why this is so remains unknown.

Table 1. To solubilize 1 mole of cholesterol[9]

---

14 moles Deoxycholate
30 moles Cholate
324 moles Ursodeoxycholate

>1 moles   Phospholipid

MAIN CHOLESTEROL SOLUBILIZERS: PHOSPHOLIPIDS AND NOT BILE SALTS

Bile salts are the major biliary lipid. The secretion of the bile salts drives the secretion of bile, and the concentration of bile salts affects many other biliary constituents, including the proportion of vesicles and micelles in bile. It is not widely appreciated that phospholipids, and not bile salts, are the main cholesterol solubilizers in bile (Table 1). Bile salts may be removed from bile by dialysis, or separated from cholesterol by chromatography, yet cholesterol does not precipitate. Cholesterol is believed to be secreted into bile in phospholipid vesicles, and phospholipid vesicles can solubilize all the biliary cholesterol even in the absence of bile salts[10,11]. It is not possible to separate phospholipids from cholesterol in solution. Jungst et al.[12] have shown that the addition of increasing quantities of phospholipid to bile progressively prolonged and eventually normalized the initially short nucleation time of bile from patients with cholesterol gallstones. Conversely, the stepwise addition of equimolar amounts of bile salts did not prolong the nucleation time; but slightly shortened it. This is because increasing bile salt concentration moves lipids, particularly phospholipids, from vesicles to micelles: the cholesterol:phospholipid ratio of the remaining vesicles rises, and this shortens the nucleation time[13].

PHOSPHOLIPID MOLECULAR SPECIES

In equilibrium phase diagrams, as well as in most other experiments, phospholipids have usually been treated as a single entity (egg lecithin, which is a mixture of phospholipids, was often used) and only the total amount considered. It is now becoming apparent that minute changes in the phospholipid molecule, as with bile salts, produce considerable changes in function. Changes in the head group or in the saturation or chain length of the fatty acids have major effects on cholesterol solubility and crystallization. Since the sn-1 fatty acid is mostly the saturated (palmitic or stearic) acid, most variations relate to the sn-2 fatty acid.

A saturated fatty acid (18:0) in the sn-2 position almost abolished cholesterol crystallization in model bile during 14 days of incubation. The effects on several aspects of the crystallization process were similar: nucleation time was prolonged, crystal growth greatly slowed, and the total crystal mass at the end of the incubation period was markedly reduced (Figure 1). The introduction of one

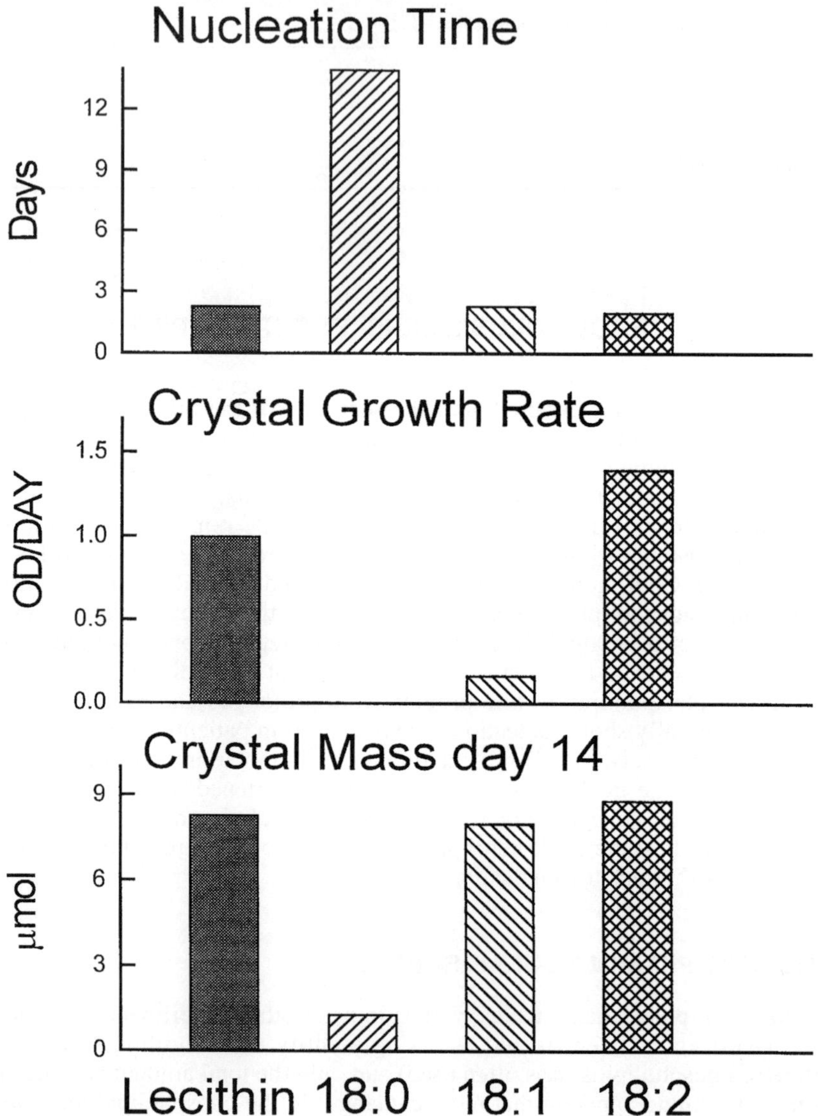

Figure 1.

double bond or two double bonds (in the sn-2 fatty acid) abolished these effects[14]. When the chain length of the sn-2 fatty acid was progressively increased (from 12 to 16 carbon atoms) using saturated fatty acids, cholesterol crystallization was progressively reduced, as above (Figure 2). Changes in the phospholipid head group (while keeping the fatty acids constant) also induced changes in cholesterol crystallization kinetics[15]: serine (PS) as a head

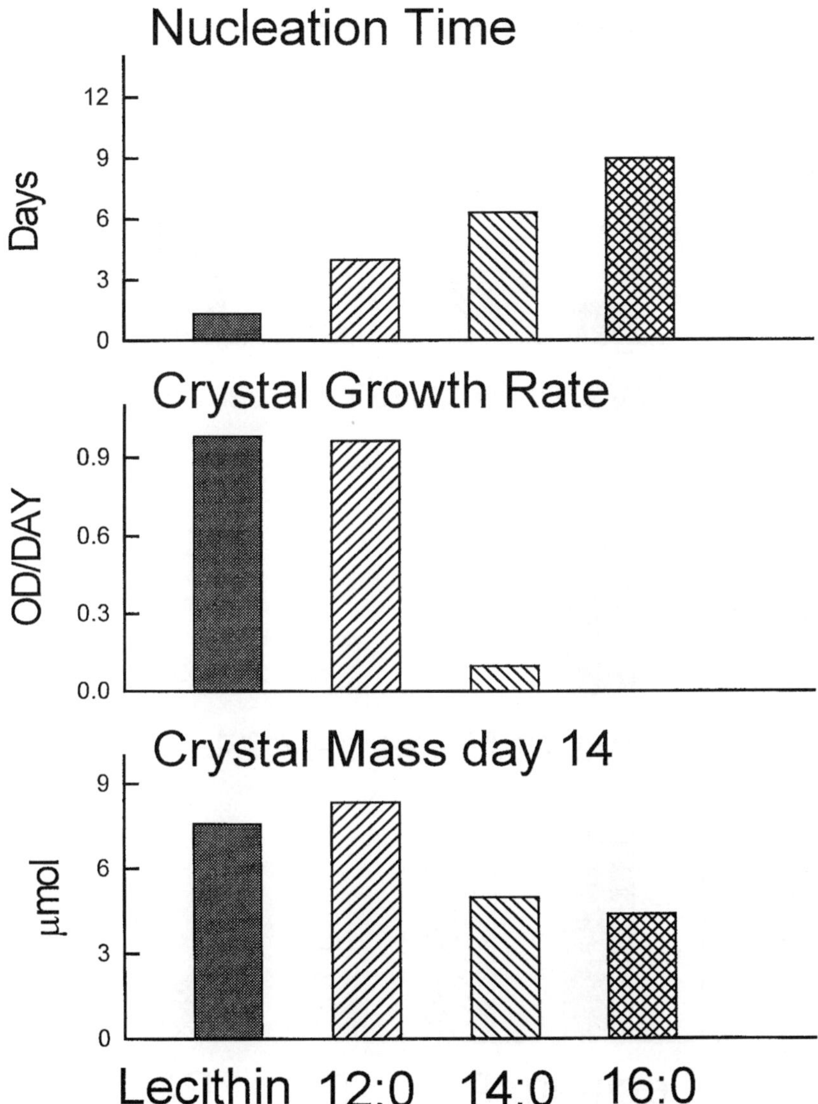

Figure 2.

group, or phosphatidyl glycerol (PG), which is devoid of a head group, inhibited all these aspects of the crystallization process (Figure 3). Phosphatidyl ethanolamine (PE) had little effect.

In all the above experiments the total amount of phospholipid and its proportion in the model bile were kept constant. The control bile contained egg lecithin

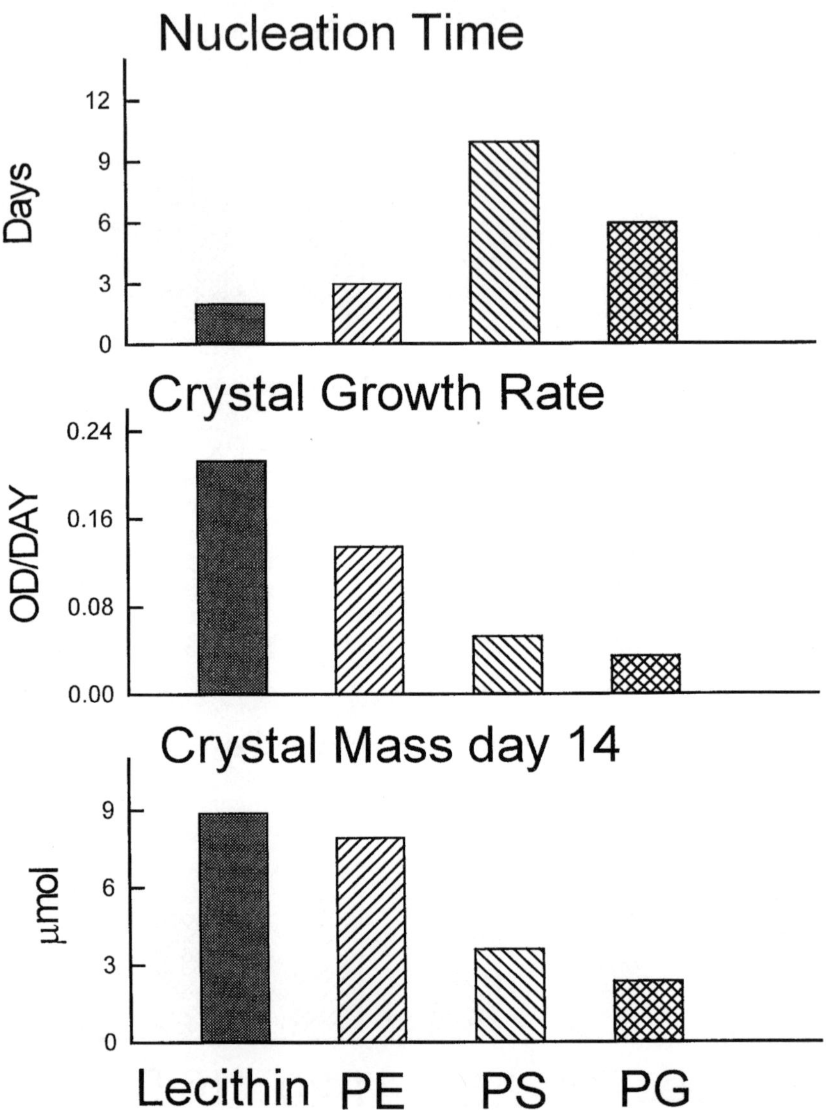

Figure 3.

which is a mixture of various molecular species of phosphatidyl choline. In the test biles 20% of this lecithin was replaced by the test phospholipid. These effects have also been demonstrated in human bile: 10%, or even 5%, of the test phospholipid showed anti-crystallization activity. This suggests that the findings may have physiological value and may prove of particular interest for the future modulation of the phospholipid composition of bile. A bile containing even a small proportion of the 'desired' phospholipid might prevent cholesterol crystallization during the brief residence time of bile in the gallbladder.

CHOLESTEROL CARRIERS IN BILE AND THE PRECRYSTALLIZATION PROCESS

The presence of vesicles and micelles in bile is accepted, but other putative carriers are controversial[10]. Crystallization, as observed by light microscopy, is preceded by the appearance of small vesicular aggregates which gradually increase in number and size. Eventually crystals appear in the vicinity of these vesicle aggregates ($\approx$ liquid crystals). The kinetics and characteristics of this sequential process have not been sufficiently studied. Is there a rate limiting step? Is it like a snowball rolling downhill which, once started, proceeds automatically? Are any of these steps designed or destined to slow crystallization? Dr Somjen in unpublished work has shown that the presence of a 'float' in incubated model bile markedly retards crystallization. Two model biles were incubated at 37°C for 14 days differing only in bile salt concentration: cholesterol 30 mM, phospholipids 70 mM, and bile salts 300 mM (A) or 100 mM (B). Bile A showed many cholesterol crystals and no float. Bile B showed a float, and no crystals. A float is a low density lipid rich layer composed mostly of multilamellar compounds. It is rich in phospholipids and cholesterol and poor in bile salts and, in the above experiment, markedly retarded crystallization.

Biliary proteins

The putative pronucleating and anti-nucleating activities of various biliary proteins is controversial, the crucial role of biliary proteins in stone formation and growth remains neglected. In analogy with other biomineralization processes it is most likely that gallstone formation requires scaffolding proteins (mucin?), as well as transport proteins (APF and others?). This is only beginning to be studied.

Crystallization

Here again the process turns out to be more complicated than previously thought. The typical notched, plate-like cholesterol monohydrate crystal is only the final product. Many intermediate forms have been discovered: thread-like, needle-like, spirals etc. The molecular composition of biliary phospholipids influences the morphology as well as the kinetics of this process[16].

Gallstone formation

This has been the neglected area of biliary research in recent decades: the disease is gallstones not crystals. Biliary research has focused on steps preceding and leading to the formation of crystals, but cholesterol crystals are not the end point of the disease. In fact, it is not even certain that crystal formation in solution is a prerequisite for gallstone formation. In physiological mineralization (bones, teeth, etc) no crystals are formed in solution. In pathological biomineralization crystals may form in solution and later be aggregated, or they may form directly on a 'nidus' without any crystals being in solution. Gallstones have not been sufficiently studied in this respect.

THE FUTURE

The complexity of all these processes poses hurdles as well as challenges for gallstone research. It also provides opportunities for future modulation. Inhibiting or slowing some of the processes may be sufficient to prevent cholesterol crystallization and stone formation during the brief residence time of bile in the gallbladder.

REFERENCES

1. Everson GT. Gallbladder function in gallstone disease. Pathogenesis and therapy of gallstone disease. Gastroenterol Clin N Am. 1991;20:85–110.
2. Festi D, Frabeoni R, Bazzoli F et al. Gallbladder motility in cholesterol gallstone disease: effect of ursodeoxycholic acid administration and gallstone dissolution. Gastroenterology. 1990;99:1779–1785.
3. Berr FT, Mayer MT, Sackmann MF, Sauerbruch T, Hall J, Paumgartner G. Pathogenic factors in early recurrence of cholesterol gallstones. Gastroenterology. 1994;106:215–224.
4. Roslyn JJ, Pitt HA, Mann LL, Ament ME, DenBestern L. Gallbladder disease in patients on long-term parenteral nutrition. Gastroenterology. 1983;84:148–154.
5. Hussaini SH, Pereira SP, Veysey MJ et al. Roles of gallbladder emptying and intestinal transit in the pathogenesis of octreotide induced gallbladder stones. Gut. 1996;38:775–783.
6. van Erpecum KJ, van Berge-Henegouwen GP, Stoelwinder B, Schmidt YMG, Willekens FLH. Bile concentration is a key factor for nucleation of cholesterol crystals and cholesterol saturation index in gallbladder bile of gallstone patients. Hepatology. 1990;11:1–6.
7. Shiffman LM, Sugerman HJ, Moore EW. Human gallbladder mucosal function. Gastroenterology. 1990;99:1452–1459.
8. Konikoff FM, Laufer H, Gilat T. Motion enhances cholesterol crystallization and promotes filament formation in model bile. Hepatology. 1996;24:324A.
9. Cabral DJ, Small DM. In Schultz SG, Forte G, Rauner BB (eds). Handbook of Physiology – The Gastrointestinal system III, Section 6. Waverly Press 1989;31:621–662.
10. Gilat T, Somjen GJ. Phospholipid vesicles and other cholesterol carriers in bile. Biochim Biophys Acta. 1996;1286:95–115.
11. Somjen GJ, Gilat T. Changing concepts of cholesterol solubility in bile. Gastroenterology. 1986;91:772–775.
12. Jungst D, Land T, Huber P, Lange V, Paumgartner G. Effect of phospholipids and bile acids on cholesterol nucleation time and vesicular/micellar cholesterol in gallbladder bile of patients with cholesterol stones. J Lipid Res. 1993;34:1457–1464.
13. Halpern Z, Dudley MA, Lynn MP, Nader JM, Breuer AC, Holzbach RT. Vesicle aggregation in model systems of supersaturated bile: relation to crystal nucleation and lipid composition of the vesicular phase. J Lipid Res. 1986;27:295–306.
14. Ringel Y, Somjen GJ, Konikoff FM, Rosenberg R, Gilat T. Increased saturation of the fatty acids in the sn-2 position of phospholipids reduces cholesterol crystallization in model biles. Biochim Biophys Acta. 1998;1390:293–300.
15. Ringel Y, Somjen G, Konikoff F, Rosenberg R, Michowitz M, Gilat T. The effects of phospholipid molecular species on cholesterol crystallization in model biles: the influence of phospholipid head groups. J Hepatol. 1998;28:1008–1014.

16. Konikoff FM, Cohen DE, Carey MC. Phospholipid molecular species influence crystal habits and transition sequences of metastable intermediates during cholesterol crystallization from bile salt-rich model bile. J Lipid Res. 1994;35:60–70.

21
Role of the gallbladder in the pathogenesis of gallstone disease

R.P. JAZRAWI, P. PAZZI, M.L. PETRONI, H.A. AHMED and T.C. NORTHFIELD

INTRODUCTION

Normal gallbladder (GB) motor functions play a vital role in the maintenance of an intact enterohepatic circulation in health, and abnormalities of GB motor functions contribute to several diseases of the gastrointestinal tract. Despite improvement in the techniques used for measuring GB motor functions, the old concept that the GB empties gradually after meals and fills between meals is still believed by many. The goals of this chapter are to describe the techniques used in measurement of GB motor functions and to discuss the information provided by these techniques; to highlight controversies in the available data; and to present a new concept of the role of GB motor functions in health and in pathogenesis of cholesterol gallstone disease. Other pathogenic factors for gallstone disease, such as abnormalities in hepatic cholesterol secretion, biliary cholesterol nucleation and intestinal transit, will be discussed elsewhere in this book.

ROLE OF GB MOTOR FUNCTIONS IN GALLSTONE PATHOGENESIS

A historical review

The earliest attempts at understanding gallstone formation focused on phenomena occurring within the gallbladder. Meckel Von Helmbach in 1856[1] suggested that stasis allows cholesterol to form stones. This idea was supported by Ord in 1879[2]. Naunyn in 1898[3] suggested that stones are formed by inflammation of the gallbladder resulting in desequamation of cells and the production of abnormal substances. These substances later become invaded with cholesterol crystals by a process which he called 'cholesterolization'. Others suggested that infection of the gallbladder wall results in exfoliation of inflammatory cells and the production of abnormal protein, creating a milieu in which gallstone formation could occur.

The importance of the physicochemical properties of gallbladder bile in the pathogenesis of cholesterol gallstones was appreciated in 1954[4] by Isaksson who recognized the role of biliary phospholipids in keeping cholesterol in solution. In 1967 Cladwell and Levitsky[5] produced gallstones in mice by feeding them a lithogenic diet. As a result of these studies, the cholesterol-holding capacity of bile became accepted as the focal point in gallstone pathogenesis. However, this realization has not undermined the importance of alteration of gallbladder motor function as an initiating factor in gallstone formation. The cholesterol nucleation theory postulated at the end of the 1970s[6] provides a rationale that stasis of GB bile plays an important role in the development of gallstones by providing the time necessary for precipitation of cholesterol crystals.

Role of GB in the enterohepatic circulation of bile acids

The integrity of the enterohepatic circulation is said to depend on the intact function of two physical pumps (GB and intestinal motility) and two chemical pumps (active bile acid uptake by the terminal ileum and the liver). During fasting, a large proportion of the bile acid pool collects in the GB and is concentrated there by removal of water and electrolytes[7]. The proportion of hepatic bile handled in the GB prior to delivery into the duodenum has been estimated to be 35–50% in animals and in humans[8,9]. The GB is able to react to the stimulus of eating by contracting and discharging its content into the duodenum. In contracting, the GB acts as a motor driving the enterohepatic circulation[10].

The increased postprandial bile acid concentration, by comparison with the fasting state[11–15], implies a role for the mechanical pumps (GB and intestinal motility) in the diurnal variation of bile acid pool distribution: the role of GB emptying in the regulation of the bile acid pool size in man has been demonstrated previously[16,17]. Evreson et al.[18] demonstrated that more complete GB emptying and faster intestinal transit increased hepatic secretion and enterohepatic cycling of all biliary lipids, and reduced the molar percent cholesterol in bile. The above studies have provided the rationale that GB motor functions are important for maintaining the integrity of the enterohepatic circulation, and that abnormalities in these are instrumental in the pathogenesis of gallstone disease.

Gallbladder motor function defects and gallstone disease

Several studies have reported that GB emptying is abnormal in patients with gallstones[19–24]. Impaired GB emptying has also been implicated in the increased risk for gallstone formation during pregnancy[25,26], in patients taking female sex hormones[26,27], following parenteral nutrition[28,29] and in acromegalics on octreotide therapy[30]. Other conditions such as rapid weight loss, idiopathic slow transit constipation, diabetes mellitus, Crohn's disease, cirrhosis and following certain surgical procedures (e.g. vagotomy, biliopancreatic bypass, gastrectomy and colectomy) have also been implicated in the increased risk of gallstone pathogenesis due to defects in GB motor functions.

Although most studies mentioned above cannot distinguish whether abnormal GB emptying is caused by the presence of gallstones or vice versa, there are several reports on humans and animals that propose that abnormal GB emptying precedes the developments of gallstones[23,24,31,32].

There are several mechanisms by which impairment of GB motor functions leads to the formation of gallstones. Impairment in GB emptying leads to reduced clearance of GB contents, culminating in stasis, cholesterol precipitation and stone growth. It might also lead to selective absorption of solvents and concentration of solutes, culminating in stratification of GB and change in bile composition. Defects in postprandial GB refilling lead to a reduced washout effect of GB contents by hepatic bile.

MEASUREMENT OF GB MOTOR FUNCTIONS

Four techniques have been used for measuring GB motor functions. These are oral cholecystography, ultrasonography, cholescintigraphy and duodenal perfusion. The advantages and disadvantages of each of these techniques will be discussed separately.

Oral cholecystography was first applied by Boyden[33,34], and the method for measuring GB volume[34] was later improved by DePaula ESilva[35]. It is no longer used as a research method due to the radiation hazards, and pitfalls in the method itself (see below).

The use of ultrasonography for measuring GB motor functions was first reported by Ornstein et al.[36], and quickly became the method of choice for measuring GB volume because, unlike cholecystography, it involves no radiation hazards and can therefore be used to carry out repeated measurements[37,38]. Quantitatively, the information provided by both ultrasonography and cholecystography is similar, but measurements by ultrasonography are more accurate due to lack of magnification errors. The specific disadvantage of ultrasonography, however, is its dependence on personal operator skills, resulting in a high intra- and interobserver error[39]. Disadvantages inherent in both techniques include the following:

1. Errors in calculation of GB volume can arise from assumptions made regarding GB shape (both techniques), distance from X-ray tube (cholecystography) or phase of respiration (ultrasonography).
2. If GB emptying and refilling both occur within one observation period these techniques can detect only the net result of both events.
3. The information obtained may differ according to the length of the observation period and the frequency of observations.
4. Obesity, intra-abdominal gas, blocked cystic duct and thickened GB wall are among many factors that can cause poor GB visualization by both techniques

It is necessary, therefore, to be prudent when interpreting or comparing results of studies using these techniques.

Englert and Chiu[40] were the first to report that the use of a gamma labelled radio-isotope ([^{113m}I]iopanoic acid) in combination with external scanning using a scintillation counter, could overcome many of the problems inherent in other methods. Harvey et al.[41,42] described the use of ^{99m}TcHIDA, one in a family of improved hepatobiliary agents. These, due to their high specificity for hepatic uptake and excretion, short half life, and low radiation exposure, rapidly became the most suitable substances for hepatobiliary scintigraphy. More recently, a synthetic gamma-labelled bile acid analogue, ^{75}SeHCAT, has become available for hepatobiliary scintigraphy. This substance behaves like a natural bile acid with regard to its overall enterohepatic circulation, ileal absorption and hepatic uptake[43-46]. With regard to measuring GB motor functions, the main difference between [99m]TcHIDA and [75]SeHCAT is that the former is not reabsorbed in the intestine, whereas the latter is reabsorbed in the terminal ileum and undergoes enterohepatic recycling[47]. Thus, following a bolus injection of both isotopes, the postprandial GB activity measurement of [99m]TcHIDA provides an index of GB emptying only, whereas that of [75]SeHCAT provides an index of GB emptying plus refilling.

The main advantages of cholescintigraphy are that the technique is non-invasive, quantitative, reproducible, has a low inter-observer error[48] and enables accurate observations to be carried out at a high sampling frequency.

The main disadvantages of cholescintigraphy are:

1. Unknown GB volume so that all results are expressed in percentage terms.
2. The technique is based on the assumption that [99m]TcHIDA mixes homo-generously with GB contents; there is some evidence in support of this assumption[49].
3. Varying distance between the region of interest and the gamma camera crystal whether situated anteriorly or posteriorly can introduce errors in radioactivity counting[49,50]. Ideally, a combination of anterior and posterior recording of activity, and calculation of the geometric means, should be carried out[49,51].

Duodenal perfusion techniques provide an alternative method of measuring GB storage and emptying. Whether they provide information on net or absolute GB storage or emptying depends on the experimental conditions, and particularly whether a hepatic bile marker, a GB bile marker or both are used in addition to a duodenal recovery marker[52,53].

The main disadvantages of these techniques are:

1. They are quite invasive.
2. They have a very low sampling frequency.
3. They may provide inaccurate information as large errors may be introduced due to inadequate mixing of intestinal and GB contents, incomplete recovery of samples and use of large correction factors.
4. Aspiration techniques assume a steady state.
5. They are unable to differentiate in the duodenal aspirate between duodenal and GB bile.
6. The hepatic marker indocyanine green can itself alter GB motor functions by its choleretic effect[54]. Similarly, depleting the duodenum of bile acids during aspiration, and reinfusion of part of the aspirate as boluses, may affect GB motility through its marked influence on intestinal motility[55,56].

VARIABILITY OF GB MOTOR FUNCTIONS IN HEALTH AND DISEASE

In health, there is no established physiological range for any of the kinetic parameters of GB motor functions described above. Furthermore, studies on GB motor function in patients with gallstones have yielded conflicting results. Increased[57–59], normal[60] and impaired gallbladder emptying have all been described[21–24,61–63]. Several factors are implicated in the wide variability in results obtained in the different studies.

Subject related differences[64–70]

Large intra-individual variations have been reported in both healthy controls and gallstone subjects, especially in cholescintigraphic studies. Furthermore, the effects of age, sex and body mass index on GB motor functions must be taken into consideration when comparing the results of different studies.

Methodological differences[71–76]

The type of stimulus (hormones, prokinetic agents or meals), the dose of stimulus (physiological or pharmacological), meal consistency (solid, liquid or mixed), caloric value and composition (fat, protein or amino acid content), the route of administration (intravenous, intramuscular or oral), the rate of stimulus administration (bolus or infusion) are all factors that should be considered when comparing results from different studies because they affect both the pattern and the extent of GB emptying and filling. Difficulties may also arise from the differences in methods used for the assessment of GB emptying and for expression of results. Thus, ultrasonography and cholescintigraphy (the techniques most commonly used) measure different aspects of GB motor functions, as the former measures changes in GB volume whereas the latter measures GB ejection of isotope. Duration of procedures can vary widely, especially with ultrasound studies. Some studies have lasted as little as 30 minutes, whereas others have lasted 3–4 hours. Similarly, the observation frequency has varied between one per minute and one to two per hour. Finally, results from previously reported, studies, especially on GB emptying, have been expressed in a number of ways, thus making comparisons between studies difficult. Terms such as 'Ejection fraction, ejection rate and ejection volume; % emptying, rate of emptying, emptying volume; time to maximum emptying, time to 50% emptying; slope of emptying, area under the curve for emptying etc.' are among those used in both ultrasound and cholescintigraphy based studies.

Conceptual problems

Qualitatively, the response of the GB to food or hormones has been conventionally described as a continuous progressive emptying curve, followed by progressive filling (Figure 1)[16,39,52,53,64,77–81]. This concept was originally challenged by studies using dual isotope scintigraphy[47]. These demonstrated that both emptying and refilling occurred simultaneously during the postprandial period, and that observation was later confirmed by measuring simultaneous postprandial emptying and refilling using a combination of duodenal perfusion and scintigraphy[8]. The observation of rapidly alternating postprandial emptying and refilling has also been reported in humans using modifications of conventional cholecystography and ultrasonography[34,82,83], and also supported by evidence from animal studies[84–86]. On the basis of these observations, a new

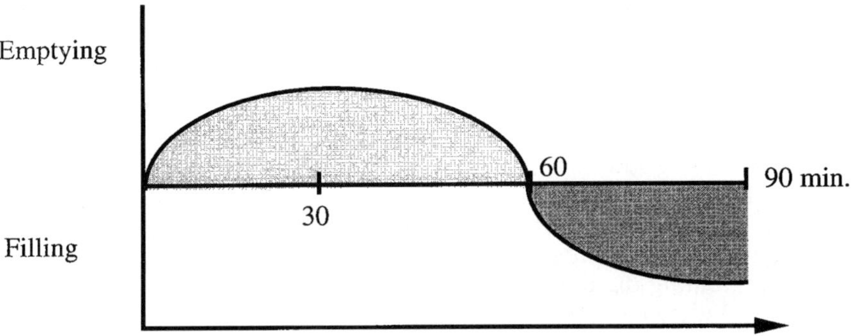

Figure 1. The old concept of the behaviour of the GB to a stimulus, which is in the form of continuous emptying over a period of time followed by continuous filling.

concept of GB response to a stimulus was proposed (Figure 2), in which the continuous emptying and refilling phases (Figure 1) are composed of several small rapidly alternating phases of emptying and refilling.

None of the previous studies of gallbladder motor function in health and gallstone disease, has been designed to enable assessment of both emptying and refilling since neither ultrasonography nor scintigraphy, when used alone, is capable of assessing both events simultaneously. We have employed both techniques simultaneously to measure GB emptying in healthy subjects and gallstone patients[87]. This enabled us to quantify for the first time postprandial GB refilling, and to calculate turnover of bile within the GB (being the sum of postprandial GB emptying and refilling) which was more than five times the fasting GB volume in health, confirming that the GB is a dynamic organ with complex motor functions and not a mere storage sac for bile that empties postprandially. We have also demonstrated that in both GB refilling and turnover were markedly

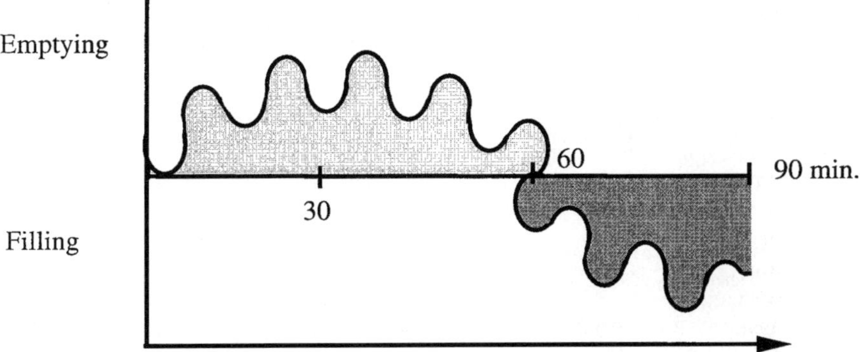

Figure 2. The new concept of rapidly alternating short periods of emptying and refilling occurring during the whole postprandial period.

impaired in gallstone patients[87]; and that they are useful measures to distinguish between those with and those without gallstone recurrence[62,88].

SUMMARY

Normal GB motor functions are of importance in health. The concept of GB emptying during meals, and refilling between meals is not accurate. GB response to a stimulus is more complex, involving rapid alternation of emptying and refilling during the postprandial period. Present methodology (ultrasonography or scintigraphy alone) is not capable of evaluating both emptying and refilling in a quantitative manner, and previous studies employing these techniques have yielded a large variation of results in health, and conflicting results in gallstone patients. Hence, there is a need for improved methodology. Postprandial refilling and turnover of bile are important parameters, which need to be assessed when addressing gallbladder motor function and its role in the pathogenesis of cholesterol gallstone disease.

REFERENCES

1. von Helmsbach M. Mikrogeologie. Berlin: Reimer, 1856.
2. Ord W. On the influence of colloids upon crystalline form and cohesion with observations on the structure and mode of formation of urinary and other calculi. London: Stanford, 1879.
3. Naunyn B. A treatise on cholelithiasis. Johns Hopkins Med J. 1898;9:91–96.
4. Isaksson B. A method for spectrophotometric determination of chenodeoxycholic acid in bile. Acta Chem Scand. 1954;8:889–897.
5. Caldwell FT, Levitsky K. The gallbladder and gallstone formation. Ann Surg. 1967;166: 753–758.
6. Holan KR, Holzbach RT, Hermann RE, Cooperman AM, Claffey WJ. Nucleation time: a key factor in the pathogenesis of cholesterol gallstone disease. Gastroenterology. 1979;77:611–617.
7. Davenport HW. Physiology of the Digestive Tract, 2nd edn. Chicago: Year Book Medical Publishers, 1966.
8. Lanzini A, Jazrawi RP, Northfield TC. Simultaneous quantitative measurements of absolute gallbladder storage and emptying during fasting and eating in humans. Gastroenterology. 1987;92:852–861.
9. Shaffer EA, McOrmond P, Duggan H. Quantitative cholescintigraphy: Assessment of gallbladder filling and emptying and duodenogastric reflux. Gastroenterology. 1980;79:899–906.
10. Low-Beer TS, Heaton KW, Heaton ST, Read AE. Gallbladder inertia and sluggish enterohepatic circulation of bile salts in coeliac disease. Lancet. 1971;1:991–994.
11. Lindblad L, Lundholm K, Schersten T. Bile acid concentration in systemic and portal serum in presumably normal man and in cholestatic and cirrhotic conditions. Scand J Gastroenterol. 1977;12:395–400.
12. Angelin B, Bjorkhem I, Einarsson K, Ewerth S. Hepatic uptake of bile acids in man. Fasting and postprandial concentrations of individual bile acids in portal venous and systemic blood serum. Clin Invest. 1982;70:724–731.
13. Hepner GW, Deemers LM. Dynamics of the enterohepatic circulation of the glycine conjugates of cholic, chenodeoxycholic, deoxycholic and sulfolithocholic acid in man. Gastroenterology. 1977;72:499–501.
14. Pennington CR, Ross, PE, Bouchier IAD. Influence of the gallbladder on serum bile acids. J Clin Pathol. 1982;35:754–756.
15. Setchell KDR, Lawson AM, Blackstock RJ, Murphy GM. Diurnal changes in serum unconjugated bile acids in normal man. Gut. 1982;23:637–642.

16. Duane WC, Hanson KC. Role of gallbladder emptying and small bowel transit in regulation of bile acid pool size in man. J Lab Clin Med. 1978;92:858–872.
17. Jazrawi RP, Northfield TC. Effects of a pharmacological dose of cholecystokinin on bile acid kinetics and biliary cholesterol saturation in man. Gut. 1986;27:355–362.
18. Everson TG, Lawson MJ, McKinley C, Showalter R, Kern F Jr. Gallbladder and small intestinal regulation of biliary lipid secretion during intraduodenal infusion of standard stimuli. J Clin Invest. 1983;71:596–603.
19. Forgacs JC, Maisey MN, Murphy GM, Dowling RH. Influence of gallstone and ursodeoxycholic acid therapy on gallbladder emptying. Gastroenterology. 1984;87:229–307.
20. Pomeranz IS, Shaffer EA. Abnormal gallbladder emptying in a subgroup of patients with gallstones. Gastroenterology. 1985;88:787–791.
21. Sylvestrowics TA, Shaffer EA. Gallbladder function during gallstone dissolution. Effect of bile acid therapy in patients with gallstones. Gastroenterology. 1988;95:740–748.
22. Masclee AAM, Jansen JBMJ, Driessen WMM, Geuskens LM, Lamers CBHW. Plasma cholecystokinin and gallbladder responses to intraduodenal fat in gallstone patients. Dig Dis Sci. 1989;34:353–359.
23. Festi D, Frabboni R, Bazzoli F et al. Gallbladder motility in cholesterol gallstone disease. Effect of ursodeoxycholic acid administration and gallstone dissolution. Gastroenterology. 1990;99:1779–1785.
24. Spengler U, Sackmann M, Sauerbruch T, Holl J, Paumgartner G. Gallbladder motility before and after extracorporeal shock-wave lithotripsy. Gastroenterology. 1989;96:860–863.
25. Braverman DZ, Johnson ML, Kern F. Effect of pregnancy and contraceptive steroids on gallbladder function. N Engl J Med. 1980;302:362–364.
26. Everson GE, McKinley C, Lawson M, Johnson M, Kern F. Gallbladder function in the human female: effect of the ovulatory cycle, pregnancy, and contraceptive steroids. Gastroenterology. 1982;82:711–719.
27. Shaffer EA, Taylor PJ, Logan K, Gadomski S, Corenblum B. The effect of progestin on gallbladder function in young women. Am J Obstet Gynecol. 1984;148:504–507.
28. Holzbach RT. Gallbladder stasis: consequence of long-term parenteral hyperalimentation and risk factor for cholelithiasis. Gastroenterology. 1983;84:1055–1058.
29. Roslyn JJ, Pitt HA, Mann LL, Ament ME, DenBesten L. Gallbladder disease in patients on long term parenteral nutrition. Gastroenterology. 1983;84:148–154.
30. Hussaini SH, Pereira SP, Veysey MJ et al. Roles of gallbladder emptying and intestinal transit in the pathogenesis of octreotide induced gallbladder stones; Gut. 1996;38:775–783.
31. LaMorte WW, Shoetz DJ, Birkett DH, Williams LF. The role of the gallbladder in the pathogenesis of cholesterol gallstone. Gastroenterology. 1979;77:580–592.
32. Pellegrini CA, Ryan T, Broderick W, Way LW. Gallbladder filling and emptying during cholesterol gallstone formation in the prairie dog. A cholescintigraphic study. Gastroenterology. 1986;90:143–149.
33. Boyden EA. A study of the behaviour of the human gallbladder in response to the ingestion of food; together with some observations on the mechanism of expulsion of bile in experimental animals. Anat Rec. 1926;40:201–256.
34. Boyden EA. An analysis of the reaction of the human gallbladder to food. Anat Rec. 1928;40:147–189.
35. DePaula E, Silva GS. A simple method for computing the volume of human gallbladder. Radiology. 1949;52:94–102.
36. Ornstein MH, Palframan A, Meire H. Real time ultrasound – a new method for investigating gallbladder dynamics. Gut. 1978;19:971.
37. Lanzini A, Northfield TC. Gallbladder motor function in man. In: Northfield T, Jazrawi R, Zentler-Munro P, Eds. Bile Acids in Health and Disease. Dordrecht: Kluwer Academic Publishers, 1988;83–86.
38. Dodds W, Groh W, Darweesh R, Lawson T, Kishk S, Kern M. Sonographic measurement of gallbladder volume. Am J Roentgenol. 1985;145:1009–1011.
39. Everson GT, Braverman DZ, Johnson L, Kern F Jr. A critical evaluation of real-time ultrasonography for the study of gallbladder volume and contraction. Gastroenterology. 1980;79:40–46.
40. Englert E, Chiu VSW. Quantitative analysis of human biliary evacuation with a radioisotope technique. Gastroenterology. 1966;50:506–518.

41. Harvey E, Loberg M, Cooper M. Tc-99mHIDA: A new radiopharmaceutical for hepatobiliary imaging. J Nucl Med. 1975;16:533–538.
42. Harvey E, Loberg M, Ryan J, Sikorski S, Faith W, Cooper M. Hepatic clearance mechanism of Tc-99m-HIDA and its effect on quantitation of hepatobiliary function. J Nucl Med. 1979;20:310–313.
43. Jazrawi RP, Ferraris R, Bridges C, Northfield TC. Kinetics of the synthetic bile acid [75]SeHCAT in man: Comparison with ^{14}C taurocholate. Gastroenterology. 1988;95:164–169.
44. Jazrawi RP, Ferraris R, Northfield TC. [75]SeHCAT: an overview of its physiological properties and clinical value. In: Northfield TC, Jazrawi RP, Zentler-Munro PL (eds). Bile Acids in Health and Disease. Dordrecht: Kluwer, 1988:277–289.
45. Galatola G, Jazrawi RP, Bridges C, Joseph AEA, Northfield TC. Direct measurement of first-pass ileal clearance of a bile acid in humans. Gastroenterology. 1991;100:1100–1105.
46. Galatola G, Jazrawi RP, Bridges C, Joseph AEA, Northfield TC. Hepatic handling of the synthetic g-labeled bile acid ([75]SeHCAT). Gastroenterology. 1988;94:771–778.
47. Jazrawi RP, Lanzini A, Britten A, Meller St, Northfield TC. Dynamic of gallbladder function and of the enterohepatic circulation of bile acids studied by a gamma labelled bile acid. Clin Sci. 1984;66:10P.
48. Krishnamurthy GT, Bobba VR, Kingston E. Radionuclide ejection fraction: A technique for quantitative analysis of motor function of the human gallbladder. Gastroenterology. 1981;80:482–490.
49. Jazrawi RP, Kupfer RM, Bridges C, Northfield TC. Isotopic assessment of gallbladder storage functions in man. Clin Sci. 1983;65:185–191.
50. Jazrawi RP, Bridges C, Joseph AEA et al. Effects of artificial depletion of the bile acid pool in man. Gut. 1986;27:771-777.
51. Oster-Jorgensen E, Gerner T, Pedersen SA. The determination of gastric emptying rate. Eur J Surg. 1991;564(suppl):32–43.
52. Mok HYI, Von Bergman K, Grundy SM. Kinetics of the enterohepatic circulation during fasting: biliary lipid secretion and gallbladder storage. Gastroenterology. 1980;78:1023–1033.
53. Van Berge Henegouwen G, Hofmann AF. Nocturnal gallbladder storage and emptying in gallstone patients and healthy controls. Gastroenterology. 1978;75:879–885.
54. Loeb PM, Berk RN, Lobo-Frenkel A, Barnhart JL. The biliary and urinary excretion and the choleretic effect of ioglycamide in dogs. Invest Radiol. 1976;11:449–458.
55. Penagini R, Misiewicz JJ, Frost PG. Effect of jejunal infusion of bile acids on small bowel transit and fasting jejunal motility in man. Gut. 1988;29:789–794.
56. Nilsson BI, Svenberg T, Tollstrom T, Hellstrom PM, Samuelson K, Schnell PO. Relationship between interdigestive gallbladder emptying, plasma motilin and migrating motor complex in man. Acta Physiol Scand. 1990;139:55–61.
57. Maudgal DP, Kupfer RM, Zentler-Munro PL, Northfield TC. Postprandial gallbladder emptying in patients with gallstones. Br Med J. 1980;280:141–143.
58. Pauletzki J, Cicala M, Holl J, Sauerbruch T, Schafmayer A, Paumgartner G. Correlation between gallbladder fasting volume and postprandial emptying in patients with gallstones and healthy controls. Gut. 1993;34:1443–1447.
59. Howard PJ, Murphy GM, Dowling RH. Gallbladder emptying patterns in response to a normal meal in healthy subjects and patients with gallstones: ultrasound study. Gut. 1991;32:1406–1411.
60. Van Erpecum KJ, Van Berge Henegouwen GP, Stolk MFJ, Hopman WPM, Jansen JBMJ, Lamers CBHW. Effect of ursodeoxycholic acid on gallbladder contraction and cholecystokinin release in gallstone patients and normal subjects. Gastroenterology. 1990;3:836–842.
61. Krishnamurthy GT, Bobba VR, McConnell D, Mesgarzadeh M, Kingstone E. Quantitative biliary dynamics: Introduction of a new noninvasive scintigraphic technique. J Nucl Med. 1983;24:217–223.
62. Pauletzki J, Althaus R, Holl J, Sackmann M, Paumgartner G. Gallbladder emptying and gallstone formation: a prospective study on gallstone recurrence. Gastroenterology. 1996;111:765–771.
63. Pomeranz IS, Shaffer EA. Abnormal gallbladder emptying in a subgroup of patients with gallstones. Gastroenterology. 1985;88:787–791.
64. Mackie CR, Baxter JN, Grime JS, Hulks G, Cushieri A. Gallbladder emptying in normal subjects: a data base for clinical cholescintigraphy. Gut. 1987;28:137–141.

65. Khalil T, Walker JP, Weiner I et al. Effect of ageing on gallbladder contraction and release of cholecystokinin-33 in humans. Surgery. 1985;98:423–429.
66. Portis SA, King JC. The gastrointestinal tract and the gallbladder in the aged. JAMA. 1952;148:73–79.
67. Palasciano G, Serio G, Portincassa P et al. Gallbladder volume in adults, and relationship to age, sex, body mass index, and gallstones: A sonographic population study. 1992;87:493–497.
68. Marzio L, Capone F, Neri M, Mezzetti M, De Angelis C, Cuccurullo F. Gallbladder kinetics in obese patients. Effect of regular mean and low-calorie meal. Dig Dis Sci. 1988;33:4–9.
69. Bonfissuto G, Soresi M, Amato S et al. Ultrasonographic assessment of gallbladder motility in obese subjects. Recenti Prog Med. 1996;87:338–341.
70. Gourtsoyiannis NC, Damilakis JE, Charoulakis NZ et al. Relationship of gallbladder contour, fasting volume and emptying to body size indices in normal subjects and patients with gallstones. Digestion. 1995;56:395–399.
71. Spellman SJ, Shaffer EA, Rosenthal L. Gallbladder emptying in response to cholecystokinin. A cholescintigraphic study. Gastroenterology. 1979;77:115–120.
72. Krishnamurthy GT, Bobba VR, Kingston E, Turner F. Measurement of gallbladder emptying sequentially using a single dose of 99mTc labelled hepatobiliary agent. Gastroenterology. 1982;83:773–776.
73. Go VLW, Hofmann AF, Summerskill WHJ. Pancreozymin bioassay in man based on pancreatic enzyme secretion: potency of specific amino acids and other digestive products. J Clin Invest. 1970;49:1558–1564.
74. Fisher RS, Rock E, Malmud LS. Effects of meal composition on gallbladder and gastric emptying in man. Dig Dis Sci. 1987;32:1337–1344.
75. Fried M, Jansen JB, Harpole T et al. Pancreatobiliary response to an intragastric amino acid meal. Comparison to albumin, dextrose, and a maximal cholecystokinin stimulus. Gastroenterology. 1989;97:1544–1549.
76. Sarva RP, Shreiner DP, Van-Thiel D, Yingvorapant N. Gallbladder function: methods of measuring filling and emptying. J Nucl Med. 1985;26:140–144.
77. Baxter JN, Grime JS, Critchley M, Shields R. Relationship between gastric emptying of solids and gallbladder emptying in normal subjects. Gut. 1985;26:342–351.
78. Sacchetti G, Mandelli V, Roncoroni R, Motanari C. Influence of age and sex on gallbladder emptying induced by a fatty meal in normal subjects. Am J Roentgenol. Radium. Ther Nucl Med. 1973;119:40–45.
79. Morewood DJW, Whitehouse GH. Ceruletide cholecystography dose-response and gallbladder function. Br J Radiol. 1984;57:439.
80. Hansen WE, Maurer H, Vollmar J, Brauning C. Guar gum and bile: effects on postprandial gallbladder contraction and on serum bile acids in man. Hepatogastroenterology. 1983;30:131–133.
81. Hopman WPM, Rosenbusch G, de Long AJL, Lamers CBHW. Gallbladder contraction: effects of fatty meals and cholecystokinin. Radiology. 1985;157:37–39.
82. Boyden EA, Bergh GS, Layne JA. An analysis of the reaction of the human gallbladder and sphincter of Oddi to magnesium sulphate. Surgery. 1943;723–733.
83. Torsoli A, Ramorino ML, Colagrande C, Demaio G. Experiments with cholecystokinin. Acta Radiol. 1960;55:193–205.
84. Takahashi I, Suzuki T, Aizawa I et al. Comparison of gallbladder contractions induced by motilin and cholecystokinin in dogs. Gastroenterology. 1982;82:419–424.
85. Traynor OJ, Dozois RR, DiMagno EP. Canine interdigestive and postprandial gallbladder motility and emptying. Am J Physiol. 1984;246:G426–431.
86. Takahashi I, Kern MK, Dodds WJ et al. Contraction pattern of opossum gallbladder during fasting and after feeding. Am J Physiol. 1986;250:G227–235.
87. Jazrawi RP, Pazzi P, Petroni ML et al. Postprandial gallbladder motor function: Refilling and turnover of bile in health and cholestasis. Gastroenterology. 1995;109:582–591.
88. Pazzi P, Petroni ML, Prandini N et al. Postprandial refilling and turnover: Specific gallbladder motor function defects in patients with gallstone recurrence. ELGH, 1999;(in press).

22
The role of the large intestine in cholesterol gallstone formation

K.W. HEATON

The idea that the colon has a role in gallstone formation may be novel to some, but it has a long history. Its origins lie in several observations made during the 1960s and early 1970s, summarized previously[1].

1. The deoxycholic acid (DCA) in bile, which constitutes 10–40% of the pool, derives from dehydroxylation of cholic acid by anaerobic bacteria in the colon. The enzyme responsible is less active at lower pH. DCA is by far the most important of the bacterially altered bile acids which are absorbed and recirculate alongside the primary bile acids, cholic and chenodeoxycholic.

2. The absorption of DCA from the colon is slow and incomplete despite the long time taken by ileal effluent to traverse the colon (20–60 h). There are probably several reasons: having a high pKa, DCA is unionized and poorly soluble at acid pH as found in the caecum; DCA binds to solid matter and throughout the colonic lumen the ratio of solid to liquid is high, the solids consisting of bacteria and food residues, chiefly dietary fibre; the only mode of absorption available to bile acids in the colon is passive diffusion, and this is slow.

3. The bile of patients with cholesterol gallstones was repeatedly found to contain an excess of DCA. This might be due in part to the presence of the gallstones since loss of the gallbladder's reservoir function results in more frequent exposure of the circulating bile acid pool to intestinal bacteria. However, it cannot be the whole story because of the many relationships between DCA and cholesterol levels in bile.

4. In the pioneering experiment, Low-Beer and Pomare fed DCA in physiological amounts (2 mg/kg/day) to normal volunteers and their duodenal bile became enriched with cholesterol as well as DCA[2]. At first this was attributed to displacement of the other dihydroxy bile acid chenodeoxycholic acid, with loss of its beneficial effects on cholesterol secretion, but the Modena group showed that DCA can have a direct effect, leaching out more cholesterol than other bile acids do from the canalicular membrane as they are secreted into bile[3].

We in Bristol were excited by these effects of feeding DCA since they were the mirror image of what we had found when we fed wheat bran[4,5]. However, the findings were not widely accepted because three other groups tried to replicate them and failed to do so[1]. Unfortunately, in those studies much larger doses of DCA were used (7–15 mg/kg/day). Such unphysiological doses may have had toxic effects on the liver and/or intestine[6]. The Modena group appreciated this point, tried a lower dose of DCA, and found it did indeed raise the cholesterol content of bile[7], as did enriching DCA in a more 'natural' way – by feeding its precursor cholic acid[8].

RELATIONSHIP BETWEEN DCA LEVELS AND CHOLESTEROL LEVELS IN BILE

Given that DCA can influence bile cholesterol levels, the question arises whether it does so in real life. In other words, does it account for any of the natural variation in levels of cholesterol in bile? A statistically significant correlation between these variables has been found in several groups of subjects including gallstone patients[9–11], mixed gallstone patients and healthy controls[3,12], and the same mix also including acromegalic patients[13]. It was not apparent in two other groups: men of the US National Cooperative Gallstone Study[10] and a mix of Japanese gallstone and cancer patients[14]. All these studies suffer from possible selection bias. To be truly valid a correlation study should be done on a random sample of the general population. Such a study has not been reported and perhaps never will, for logistical reasons. Meanwhile, some variability in the results of correlation studies must be expected because, of course, DCA is not the only determinant of cholesterol levels in bile.

OTHER INDUCED CHANGES IN DCA AND THEIR EFFECTS ON BILE CHOLESTEROL

The case for the DCA–cholesterol relationship being meaningful would be strengthened if changes induced in DCA levels by less artificial means than feeding DCA had the predicted effect on bile cholesterol, and consistently so. In fact, DCA levels have been manipulated upwards or downwards by a wide variety of means other than feeding DCA (Table 1). All of 14 such studies found that bile cholesterol levels changed in the same direction as DCA[1,15]. The unanimity of these results encourages the conclusion that DCA levels influence the cholesterol content of bile in the natural situation, especially as one of the measures used to reduce DCA was a dietary change – increased intake of wheat fibre. This raises the possibility that spontaneous variations in fibre intake could influence the risk of cholesterol gallstones.

FACTORS DETERMINING INPUT OF DCA FROM THE COLON

Theoretically the input of DCA could increase for a reason that lies outside the colon, viz. that there is more substrate available to the dehydroxylating bacteria,

Table 1. Agents which simultaneously raise or lower bile % DCA and cholesterol content (moles % or cholesterol saturation index)[1,15]

Bile DCA and cholesterol raised	Bile DCA and cholesterol lowered
DCA in physiological doses	senna laxative
cholic acid	metronidazole
loperamide	ampicillin
octreotide[46]	*Strep. faecium*
	thyroxine
	lactulose
	wheat fibre (bran etc)

i.e. more cholic acid entering the colon. A possible cause for this is more frequent circulation of the bile acid pool secondary to impaired gallbladder function, an idea favoured by Carey[16]. However, in coeliac disease, where the gallbladder is exceedingly sluggish, there is less, not more, bacterial breakdown of cholate[17].

Possible colonic factors are:

(a) greater proportion of bacteria able to dehydroxylate bile acids;
(b) bacterial enzymes (dehydroxylases) more active, e.g. because luminal pH is higher;
(c) DCA partitioned more into the water phase so that more is available for absorption; this could happen if intraluminal pH rose, allowing more DCA to be ionized, or if there were less solid matter in the lumen to which DCA can bind (or if the solid matter had a lower binding capacity);
(d) more time for absorption, and slower transit of colonic contents.

These factors interact in a complex way. For example, faster transit results in more solids available to bind DCA, at least in the distal colon (bulkier faeces), which should discourage absorption. At the same time, faster transit results in lower pH, at least in the mid- and left colon[18], and this should discourage DCA production; it should also mean that less DCA is soluble and available for absorption. On the other hand, at lower pH more DCA is unionized and this should encourage absorption.

Similarly, extra solids in the colonic lumen, e.g. from increased dietary fibre (non-starch polysaccharide), mean more binding sites for bile acids[19] which should reduce DCA absorption, as should the faster transit which results from most forms of fibre; moreover, by being fermented to short chain fatty acids, fibre reduces colonic pH which should reduce DCA formation. However, again, lower pH means DCA is more protonated and therefore more easily absorbed.

In practice, it seems that insoluble fibre products like wheat bran deplete the circulating DCA pool (and lower cholesterol saturation) whereas soluble fibre such as pectin can even increase biliary DCA[20,21]. A mixed diet of fibre-rich foods seems to have a modest or transient effect on DCA[22,23]. The effect of dietary fibre may depend on its effect on colonic transit time and this varies greatly between individuals[18,24,25].

EPIDEMIOLOGICAL EVIDENCE

All the above point to the likelihood of a colonic factor in cholesterol gallstone formation. What was lacking for a long time was evidence that a colonic factor exists in real life, that is, epidemiological evidence.

Evidence that high DCA levels precede formation of gallstones

Berr et al. looked for predictors of gallstone recurrence after stone dissolution (oral bile acid therapy after extracorporeal lithotripsy) by comparing biliary composition, bile acid kinetics and gallbladder emptying in response to cholecystokinin in patients with and without recurrence, the two groups being well matched for sex, age, body mass index, and the size and number of original gallstones[26]. Predictors of recurrence were excess DCA, defined as a DCA pool larger than that of cholic acid, and incomplete gallbladder emptying. The combination of the two was present in seven of patients with recurrent disease but in none of those without recurrence. No studies were made of colonic variables but, in another study by the same group, DCA excess was blamed on increased dehydroxylating activity by faecal bacteria rather than on slow transit[15].

Evidence that slow colonic transit predisposes to gallstones

The East Bristol Gallstone Survey was designed to test *inter alia* the hypothesis that, in a random sample of the population, colonic transit is slower in women with newly discovered, unsuspected gallstones, who would not, therefore, have changed their diet, than in women with ultrasonically normal gallbladders. To this end, we measured transit time by the best practicable method, using swallowed radio-opaque plastic pellets and X-raying the stools, in all cases of gallstones and in controls matched for age and sex. (In a few women who refused to have this done transit time was estimated from the form or appearance of the stools on a 7-point scale and defaecation frequency, using a validated method.) When obese women were excluded, which left 15 women with no obvious cause for their gallstones, it was found that their transit time was

Table 2. Bowel function of non-obese women with gallstones and matched stone-free controls in a population study[27]

Measurement	Unsuspected gallstones ($n = 15$)	Stone-free controls ($n = 15$)
whole-gut transit-time (h)	82 ± 35*	63 ± 16
faecal output (g/24 h)	74 ± 54**	141 ± 56

Values are mean ± SD.
*$p = 0.032$ vs. controls
**$p = 0.015$ vs. controls

on average 19 h slower than that of controls. They also had a low stool output, consistent with slow transit[27] (Table 2).

This was a relatively small study and needs to be confirmed. To date, no other prevalence or incidence studies of gallstones have included measurement of intestinal transit time or stool output.

Laxative usage can be considered as a proxy for constipation and a group in southern Italy has reported laxative use to be an independent risk factor for the development of gallstones, increasing the risk by 2.35 (95% CI 1.40–3.96)[28]. This was the first incidence study to make any attempt to assess large bowel function.

Co-existence of gallstones and constipation

Heaton et al. reported a population survey in a remote mountainous area of northern India where obesity is virtually absent in women yet gallstones are common. Against what would be expected in a 'primitive' society with a high fibre intake, the women in the community were found to have slow intestinal transit as judged by stool form (the only practicable method of assessing transit time), though there was no difference between those with and without gallstones[29].

If slow transit is a risk factor for gallstones, conditions where constipation is common should be associated with a high prevalence of gallstones. Though rigorous data are not available, it seems likely that the following conditions can be categorized in this way: pregnancy, crash dieting, use of phenothiazine drugs, extreme old age[30], Parkinson's disease[31] and, perhaps, physical inactivity in men[32–34].

More speculatively, alcohol's protective effect against gallstones[34–36] might be explained in part by its role in accelerating intestinal transit[37].

Evidence that dietary fibre protects against gallstones

Dietary fibre has many effects on colonic function including some which would be expected to reduce the risk of gallstones – faster transit, lower pH, more binding matter for DCA. However, dietary studies have had inconsistent results in gallstone disease[38,39]. All the same, one would expect a large enough cross-sectional, population-based study to show some relationship. In fact the huge MICOL study did show a significant negative relationship between gallstones and total fibre intake (divided into five levels; $p = 0.02$) in the 11 850 female participants[34].

Prospective studies have also given mixed results. In southern Italy, incident gallstones were reduced by 60% in eaters of wholemeal bread[28] and, in southern Germany, recurrence after dissolution was almost abolished by a high fibre diet[40]. However, in a British–Belgian study recurrence was unaffected in subjects eating a similar diet supplemented with wheat bran [41].

These mixed results may simply reflect the methodological difficulties which bedevil nutritional studies. But it must also be borne in mind that fibre is a diverse group of substances and total fibre intake is a poor predictor of bowel function[37]. Therefore, the inconsistency of fibre studies does not necessarily undermine the hypothesis that slow transit or some related aspect of colonic function is a determinant of gallstone formation.

OTHER DETERMINANTS OF COLONIC FUNCTION AND SO, PERHAPS, OF GALLSTONES

Many factors affect bowel function and colonic transit time besides dietary fibre intake. Factors demonstrably speeding up transit are starch intake[37], alcohol intake[37], particulate matter in food[42], anxiety[43] and, probably, having an extrovert personality[44]. Factors slowing down transit are female sex hormones[37], depression[43], suppressing the call to stool (urge to defaecate)[45] and the use of common drugs like analgesics and antidepressants. Other likely factors are travel and irregular habits and, of course, genetic factors. Much work is needed to unravel the relative importance of these factors but they are likely to vary greatly from person to person.

SUMMARY, CONCLUSIONS AND RECOMMENDATIONS

Several lines of evidence, both epidemiological and experimental, converge on the hypothesis that enrichment of bile with deoxycholic acid, the colonic bile acid, leads to enrichment of bile with cholesterol. Biliary DCA can be raised and lowered by slowing down and speeding up colonic transit respectively. Slow transit is characteristic of non-obese British women with gallstones and, surprisingly, of non-obese peasants in a gallstone-prone mountain community. High biliary DCA predicts recurrence of gallstones and so does laxative usage, a pointer to constipation and, therefore, to slow transit. In some studies, at least, a high fibre intake is protective against gallstones. Much else besides fibre influences colonic function. Future studies of gallstone aetiology should include measurements of colonic function. Measures which speed up colonic transit should be tested for their ability to prevent gallstone formation in high-risk individuals.

REFERENCES

1. Marcus SN, Heaton KW. Deoxycholic acid and the pathogenesis of gallstones. Gut. 1988;29:522–533.
2. Low-Beer TS, Pomare EW. Can colonic bacterial metabolites predispose to cholesterol gallstones? Br Med J. 1975;1:438–440.
3. Carulli N, Loria P, Bertolotti M et al. Effects of acute changes of bile acid pool composition on biliary lipid secretion. J Clin Invest. 1984;74:614–624.
4. Pomare EW, Heaton KW. Alteration of bile salt metabolism by dietary fibre (bran). Br Med J. 1973;4:262–264.
5. Pomare EW, Heaton KW, Low-Beer TS, Espiner HJ. The effect of wheat bran upon bile salt metabolism and upon the lipid composition of bile in gallstone patients. Am J Dig Dis 1976;21:521–526.
6. Carulli N, Ponz de Leon M, Zironi F et al. Bile acid feeding and hepatic sterol metabolism: effect of deoxycholic acid. Gastroenterology. 1980;79:637–641.
7. Di Donato P, Carubbi F, Ponz de Leon M et al. Effect of small doses of deoxycholic acid on bile cholesterol saturation in patients with liver cirrhosis. Gut. 1996;27:23–28.
8. Carulli N, Ponz de Leon M, Loria P et al. Effect of the selective expansion of the cholic acid pool on bile lipid composition: possible mechanism of bile acid induced biliary cholesterol desaturation. Gastroenterology. 1981;81:539–546.
9. Van der Linden W, Bergmann F. An analysis of data on human hepatic bile. Relationship between main bile components, serum cholesterol and serum triglycerides. Scand J Clin Lab Invest. 1977;37:741–747.

10. Hofmann AF, Grundy SM, Lachin JM et al. Pretreatment biliary lipid composition in white patients with radiolucent gallstones in the National Cooperative Gallstone Study. Gastroenterology. 1982;83:738–752.
11. Alvaro D, Angelico F, Attili AF et al. Plasma lipid lipoproteins and biliary lipid composition in female gallstone patients. Biomed Biochem Acta. 1986;45:761–768.
12. Shoda J, He B-F, Tanaka N et al. Increase of deoxycholate in supersaturated bile of patients with cholesterol gallstone disease and its correlation with de novo synthesis of cholesterol and bile acids in liver, gallbladder emptying, and small intestinal transit. Hepatology. 1995;21:1291–1302.
13. Hussaini SH, Pereira SP, Murphy GM et al. Deoxycholic acid influences cholesterol solubilization and microcrystal nucleation time in gallbladder bile. Hepatology. 1995;22:1735–1744.
14. Noshiro N, Chijiwa K, Makino I et al. Deoxycholic acid in gall bladder bile does not account for the shortened nucleation time in patients with cholesterol gallstones. Gut. 1995;36:121–125.
15. Berr F, Kullak-Ublick GA, Paumgartner G et al. 7α-dehydroxylating bacteria enhance deoxycholic acid input and cholesterol saturation of bile in patients with gallstones. Gastroenterology. 1996;111:1611–1620.
16. Carey MC. Formation and growth of cholesterol gallstones: the new synthesis. In: Fromm H, Leuschner U, eds. Bile Acids – Cholestasis – Gallstones (Falk Symposium No. 84). Dordrecht: Kluwer, 1996;147–175.
17. Low-Beer TS, Heaton KW, Heaton ST et al. Gallbladder inertia and sluggish enterohepatic circulation of bile-salts in coeliac disease. Lancet. 1971;1:991–994.
18. Lewis SJ, Heaton KW. Increasing butyrate concentration in the distal colon by accelerating intestinal transit. Gut. 1997;41:245–251.
19. Kritchevsky D. In vitro binding properties of dietary fibre. Eur J Clin Nutr. 1995;49:S113–115.
20. Nagengast FM. Dietary fibre and bile acid metabolism. In: Schweizer TF, Edwards CA, eds. Dietary Fibre – A Component of Food. London: Springer-Verlag, 1992;215–231.
21. Pomare EW. Fibre and bile acid metabolism. In: Wallace G, Bell L, eds. Fibre in Human and Animal Nutrition. Wellington: Roy. Soc. N.Z. 1983;179–182.
22. Thornton JR, Emmett PM, Heaton KW. Diet and gallstones: effects of refined and unrefined carbohydrate diets on bile cholesterol saturation and bile acid metabolism. Gut. 1983;24:2–6.
23. Nagengast FM, van den Ban G, Ploeman JP et al. The effect of a natural high-fibre diet on faecal and biliary bile acids, faecal pH and whole-gut transit time in man. A controlled study. Eur J Clin Nutr. 1993;47:631–639.
24. Marcus SN, Heaton KW. Intestinal transit, deoxycholic acid and the cholesterol saturation of bile – three inter-related factors. Gut. 1986;27:550–558.
25. Müller-Lissner SA. Effect of wheat bran on weight of stool and gastrointestinal transit time: a meta-analysis. Br Med J. 1988;296:615–617.
26. Berr F, Mayer M, Sackmann MF et al. Pathogenic factors in early recurrence of cholesterol gallstones. Gastroenterology. 1994;106:215–224.
27. Heaton KW, Emmett PM, Symes CL et al. An explanation for gallstones in normal-weight women: slow intestinal transit. Lancet. 1993;341:8–10.
28. Misciagna G, Leoci C, Guerra V et al. Epidemiology of cholelithiasis in Southern Italy. Part II: Risk factors. Eur J Gastroenterol Hepatol. 1996;8:585–593.
29. Spathis A, Heaton KW, Emmett PM et al. Gallstones in a community free of obesity but prone to slow intestinal transit. Eur J Gastroenterol Hepatol. 1997;9:201–206.
30. Heaton KW. Epidemiology and prevention [of gallstones]. Eur J Gastroenterol Hepatol. 1994;6:852–856.
31. Modaine P, Levy S, Masmoudi K et al. Parkinson's disease: a new risk factor for gallstone disease? J Hepatol 1995;23:484.
32. Heaton KW, Braddon FEM, Emmett PM et al. Why do men get gallstones? Roles of abdominal fat and hyperinsulinaemia. Eur J Gastroenterol Hepatol. 1991;3:745–751.
33. Leitzmann MF, Giovannucci EL, Rimm EB et al. The relation of physical activity to risk for symptomatic gallstone disease in men. Ann Intern Med. 1998;128:417–425.
34. Attili AF, Scafato E, Marchioli R et al. Diet and gallstones in Italy: the cross-sectional MICOL results. Hepatology. 1998;27:1492–1498.
35. Diehl AK. Epidemiology and natural history of gallstone disease. Gastroenterol Clin N Am. 1991;20:1–20.
36. Maclure KM, Hayes KC, Colditz G A et al. Weight, diet and the risk of symptomatic gallstones in middle-aged women. N Engl J Med. 1989;32:563–569.

37. Probert CSJ, Emmett PM, Heaton KW. Some determinants of whole-gut transit-time: a population-based study. Q J Med. 1995;88:311–315.
38. Sama C, Labate AMM, Taroni F et al. Epidemiology and natural history of gallstone disease. Semin Liver Dis. 1990;10:149–158.
39. Hayes KC, Livingston A, Trautwein EA. Dietary impact on biliary lipids and gallstones. Annu Rev Nutr. 1992;12:299–326.
40. Tudyka J, Wechsler JG, Kratzer W et al. Gallstone recurrence after successful dissolution therapy. Dig Dis Sci. 1996;41:235–241.
41. Hood KA, Gleeson D, Ruppin DC et al. Gallstone recurrence and its prevention: the British/Belgian Gallstone Study Group's post-dissolution trial. Gut. 1993;34:1277–1288.
42. Lewis SJ, Heaton KW. The intestinal effects of bran-like plastic particles: is the concept of "roughage" valid after all? Eur J Gastroenterol Hepatol. 1997;9:553–558.
43. Gorard DA, Gomborone JE, Libby GW et al. Intestinal transit in anxiety and depression. Gut. 1996;39:551–555.
44. Tucker DM, Sandstead HH, Logan GM et al. Dietary fiber and personality factors as determinants of stool output. Gastroenterology. 1981;81:879–883.
45. Klauser AG, Voderholzer WA, Heinrich SA et al. Behavioral modification of colonic function: can constipation be learned? Dig Dis Sci. 1990;35:1271–1275.
46. Hussaini SH, Murphy GM, Kennedy C et al. The role of bile composition and physical chemistry in the pathogenesis of octreotide-associated gallbladder stones. Gastroenterology. 1994;107:1503–1513.

23
The octreotide model

R.H. DOWLING, S.H. HUSSAINI, M.J. VEYSEY, L.A. THOMAS,
G.L. FRENCH, J.A.H. WASS and G.M. MURPHY

INTRODUCTION

The first reports of gallstones occurring in patients treated with octreotide (OT) appeared some ten years ago[1,2]. These included a letter[2] from
St Bartholomew's and Guy's Hospitals which proved to be a catalyst for a
decade of fruitful collaboration between the Endocrinology and Gastroenterology Departments of these two London Hospitals. However, in 1989
ultrasonographic examination of the gallbladder was not performed routinely
before OT treatment began. Therefore, the detection of gallbladder stones
(GBS) during OT therapy was always open to the criticism that, in some patients
at least, the stones could have antedated treatment with the somatostatin
analogue.

The pathogenesis of cholesterol-rich gallstones is fundamentally different
from that of 'non-cholesterol' brown or black pigment stones containing variable
amounts of calcium salts. When we first began working in this area, the composition of octreotide-induced GBS had not been studied fully, although anecdo-
tal reports[3-5] had suggested that most of these iatrogenic stones were cholesterol
rich. Therefore, before attempting to unravel the pathogenesis of OT-induced
GBS (and, based on our findings, to develop strategies for their prevention), we
first had to establish whether or not the somatostatin-associated stones were
indeed cholesterol rich.

The initial aims of the Guy's–St Bartholomew's study[6] were to:

(1) Define more fully the prevalence and incidence of GBS during OT
    treatment.
(2) Study the composition of these iatrogenic stones.
(3) Assess their dissolvability with oral bile acid treatment.
(4) Determine their pathogenesis.
(5) Develop scientifically based strategies for countering the adverse effects of
    OT, and for preventing the iatrogenic stones.

COMPOSITION OF OCTREOTIDE-ASSOCIATED GALLBLADDER STONES

Since most patients with stones induced by octreotide had no symptoms, very few came to cholecystectomy. However, four such patients did undergo surgical removal of the gallbladder, when the stones were retrieved and analysed directly for their composition. In all four cases, the stones were cholesterol rich with cholesterol values ranging from 71% to 87% by weight[7].

In those who did not undergo cholecystectomy, we used a variety of indirect methods to assess gallstone composition[7] including:

(1) Computerized tomography of the stones in vivo. Maximum gallstone attenuation scores, measured in Hounsfield Units, predict stone composition and dissolvability[8,9].
(2) Obtaining samples of fresh gallbladder bile, which we examined by microscopy for evidence of cholesterol micro-crystals, and in which we determined bile lipid composition and calculated biliary cholesterol saturation indices.
(3) The gallstone dissolution response to oral ursodeoxycholic acid.

The results of these studies[7] showed that most of the iatrogenic stones were cholesterol rich although, like conventional GBS (unrelated to acromegaly or OT treatment), some (four of 16) contained considerable amounts of calcium and had CT attenuation scores of > 100 HU. For this reason, our subsequent studies in acromegalic patients treated with octreotide focused on the pathogenesis and prevention of cholesterol stones.

EFFECT OF OCTREOTIDE ON GALLBLADDER EMPTYING

Octreotide reduces circulating growth hormone (GH) and insulin-like growth factor-1 (IGF-1) levels: it is, therefore, an effective treatment for acromegaly. However, the inhibitory effects of octreotide are non-specific: it also inhibits the release of peptide hormones from the intestine, including cholecystokinin (CCK)[10–13]. This is the principal, but not the sole, mechanism whereby OT treatment inhibits meal-stimulated gallbladder emptying, a phenomenon which has been shown repeatedly[11–14] since it was first reported in 1987[10]. We certainly confirmed that OT treatment 'paralyses' the gallbladder and abolishes its emptying response to a fat-rich liquid test meal[14]. However, given the fact that at least three abnormalities contribute to the pathogenesis of cholesterol-rich GBS – the so-called triple defect[15,16], we were reluctant to accept that GB stasis was the sole mechanism whereby OT induced cholesterol gallstones to form. We therefore proceeded to study bile composition in acromegalic patients with and without gallstones, before and during OT treatment[17].

EFFECT OF OCTREOTIDE ON THE LIPID AND BILE ACID COMPOSITION OF GB BILE

In samples of fresh bile obtained by percutaneous, transhepatic, ultrasound-guided puncture of the gallbladder[18,19] Hussaini et al.[17] showed that acromegalic patients with OT-induced GBS had:

(1) Bile supersaturated with cholesterol;
(2) Excess biliary cholesterol in vesicles;
(3) A high molar ratio of cholesterol:phospholipids in the vesicular fraction;
(4) Rapid nucleation of cholesterol micro-crystals;
(5) Approximately twice as much deoxycholic acid (DCA; expressed as a percentage of total biliary bile acids) as normal.

To ensure that these changes in bile composition and physical chemistry were due to the octreotide treatment, and that they did not develop as a consequence of induced gallstones, a small number of patients was studied on two occasions, before and during OT therapy[17]. The results of this study showed that treatment with the somatostatin analogue led to a doubling of the mean percentage DCA in bile, independent of stone formation. At the same time, the biliary cholesterol saturation increased and the bile composition changed from being unsaturated in cholesterol before treatment, to supersaturated during OT therapy.

MECHANISM FOR THE INCREASE IN PERCENTAGE DCA IN BILE DURING OT TREATMENT

Previous studies had shown that a single 50 μg injection of OT markedly prolongs small bowel transit in control subjects and patients with the irritable bowel syndrome[20–22]. At that time, however, there was no information about the effects of OT on large bowel transit. This is of importance since the caecum and ascending colon are the principal sites for DCA formation[23–25].

In our initial studies[14], we confirmed that octreotide significantly prolongs mouth-to-caecum transit time (MCTT) both in control subjects and in acromegalic patients. However, it required the power of paired studies (Figure 1) in the same individual patients examined before and during OT treatment, to show that the somatostatin analogue significantly, and consistently, increased LBTT – by a mean of approximately 15 h[26]. In this same study, we again measured the percentage DCA, but this time in fasting serum rather than in bile. Once more, we showed that OT treatment doubled the mean proportion of DCA in serum (and, by implication, in bile). This 'guilt by association' linkage of percentage DCA with intestinal transit is supported by the results of separate studies[26–31] in 207 individuals (control subjects, acromegalic patients untreated and treated with octreotide, and patients with simple constipation). In these 207 individuals, there was a highly significant linear relationship between the percentage DCA in serum (and again by inference, in bile) and LBTT (Figure 2). More important, using serum sampling and isotope dilution, Veysey et al.[28] went on to show that LBTT was significantly linearly related to the DCA pool size and to the DCA formation rate (input into the enterohepatic circulation).

ROLE OF PROLONGED INTESTINAL TRANSIT IN THE PATHOGENESIS OF CONVENTIONAL CHOLESTEROL GALLSTONES

If prolongation of colonic transit were relevant only to acromegalic patients treated long-term with octreotide who developed iatrogenic stones, the observa-

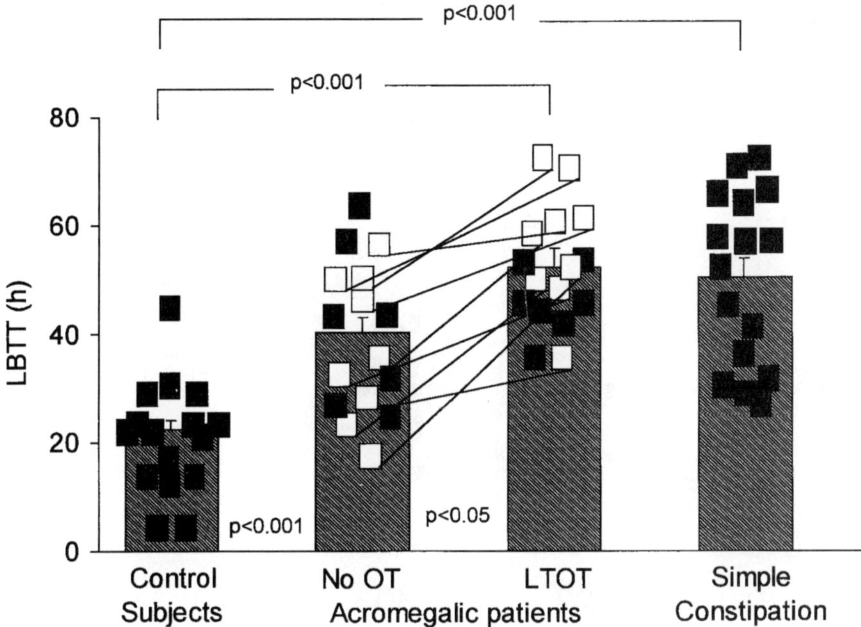

Figure 1. Group data for LBTT in non-acromegalic control subjects, acromegalic patients untreated with octreotide (OT), acromegalic patients on long term octreotide treatment (LTOT), and patients with simple constipation. Reproduced with kind permission of BMJ Publishing Group (Gut, 1999;44:675–681).

tions described above would have limited value. Fortunately, this does not seem to be the case and, although there is relatively little information about the importance of intestinal transit in the pathogenesis of sporadic gallstone disease, the results of four separate studies[29,32–34] on this topic, all point in the same direction. However, in one study[32] the authors measured whole gut transit time; in two others[33,34] they measured only small (and not large) bowel transit time while in the fourth[29] the authors studied both MCTT and LBTT. Thus, in the study from Bristol[32], Heaton et al. showed that in normal weight women with gallstones but no other risk factors, whole gut transit time was prolonged and faecal wet weight reduced, compared to results in matched controls. To paraphrase their findings, the gallstone carrying women 'suffered' from slow transit constipation.

At Guy's Hospital, Thomas et al.[29] not only wished to compare results in control subjects and gallstone carriers: they also wished to define, in more detail, how prolongation of colonic transit might affect DCA metabolism.

EFFECT OF PROLONGED COLONIC TRANSIT ON DCA FORMATION, SOLUBILIZATION/BIOAVAILABILITY AND ABSORPTION

The results of the study by Thomas et al. were presented at the 1998 international bile acid meeting in Titisee[35]. Therefore, they are summarized only briefly here.

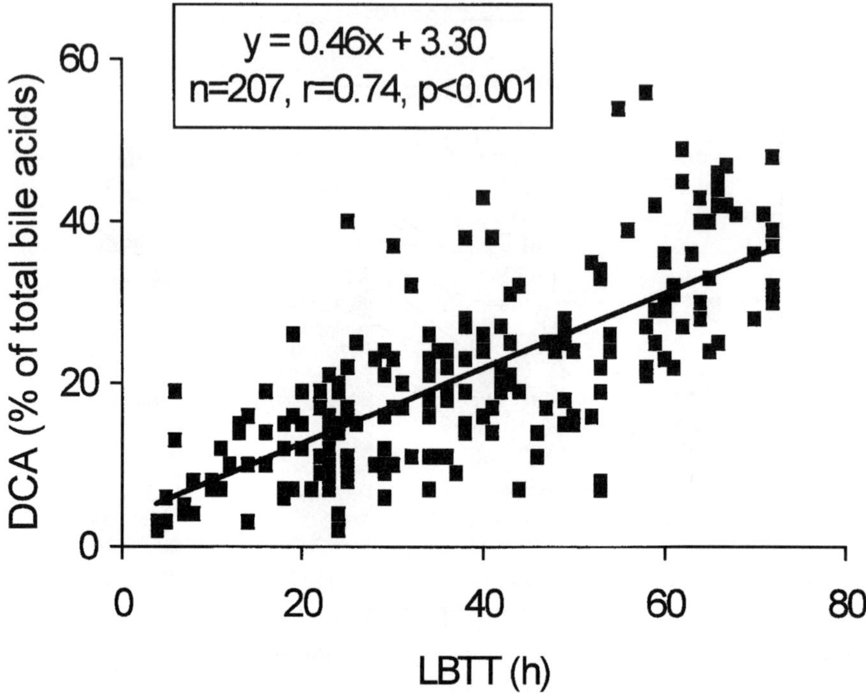

Figure 2. Relationship between the proportion of deoxycholic acid (DCA; expressed as a percentage of total serum bile acids) in fasting serum, measured by gas chromatography-mass spectrometry, and large bowel transit time (LBTT), assessed by recording the progress of radio-opaque marker shapes through the intestine. The data in these 207 individuals come from five separate studies[26,28–31] in which a similar pattern of results was found.

In 20 gallstone-free controls and 20 patients with presumed cholesterol-rich gallbladder stones, the authors compared LBTT, intracolonic pH, the percentage DCA in fasting serum and, in caecal aspirates obtained during clinically indicated colonoscopy, the numbers of total and Gram positive anaerobes, and the activities of the bacterial enzymes responsible for bile acid deconjugation (cholyl glycine hydrolase; CGH) and dehydroxylation (cholic acid 7α-dehydroxylase; 7α DH).

With the exception of CGH (where the two-fold increase in mean enzyme activity in the gallstone patients was not statistically significant), the mean values for all the other variables were significantly greater in the gallstone carriers than in the matched controls. In other words, the prolonged LBTT, the increased numbers of caecal anaerobes and the increased activities of their deconjugating and dehydroxylating enzymes, all favour increased DCA formation.

The associated increase in colonic luminal pH (probably as a result of more time for short chain fatty acid absorption from the colon), favours increased solubilization of the newly formed/nascent DCA. This conclusion is supported by the results of a separate but related study[36] which showed that the solubility of nascent DCA is critically dependent on small changes in intracolonic pH between 5.0 and 7.0 – the range of pH values found as the radiotelemetry capsule passed from the caecum to the distal colon[35].

Deoxycholic acid is absorbed from the human colon, mainly by passive non-ionic diffusion[37,38]. Thomas et al. did not study this, nor did they measure segmental colonic absorption directly, in their patients. However, the net result of the multiple events described above was a clear-cut, and significant, increase in the percentage DCA in serum[35,36]. The implication of these observations is that the percentage DCA in serum is, indeed, a valid surrogate marker for the percentage DCA in bile and that this, in turn, is related to biliary cholesterol saturation and, ultimately, to the risk of cholesterol gallstone formation. While these assumptions remain unproven, the indirect evidence in support of the working hypothesis is strong (Figure 3).

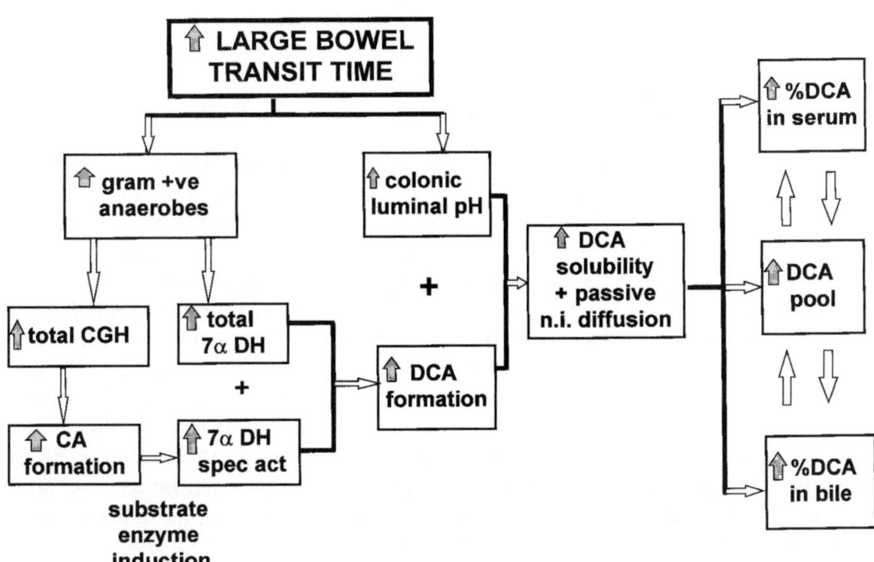

Figure 3. Flow diagram summarizing the results of several studies from the authors' department[14,15,27,31,36,61–63] showing how prolongation of large bowel transit might increase the proportion of deoxycholic acid (DCA) in the bile acid pool, and in serum and bile. Thus, an increase in large bowel transit time favours an increase in the numbers of Gram positive (+ve) anaerobes in the proximal colon. This increase in the numbers of anaerobes leads to increases in the total amounts (masses) of the intestinal bacterial bile acid metabolizing enzymes responsible for deconjugation (cholylglycine hydrolase: CGH) and 7α-dehydroxylation (7α-dehydroxylase: 7α-DH) of the conjugated bile acids, in the caecum and colon. The resultant increase in deconjugation means that more cholic acid (CA) is formed in the proximal colon and this, in turn, may increase the specific activity (spec act) of 7α-DH. The combination of increased total amounts of 7α-DH and increased 7α-DH specific activity, favours enhanced DCA formation. At the same time, the prolongation in large bowel transit time increases colonic luminal pH which ensures that the newly-formed unconjugated DCA is solubilized in, and is therefore made bioavailable for passive non-ionic (n.i.) diffusion from, the colon. This expands the proportion of DCA in the bile acid pool which is in dynamic equilibrium with the %DCA in serum and bile. Reproduced, with permission, from Dowling RH, Ulster Med J. 1998;67:20–24.

COUNTERING THE ADVERSE EFFECTS OF OCTREOTIDE – THEORETICAL OPTIONS

Having broadened the discussion from OT-induced gallstones to sporadic gall-stone disease, we now return to the specific example of iatrogenic gallstones and the OT model.

If the sequence of events described above (see Figure 3) is correct, it should be possible to counter the adverse effects of OT on bile composition, and the attendant risk of cholesterol gallstone formation. Thus, if prolonged colonic transit is the critical step in this complex process, in theory it should be possible to prevent the unwanted chain of events with the use of prokinetic regimens designed to counter the transit-prolonging effects of OT. Possible candidate regimes (Table 1) include the use of cisapride[39,40] (see below), senna[41], high-fibre diets[42,43], erythromycin[44,45], non-antibiotic analogues of erythromycin[46] cholecystokinin, which is prokinetic to both the GB and the intestine[47], the related peptide caerulin[48], and lactulose[49,50] (which also affects intracolonic pH).

Alternatively, if anaerobic bacterial proliferation in the colon is considered to be the major culprit, it should be possible to prevent the increase in the percentage DCA in bile, and in biliary cholesterol saturation, with the use of broad-spectrum antibiotics[51–53].

If, however, 7α-dehydroxylation is the most critical step, the exciting possibility of manipulating the gene for this intracellular bacterial enzyme is a tantalizing dream. Cholic acid 7α-dehydroxylation is a complex, seven-step pathway which has been studied in a single bacterial strain (*Eubacterium* sp. strain VPI 12708)[54–57]. In this strain, Hylemon and colleagues have identified seven different genes, each coding for a different protein in the 7α dehydroxylase reaction. These genes have now been cloned and sequenced[58]. Most are found on a large bile acid-inducible operon[56]. We (Sarsam, French, Murphy and Dowling, unpublished observations), and others[57] are currently using this information and are applying genetic engineering techniques to modify the genes encoding 7α-dehydroxylase activity. The ultimate aim of these studies is to splice the modified genes into anaerobic bacteria that may then be used as probiotics to re-populate the colon of individuals at risk of developing gallstones or colorectal cancer.

It remains possible, however, that if we could render the newly formed DCA insoluble (and therefore unavailable for absorption), we could prevent the rise in serum and biliary DCA, the increase in biliary cholesterol saturation and the risk of gallstone formation. We have known for many years that the administration of synthetic disaccharides, such as lactulose, will lower colonic luminal and/or faecal pH and reduce the percentage DCA in bile and biliary cholesterol saturation[49,50,59].

COUNTERING THE ADVERSE EFFECTS OF OT: EXPERIMENTAL RESULTS

Given the theoretical possibilities discussed above (Table 1), when considering which approach to adopt we were spoilt for choice. In the end, however, we opted for cisapride, the 5HT-4 agonist which has a good safety record and is

Table 1.   Candidate regimes to counter OT effect on large bowel transit time (LBTT)

Cisapride[39,40]

Senna[41]

High-fibre diets[42,43]

Erythromycin[44,45]

Non-antibiotic analogues of erythromycin[46]

Cholecystokinin[47]

Caerulin[46]

Lactulose[49,50]

widely used in the treatment of gastro-oesophageal reflux. To study its efficacy in countering the adverse effects of octreotide on mouth-to-caecum and large bowel transit times, and the percentage DCA in fasting serum, Veysey et al.[30,60] adopted a prospective double-blind random allocation study design. They studied acromegalic patients taking long-term octreotide plus either cisapride, in an oral dose of 10 mg four times daily, or placebo. The results were then compared with those in a historic disease control group of acromegalic patients who had not been treated with octreotide.

Once again, the results of the studies were presented, in preliminary form[30], at an International Bile Acid meeting (1996). In brief, however, the result of these studies confirmed that in acromegalic patients, long-term octreotide significantly prolongs both small and large bowel transit times, and increases the percentage DCA in serum. However, the addition of the intestinal prokinetic drug, cisapride, reversed/overcame the increase in these parameters seen during chronic OT treatment. In theory, therefore, the use of intestinal prokinetic regimes should prevent cholelithiasis in individuals at high risk of gallstone formation (including patients on long-term OT). In practice, proof that they can do so will require prospective double-blind trials. To date, such information is lacking but, nonetheless, for the first time we now have logical, scientifically based strategies for gallstone prevention.

REFERENCES

1. McKnight JA, McCance DR, Crothers JG, Atkinson AB. Changes in glucose tolerance and development of gall stones during high dose treatment with octreotide for acromegaly. Br Med J. 1989;299:604–605.
2. Wass JAH, Anderson JV, Besser GM, Dowling RH. Gall stones and treatment with octreotide for acromegaly. Br Med J. 1989;299:1162–1163.
3. Souquet JC, Girard I, Valette PJ, Chayvialle JA. Sandostatin and gallbladder lithiasis. In: Sandostatin 1991: State of the Art. Proceedings of a conference held in Monte Carlo, Monaco, October 9–12, 1991.
4. Buscail LE, Puel-Bousquet C, Harris AG et al. Effets sur la lithogenese biliare du traitement au long cours pas octreotide (SMS 201–995) chez des patients acromegales. Gastroenterol Clin Biol. 1991;15:800–804.

5. Sassolas G, Harris AG, James-Deidier A, and the French SMS 291–995 acromegaly study group. Long term effect of incremental doses of the somastostatin analog SMS 201–995 in 58 acromegalic patients. J Clin Endocrinol Metab. 1990;71:391–397.
6. Dowling RH, Hussaini SH, Murphy GM, Besser GM, Wass JAH. Gallstones during octreotide therapy. Metab Clin Exp. 1992;41(Suppl. 2)22–23.
7. Hussaini SH, Pereira SP, Murphy GM et al. Composition of gall bladder stones associated with octreotide: response to oral ursodeoxycholic acid. Gut. 1995;36:126–132.
8. Rajagopal SU, Keightley A, Bills P, Walters JRF, Murphy GM, Dowling RH. Predictive value of pre-treatment CT scanning vs conventional radiology in determining composition, dissolvability and fragmentability of gallbladder stones (GBS). J Hepatol. 1989;9:S211.
9. Brakel K, Lameris JS, Nijs HGT et al. Predicting gallstone composition with CT: In vivo and in vitro analysis. Radiology. 1990;174:337–341.
10. Lembcke B, Creutzfeldt W, Schleser S et al. Effect of somatostatin analogue Sandostatin (SMS 201–995) on gastrointestinal, pancreatic and biliary function, and hormone release in normal men. Digestion. 1987;36:108–124.
11. van Liessum PA, Hopman WP, Pieters GF. Postprandial gallbladder motility during long term treatment with the long-acting somatostatin analog SMS 201–995 in acromegaly. J Clin Endocrinol Metab. 1989;69:557–562.
12. Mitsukawa T, Takemura J, Nishizono F, Nakatsuru K, Ogho S, Matsukura S. Effects of atropine, proglumide and somatostatin analogue (SMS 201–995) on bombesin-induced gallbladder contraction and CCK secretion in humans. Am J Gastroenterol. 1989;84:1371–1374.
13. Stolk MFJ, van Erpecum KJ, Koppeschaar HPF et al. Postprandial gallbladder motility and hormone release during intermittent and continuous subcutaneous octreotide therapy in acromegaly. Gut. 1993;34:808–813.
14. Hussaini SH, Pereira SP, Veysey MJ et al. The roles of gallbladder emptying and intestinal transit in the pathogenesis of octreotide induced gallbladder stones. Gut. 1996;38:775–783.
15. Dowling RH, Gleeson D, Ruppin DC, Murphy GM and the British/Belgian Gallstone Study Group. Gallstone recurrence and post-dissolution management. In: Paumgartner G, Stiehl A, Gerok W (eds). Enterohepatic Circulation of Bile Acids and Sterol Metabolism. Lancaster MTP: 1985:361–369.
16. Carey MC. Formation of cholesterol gallstones: the new paradigms. In: Paumgartner G, Stiehl A, Gerok W (eds). Trends in Bile Acid Research. Dordrecht: Kluwer Academic Publishers, 1989:259–281.
17. Hussaini SH, Murphy GM, Kennedy C, Besser GM, Wass JAH, Dowling RH. The role of bile composition and physical chemistry in the pathogenesis of octreotide-associated gallbladder stones. Gastroenterology. 1994;107:1503–1513.
18. Swobodnik W, Hagert N, Janowitz P, Wenk H. Diagnostic fine-needle puncture of the gallbladder with US guidance. Radiology. 1991;178:755–758.
19. Hussaini SH, Kenndy C, Pereira SP, Wass JAH, Dowling RH. Ultrasound-guided percutaneous fine needle puncture of the gallbladder for studies of bile composition. Br J Radiol. 1995;68:271–276.
20. Fuessl HS, Carolan G, Williams G, Bloom SR. Effect of a long-acting somatostatin analogue (SMS 201–995) on postprandial gastric emptying of 99mTc-tin colloid and mouth-to-caecum transit time in man. Digestion. 1987;36:101–107.
21. Moller N, Petrany G, Cassidy D et al. Effects of the somatostatin analogue SMS 201–995 (sandostatin) on mouth-to-caecum transit time and absorption of fat and carbohydrates in normal man. Clin Sci. 1988;75:345–350.
22. O'Donnell LJD, Watson AJM, Cameron D, Farthing MJG. Effect of octreotide on mouth-to-caecum transit time in healthy subjects and in the irritable bowel syndrome. Aliment Pharmacol Ther. 1990;4:177–182.
23. Nair PP, Gordon M, Reback J. The enzymatic cleavage of the carbon–nitrogen bond in 3α, 7α-trihydroxy-5β-cholan-24-oyl glycine. J Biol Chem. 1967;243:7–11.
24. Hill MJ, Drasar BS. The normal colonic bacterial flora. Gut. 1975;16:318–323.
25. Midtvedt T. Microbial bile acid transformation. Am J Clin Nutr. 1974;27:1341–1347.
26. Veysey MJ, Thomas LA, Mallet AI et al. Prolonged large bowel transit increases serum deoxycholic acid: a risk factor for octeotide induced gallstones. Gut. 1999;44:675–681.
27. Veysey MJ, Arraton SRD, Mallet A et al. Long-term octreotide treatment increases large bowel transit time (LBTT), the proportion of deoxycholic acid (%DCA) in serum and the risk of gallstone formation. Gut. 1996;39(Suppl. 3):A134.

28. Veysey MJ, Gathercole DJ, Mallet A et al. Large bowel transit time influences deoxycholic acid input rate and pool size – risk factors for octeotide-induced gallstones. Gastroenterology. 1997;112:A525.
29. Thomas LA, Bathgate T, Veysey MJ et al. Is cholelithiasis an intestinal disease? Gut. 1997;41(Suppl 3):A2.
30. Veysey MJ, Arraton SRD, Mallet A et al. Does cisapride overcome the effects of octreotide on intestinal transit, thereby reducing the proportion of deoxycholic acid in bile and serum? In: Paumgartner G, Stiehl A, Gerok W (eds). Bile Acids in Hepatobiliary Diseases: Basic Research and Clinical Application. Dordrecht: Kluwer Academic Publishers, 1997:82–91.
31. Veysey MJ, Arraton SRD, Gilani SS et al. The relationship between large bowel transit time (LBTT) and the proportion of deoxycholic acid (%DCA) in serum. Gut. 1996;38 (Suppl 1):A53.
32. Heaton KW, Emmett PM, Symes CL, Braddon FEM. An explanation for gallstones in normal-weight women: slow intestinal transit. Lancet. 1993;341:8–10.
33. Shoda J, He B-F, Tanaka N et al. Increase of deoxycholate in supersaturated bile of patients with cholesterol gallstone disease and its correlation with de novo syntheses of cholesterol and bile acids in liver, gallbladder emptying, and small intestinal transit. Hepatology. 1995;21:1291–1302.
34. Azzaroli F, Mazzella G, De Vegori E et al. Sluggish gallbladder and small bowel motility are associated with cholesterol gallstones. Gastroenterology. 1997;112:A499.
35. Thomas LA, Bathgate T, Veysey MJ et al. Transit-induced changes in colonic bacteriology, bile acid metabolizing enzymes and luminal pH influence deoxycholic acid formation. In: Paumgartner G (ed). Bile Acids and Cholestasis. Dordrecht: Kluwer Academic Publishers. In press.
36. Thomas LA, Bathgate T, Veysey MJ et al. Do changes in colonic luminal pH explain the increased proportions of serum and biliary deoxycholic acid seen in patients with cholesterol gallbladder stones (GBS)? Gut. 1997;41(Suppl. 3):A32.
37. Samuel P, Saypol GM, Meilman E, Mosbach EH, Chafizadehj M. Absorption of bile acids from the large bowel in man. J Clin Invest. 1968;47:2070–2078.
38. Morris JS, Low-Beer TS, Heaton KW. Bile salt metabolism and the colon. Scand J Gastroenterol. 1975;8:425–431.
39. El Oufir L, Flourie B, Bruley des Varannes S et al. Relations between transit time, fermentation products, and hydrogen consuming flora in healthy humans. Gut. 1996;38:870–877.
40. Veysey MJ, Jenkins P, Besser GM, Wass JAH, Dowling RH. The effect of cisparide on large bowel transit time: a randomized double-blind placebo-controlled study in four groups of individuals. Gut. 1997;41(Suppl. 3):A123.
41. Marcus SN, Heaton KW. Intestinal transit, deoxycholic acid and the cholesterol saturation of bile – three inter-related factors. Gut. 1986;27:550–558.
42. Pomare EW, Heaton KW, Low-Beer RS, Espiner HJ. The effect of wheat bran upon bile salt metabolism and upon the lipid composition of bile in gallstone patients. Am J Dig Dis. 1976;21:521–526.
43. Marcus SN, Heaton KW. Effects of a new, concentrated, wheat fibre preparation on intestinal transit, deoxycholic acid metabolism and the composition of bile. Gut. 1986;27:893–900.
44. Catnach SM, Fairclough PD, Trembath RC et al. Effect of oral erythromycin on gallbladder motility in normal subjects with gallstones. Gastroenterology. 1992;102:2071–2076.
45. Weber FH, Richards RD, McCallum RW. Erythromycin: a motilin agonist and gastrointestinal agent. Am J Gastroenterol. 1993;88:485–490.
46. Kawamura O, Sekiguchi T, Itoh Z, Omura S. Effect of erythromycin derivative EM523L on human interdigestive gastrointestinal tract. Dig Dis Sci. 1993;39:1026–1031.
47. Meyer BM, Beglinger C, Jansen JBMJ et al. Role of cholecystokinin in regulation of gastrointestinal motor functions. Lancet. 1989;ii:12–15.
48. Hasse C, Nielke A, Nies C, Al-Bazaz B, Gotzen L, Rothmund M. Influence of cerletid on gallbladder contraction: a possible prophylaxis of acute acalculous cholecystitis in intensive care patients. Digestion. 1995;56:389–394.
49. van Berge Henegouwen GP, van der Werf SD, Ruden AT. Effect of long term lactulose ingestion on secondary bile salt metabolism in man: potential protective effect of lactulose in colonic car-cinogenesis. Gut. 1987;28:675–680s.
50. Thornton JR, Heaton KW. Do colonic bacteria contribute to cholesterol gall stone formation? Effects of lactulose on bile. Br Med J. 1981;282:1018–1020.

51. Low-Beer TS, Nutter S. Colonic bacterial activity, biliary cholesterol saturation, and pathogenesis of gallstones. Lancet. 1978;11:1063–1065.
52. Ponz de Leon M, Carulli N, Lori R, Loria P, Romani M. Regulation of cholesterol absorption by bile acids: role of deoxycholic acid and cholic acid pool expansion on dietary cholesterol absorption. Ital J Gastroenterol. 1983;15:86–93.
53. Berr F, Kullak-Ublick GA, Paumgartner G et al. 7-alpha-dehydroxylating bacteria enhance deoxycholic acid input and cholesterol saturation of bile in patients with gallstones. Gastroenterology. 1996;111:1611–1620.
54. Bjorkhem I, Einarsson K, Melone P, Hylemon PB. Mechanism of intestinal formation of cholic acid in humans: evidence for a 3-oxo-Δ^{4} steroid intermediate. J Lipid Res. 1989;30:1033–1040.
55. Hylemon PB, Melone PD, Franklund CV, Lund E, Bjorkhem I. Mechanism of intestinal 7α-dehydroxylation of cholic acid: evidence of allo-deoxycholic acid is an inducible side product. J Lipid Res. 1991;32:89–96.
56. Mallonee DH, Hylemon PB. Sequencing and expression of a gene encoding a bile acid transporter from Eubacterium sp strain VP1 12 708. J Bacteriol. 1996;178:7053–7058.
57. Mallonee DH, Adams JL, Hylemon PB,. The bile acid inducible baiB gene from Eubacterium sp. strain VP1 12 708 encodes a bile acid-coenzyme A ligase. J Bacteriol. 1992;174:2065–2071.
58. Doerner KC, Takamine F, La Voie CP, Mallonee DH, Hylemon PB. Assessment of fecal bacteria with bile acid 7α-dehydroxylating activity for the present of *bai*-like genes. Appl Environ Microbiol. 1997;63:1185–1188.
59. Lewis SJ, Heaton KW. Increasing butyrate concentration in the distal colon by accelerating intestinal transit. Gut. 1997;41:245–251.
60. Veysey MJ, Malcolm P, Jenkins P, Murphy GM, Wass JAH, Dowling RH. Can cisapride overcome the effects of octreotide (OT) on gallbladder emptying? Gut. 1996;39(Suppl. 3):A130.
61. Veysey MJ, Mallet A, Murphy GM, Dowling RH. Deoxycholic acid pool size and input rate, measured by stable isotope dilution, are increased in patients with slow transit constipation. Clin Sci. 1997;92:3P.
62. Thomas LA, Veysey MJ, Murphy GM, Dowling RH, King A, French GR. Bile acid metabolizing intestinal bacterial enzyme activity: A novel factor in cholesterol gallstone pathogenesis. Gut. 1997;40(Suppl. 1):A67.
63. Veysey MJ, Arraton SRD, Mallet A et al. Cisapride reverses the effects of octreotide (OT) on intestinal transit and the proportion of deoxycholic acid (%DCA) in bile and serum. Gut. 1996;3:(Suppl. 3):A103.

Section VIII
Therapy

24
Oral bile acid therapy

E. RODA, A. COLECCHIA, G. MAZZELLA, A. LAROCCA,
L. SANDRI, F. ROMANO and D. FESTI

INTRODUCTION

For nearly a century conventional cholecystectomy has been the only active treatment for patients with gallstone disease. The demonstration in 1972 that oral administration of chenodeoxycholic acid[1], a naturally occurring primary bile acid, and later ursodeoxycholic acid[2], could desaturate bile and consequently induce gallstone dissolution heralded the era of non-surgical treatment of gallstone disease. Subsequently, other therapeutic approaches were developed, such as gallstone fragmentation using extra-corporeal shock-waves lithotripsy[3] or gallstone dissolution using contact solvents through a catheter placed into the gallbladder[4].

More recently laparoscopic cholecystectomy has revolutionized the surgical management of gallstone disease[5] and increased the options available. Indeed, it has been claimed that the wide availability of laparoscopic cholecystectomy has unjustifiably extended the indications for the procedure[6,7]. Reports that laparoscopic cholecystectomy carries a significant complication rate, however, have refocused attention on non-surgical treatments, particularly oral bile acid therapy, which remain important options in the management of selected gallstone patients.

RATIONALE OF ORAL BILE ACID THERAPY

The rationale of bile acid therapy of gallstones is to interfere with cholesterol supersaturation of bile, which represents the major mechanism responsible for cholesterol gallstone formation[8]. It is now accepted that only those agents able to decrease cholesterol secretion rate are also able to desaturate bile and to promote eventual gallstone dissolution[9]. To date, only two bile acids, chenodeoxycholic acid (CDCA) and ursodeoxycholic acid (UDCA), have been shown to have these properties[8]. Other bile acids such as ursocholic acid, and other agents such as the HMG CoA reductase inhibitors (statins) have been shown to reduce biliary cholesterol saturation, but there is no convincing evidence that they can promote cholesterol gallstone dissolution[10,11]. Other compounds such as lecithin, dehydrocholic acid and terpenes have proved ineffective in the treatment of cholesterol gallstones.

Pharmacology

Bile acids are considered to form a new class of therapeutic agents and, since their activity is related to their concentration in the enterohepatic rather than the systemic circulation, they have been named the first *enterohepatic* drugs[12]. After oral administration, CDCA and UDCA are rapidly absorbed in the intestine and reach the liver via the portal blood, where they are conjugated with glycine or taurine and secreted into bile[13]. Most of the ingested bile acid is absorbed in the upper intestine by passive diffusion, and absorption is then completed by an active transport mechanism in the terminal ileum. Extraction from the portal blood by the liver is extremely rapid and efficient[14], resulting in very low systemic blood concentrations[15]. The presence of high concentrations in the enterohepatic circulation and low systemic concentrations is the main peculiarity of these enterohepatic drugs: their efficacy is related to biliary and not to systemic concentrations[12].

Effects on biliary lipid secretion

The most important effect of oral CDCA and UDCA is to decrease the secretion of cholesterol into bile. Although both decrease biliary cholesterol saturation by decreasing cholesterol secretion, they achieve this effect in different ways. Studies evaluating biliary lipid secretion after acute replacement of the pre-existing bile acid pool with either one of the two cholelitholytic bile acids have shown that UDCA, but not CDCA, induces a rapid and significant decrease in cholesterol secretion[16].

UDCA is a hydrophilic bile acid with low detergency and low capacity to dissolve cholesterol in mixed micelles; its limited capacity to solubilize cholesterol and transport it through the canalicular mambrane is thought to explain its ability to decrease cholesterol secretion[17]. CDCA, on the other hand, is less hydrophilic, more detergent and very good at forming micelles, but is unable to reduce cholesterol secretion acutely. After chronic feeding, however, CDCA does reduce cholesterol secretion[18], by inhibiting HMG CoA reductase, the rate-limiting enzyme in the synthesis of cholesterol[19].

Both the main cholelitholytic bile acids also affect intestinal cholesterol absorption and hepatic bile acid synthesis. UDCA, but not CDCA, reduces cholesterol absorption in the intestine[20], but how it does this is not clear. Furthermore, CDCA, but not UDCA, inhibits 7α-hydroxylase, the rate-limiting enzyme in the conversion of cholesterol to bile acids[18]. UDCA, by contrast, seems not to affect, or may slightly increase, the synthesis of bile acid[18]. All of these effects – the decreased bile acid synthesis, decreased biliary cholesterol excretion and the lack of reduced cholesterol absorption with CDCA – may explain why total body cholesterol stores increase during therapy with CDCA but not UDCA. In other words, UDCA therapy maintains cholesterol balance by reducing cholesterol absorption and increasing bile acid synthesis, whereas

CDCA may increase body cholesterol stores slightly, as suggested by the increased LDL plasma levels[21].

CDCA and UDCA can both modify cholesterol solubilization in bile: the first by forming micelles[18] and the second by forming a liquid crystalline phase[22].

Other effects

CDCA has largely been superseded by UDCA in therapy because of its unwanted effects. Recent literature has focused on the effects of UDCA on the putative mechanisms of gallstone formation. UDCA reduced the production of nucleating agents, such as mucin[23], by the gallbladder mucosa and consequently increases cholesterol crystal nucleation time. UDCA also seems to restore the delayed intestinal transit time in gallstone patients[24] to normal[25]. It seems to affect gallbladder motility, which is defective in gallstone patients in terms of both a larger fasting gallbladder volume and a lower contractility[26]. It certainly further increases gallbladder volume[26–28], but its effect on gallbladder contractility remains controversial: some studies report no effect on gallbladder contractility[27], but others report further impairment[26,28].

EFFICACY AND SAFETY OF ORAL BILE ACID THERAPY

Comparative studies have demonstrated that UDCA acts more rapidly and achieves a higher total dissolution rate with fewer unwanted effects. Treatment with CDCA can induce diarrhoea, transient elevations of serum transaminases and a slight increase in serum LDL cholesterol[29,30] and is therefore no longer recommended.

Treatment with UDCA is unlikely to be successful unless the following generally agreed[5,31] criteria are met: patency of the cystic duct, documented by opacification of the gallbladder on oral cholecystography, lack of calcification of gallstones on X-ray or computed tomography, stone diameter < 20 mm, and lack of frequent biliary pain and complications of gallstone disease. Overall, 10–30% of patients with symptomatic gallstones fulfil these criteria. The success rate mainly depends on gallstone size, drug dose and treatment period. Complete gallstone dissolution is achieved in up to 90% of patients with pure cholesterol gallstones < 5 mm in diameter; in up to 60% of patients with stones < 10 mm, in up to 40% of patients with stones < 20 mm at a dose of 8–10 mg/kg/day given for an average period of about 12 months. There are few data on the therapeutic effects of longer treatment periods or higher doses. Rim calcification of gallstones may develop during oral bile acid treatment and definitively precludes dissolution. It was initially postulated[32] that calcification was a side effect of ursodeoxycholic acid treatment due to the formation of calcium glyco-ursodeoxycholate. It has been subsequently shown[33], however, that gallstone calcification occurs during chenodeoxycholic, ursodeoxycholic and auro-ursodeoxycholic acid administration and, although no predictive factors could be identified for gallstone calcification, it is more likely with advancing age. This, together with a report of calcification during placebo administration[21], suggests that rim calcification may simply be part of the natural history of gallstone disease rather than an unwanted effect of oral bile acid treatment.

Patients who have successfully undergone oral bile acid therapy have a stone recurrence of up to 60% after 10 years[34]. Cholesterol gallstones recur because the mechanisms which led to their formation are still present: cholesterol supersaturation of bile, cholesterol crystal nucleation and impaired gallbladder motility. A search for factors predictive of gallstone recurrence has identified only multiple gallstones before treatment[34] and > 50% impairment of gallbladder contraction[35]. Several measures have been proposed to prevent gallstone recurrence, but only continuing UDCA therapy in the long term seems to provide an effective prophylaxis.

Recent data[36], however, indicate that most patients with recurrent gallstones do not develop symptoms and therefore, do not need further treatment[31].

CONCLUSIONS

Oral bile acid therapy offers a safe and effective treatment to a selected group of cholesterol gallstone patients. According to the American College of Physicians Guidelines for Gallstone Treatment[37] and to the last Working Team on Gallstone Treatment Report[31], and in the absence of definitive cost-effectiveness studies on gallstone treatment, the medical treatment of gallstones is indicated when the patient fulfils the criteria, is at high surgical risk, and prefers a non-surgical approach.

REFERENCES

1. Danzinger RG, Hofmann AF, Schoenfield LJ, Thistle JL. Dissolution of cholesterol gallstones by chenodeoxycholic acid. N Engl J Med. 1972;286:1–8.
2. Makino I, Shinozaki K, Yoshino K, Nakagawa S. Dissolution of cholesterol gallstones by ursodeoxycholic acid. Jpn J Gastroenterol. 1975;72:690–702.
3. Sachman M, Delius M, Sauerbruch T et al. Shockwave lithotripsy of gallbladder stones: the first 175 patients. N Engl J Med. 1988;318:393–397.
4. Thistle JL, May GR, Bender CE, Williams HJ, LeRoy AJ, Nelson PE. Dissolution of cholesterol gallbladder stones by methyl ter-butyl ether administered by percutaneous transhepatic catheter. N Engl J Med. 1989;320:633–639.
5. Strasberg SM, Clavien PA. Cholecystolithiasis: lithotherapy for the 1990s. Hepatology. 1992;16:820–839.
6. Nenner RP, Imperato PJ, Rosenberg C, Ronberg E. Increased cholecystectomy rates among medicare patients after the introduction of laparoscopic cholecystectomy. J Commun Health. 1994;19:409–415.
7. Orlando R, Russell JC. Managing gallbladder disease in a cost-effective manner. Surg Clin N Am. 1996;76:117–128.
8. Roda E, Aldini R, Bazzoli F, Festi D, Mazzella G, Roda A. Pathophysiology and pharmacotherapy of cholelithiasis. Pharmacol Ther. 1992;S3:167–185.
9. Hoffmann AF. Medical treatment of cholesterol gallstones by bile desaturating agents. Hepatology. 1984;4:199S–208S.
10. Chapman BA, Burt MJ, Chisholm RJ, Allan RB, Yeo KHJ, Ross AG. Dissolution of gallstones with simvastatin, an HMG CoA reductase inhibitor. Dig Dis Sci. 1998;43:349–353.
11. Bazzoli F, Mazzella G, Zagari RM et al. HMG.CoA reductase inhibitors lower biliary cholesterol saturation, but are ineffective cholesterol gallstone dissolving agents. Gastroenterology. 1992;102:A302.
12. Hofmann AF. Pharmacology of ursodeoxycholic acid, an enterohepatic drug. Scand J Gastroenterol. 1994;29(Suppl. 204):1–15.

13. Hofmann AF. Enterohepatic circulation of bile acids. In: Schultz SG (ed). Handbook of Physiology. The Gastrointestinal System. Vol. III. Bethesda: American Physiological Society 1989;567–596.
14. Reichen J, Paumgartner G. Uptake of bile acid by perfused rat liver. Am J Physiol. 1976;231:734–742.
15. Barbara L, Roda E, Roda A et al. Diurnal variations of serum bile acids in healthy subjects and hepatobiliary disease patients. Rendic Gastroenterol. 1976;8:194–198.
16. Sama C, La Russo NP, Lopez del Pino V, Thistle JL. Effects of acute bile acids administration on biliary lipid secretion in healthy volunteers. Gastroenterology. 1982;82:51S–525.
17. Carulli N, Loria P, Bertolotti M. Effects of acute changes of bile acid pool composition on biliary lipid secretion. J Clin Invest. 1984;74:614–624.
18. Tint GS, Salen G, Shaffer S. Effect of ursodeoxycholic acid and chenodeoxycholic acid on cholesterol and bile acid metabolism. Gastroenterology. 1986;91:1007–1018.
19. Ahlberg J, Angelin B, Einarsson K. Hepatic 3-hydroxy-3-methylglutaryl coenzyme A reductase activity and biliary lipid composition in man: relation to cholesterol gallstone disease and effects of cholic and chenodeoxycholic acid treatment. J Lipid Res. 1981;22:418–422.
20. Ponz de Leon M, Carulli N, Loria P, Iori R, Zironi F. Cholesterol absorption during bile acid feeding. Effect of ursodeoxycholic acid (UDCA) administration. Gastroenterology. 1980;78:214–219.
21. Schoenfield LJ, Lachin JM. The Steering Committee and the National Cooperative Gallstone Study Group. Chenodiol (chenodeoxycholic acid) for dissolution of gallstones: the National Cooperative Gallstone Study. Ann Intern Med. 1981;95:257–282.
22. Sahlin S, Thyberg P, Ahlberg J, Angelin B, Einarsson K. Distribution of cholesterol between vesicles and micelles in human gallbladder bile: influence of treatment with chenodeoxycholic acid and ursodeoxycholic acid. Hepatology. 1991;13:104–110.
23. Kano M, Shoda J, Irimura T et al. Effect of long term ursodeoxycholate administration on expression levels of secretory low-molecular-weight phospholipase A2 and mucin genes in gallbladder and biliary composition in patients with multiple cholesterol stones. Hepatology. 1998;28:302–313.
24. Azzaroli F, Mazzella G, Montagnani M, Festi D, Colecchia A, Roda E. First evidence that UDCA can hasten small bowel transit in humans with gallbladder cholelithiasis. Hepatology. 1998;28:1839.
25. Azzaroli F, Mazzella G, Mazzeo C et al. Sluggish small bowel motility is involved in determining increased biliary deoxycholic acid in cholesterol gallstone patients. Am J Gastroenterol. 1999 (in press).
26. Festi D, Frabboni R, Bazzoli F et al. Gallbladder motility in cholesterol gallstone disease: Effect of ursodeoxycholic acid administration and gallstone dissolution. Gastroenterology. 1990;99:1779–1785.
27. Van Erpecum KJ, VanBerge-Henegouwen GP, Stolk MFJ, Hopman WPM, Jansen JBMJ, Lamers CBHW. Effects of ursodeoxycholic acid on gallbladder contraction and cholecystokinin release in gallstone patients and normal subjects. Gastroenterology. 1990;99:836–842.
28. Forgacs ICX, Maisey MN, Murphy GM, Dowling RH. Influence of gallstones and ursodeoxycholic acid therapy on gallbladder emptying. Gastroenterology. 1988;95:740–748.
29. Roda E, Bazzoli F, Morselli Labate AM et al. Ursodeoxycholic acid vs. chenodeoxycholic acid as cholesterol gallstone-dissolving agents: a comparative randomized study. Hepatology. 1982;2:804–810.
30. May GR, Sutherland LR, Shaffer EA. Efficacy of bile acid therapy for gallstone dissolution: a meta-analysis of randomized trials. Aliment Pharmacol Ther. 1993;7:139–148.
31. Paumgartner G, Cax-Locke DL, Dubois F, Roda E, Thistle JL. Strategies in the treatment of gallstone disease. Gastroenterol Int. 1993;6:65–75.
32. Bateson MC, Bouchier LAD, Trash DB et al. Calcification of radiolucent gallstones during treatment with ursodeoxycholic acid. Br Med J. 1081;283:645–646.
33. Bazzoli F, Festi D, Mazzella G et al. Acquired gallstone opacification during cholelitholytic treatment with chenodeoxycholic, ursodeoxycholic, and tauroursodeoxcholic acids. Am J Gastroenterol. 1995;90:978–981.
34. Villanova N, Bazzoli F, Taroni et al. Gallstone recurrence after successful oral bile acid treatment. A 12-year follow-up and evaluation of long term post dissolution treatment. Gastroenterology. 1989;97:726–731.

35. Berr F, Mayer M, Sackman M, Paumgartner G. Pathogenetic factors in early recurrence of cholesterol gallstones. Gastroenterology. 1994;106:215–224.
36. Bazzoli F, Festi D, Zagari RM et al. Gallstone recurrence and history of specific symptoms during a long-term postdissolution followup. Gastroenterology. 1992;102:A302.
37. American College of Physicians. Guidelines for the treatment of gallstones. Ann Intern Med. 1993;119:620–622.

25
Cholesterol solvents for topical gallstone dissolution

U. LEUSCHNER

The history of contact dissolution of cholesterol gallstones started in 1891 when Walker introduced diethyl ether for cholesterol stone dissolution. Trials since 1938 used chloroform, and later ether/alcohol mixtures to dissolve gallstones, or nitroglycerin, atropine, magnesium sulphate and olive oil to allow dissolution or expulsion from the biliary tree[1,2]. In 1975 a heparin containing solvent was developed and in 1976 Way introduced a solvent containing 0.34% chenodeoxycholic acid, and a 0.4% cholic acid solution.

Modern contact dissolution of gallstones started in 1980 when Thistle introduced monooctanoin therapy[3]. In 1982 our group combined monooctanoin with EDTA in order to enhance cholesterol stone dissolution[4,5]. In 1989 Swobodnik combined EDTA with urea and in 1985 Thistle's group published clinical results with methyl tert-butyl ether (MTBE)[6]. Finally, in 1997 Zakko introduced ethyl propionate[7].

MONOOCTANOIN (CAPMUL 8210)

Glyceryl-1-monooctanoate is a C_1 glycerol ester of octanoic acid. Monooctanoin consists of 70–85% glycerol-1-monooctanoin, 15–30% glycerol-1-2-dioctanoate and < 2.5% free glycerol. It is a viscous substance which can dissolve 11.7 g cholesterol per 100 ml. Capmul 8210 is instilled into the bile ducts via a nasobiliary tube at a rate of 5 ml/h. The common bile duct has to be patent, and the infusion pressure should not exceed the pressure of bile secretion (25 cm H_2O). A study by Palmer[8] and co-workers in 343 patients reported complete stone dissolution in about 25% of patients, and size reduction making endoscopic stone extraction possible in about 9%. This means that stones could be removed from the biliary tree in about 35%, over a mean treatment time of 10 days.

Robinson[9] reported unwanted effects in 77% of 326 patients, with multiple unwanted effects in 41%. Palmer[8] reported life threatening complications: severe haemorrhage from a duodenal ulcer in one patient, acute pancreatitis in two patients, obstructive jaundice in three patients, and pulmonary oedema and systemic acidosis in one patient each. Monooctanoin is not in use any longer.

MONOOCTANOIN/EDTA SOLVENT

Since most cholesterol stones contain a pigmented nucleus or one or more slightly pigmented or even calcified shells, we developed an EDTA-containing solvent[5,10]. The solvent was buffered with NaOH to pH 9.5, and contained the amino acids arginine and carnosine to increase the buffering capacity, and taurocholic acid and taurochenodeoxycholic acid as detergents to augment the wetting of the stone surface. The EDTA solvent was infused at a rate of 10–15 ml/h and alternated with monooctanoin infused at 5 ml/h. EDTA chelates calcium from calcium bilirubinate, and the bilirubinate then forms sodium bilirubinate with NaOH. Sodium bilirubinate is water soluble. Since calcium-EDTA and sodium bilirubinate decrease pH, and since the calcium chelating capacity of EDTA is highest at pH 9.4, the system had to be buffered and had to have a high buffer capacity. An optimal specific dissolution rate in experiments with pigment stone powder discs and complete pigment stones at pH 9.4 was obtained when EDTA was combined with the detergent sulphabetain 12 (SB 12) and urea. This solvent enabled us to enhance cholesterol gallstone dissolution significantly and even to dissolve complete calcium bilirubinate concretions in the common bile duct.

METHY TERT-BUTYL ETHER (MTBE)

MTBE is a C_5-aliphatic ether. Its boiling point is 55.2°C, and its solubilizing capacity for cholesterol is 14–18 g/100 ml. Because of its low viscosity it dissolves stones 50 times faster than monooctanoin. The vapour pressure of MTBE is 245 mmHg at 25°C. MTBE is metabolized to tert-butanol, with only very small quantities of potentially toxic methanol, formaldehyde and the non-toxic formic acid (Figure 1). In contrast to solvents containing bile acids, monooctanoin or EDTA, MTBE is instilled into the gallbladder after percutaneous transhepatic gallbladder puncture. Like the other solvents (except EDTA solution) it dissolves cholesterol from gallbladder and common bile duct stones. After a treatment time of 6 h with MTBE the ether and tert-butanol had completely disappeared from the blood, and from the urine 12–18 h later. MTBE and tert-butanol are completely eliminated from breast milk within 52 h[11]. There are no data available on MTBE concentrations in the fatty tissue.

The clinical efficacy of MTBE therapy in patients with cholesterol gallbladder stones is extremely good, unwanted effects are rare, and the costs are very low. In a European survey of 803 patients with cholesterol gallbladder stones, percutaneous transhepatic gallbladder puncture under local anaesthesia was successful in 93–98% (Table 1). Stone dissolution was achieved in 93.4–96.2% in patients with a mean of seven stones and a mean stone size of 1.6 cm. Some sludge was left in 42–44% of the patients. The mean treatment time was 9 h: 5.2 h in patients with solitary gallbladder stones, and 11.2 h in those with multiple concretions[12]. The mean duration of hospitalization was 3 days.

Minor complications, including haemolysis, nausea, somnolence, hypertension and gallbladder inflammation, occurred in 16% of patients treated with MTBE, and a bile leak after catheter removal in 5%. Elective cholecystectomy

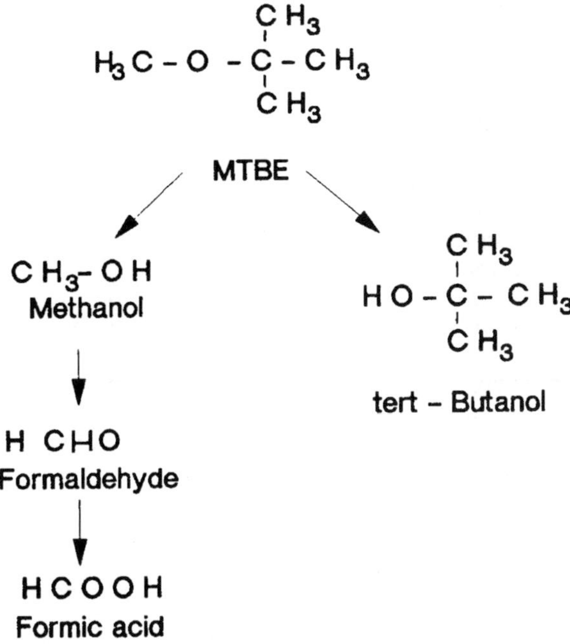

Figure 1. Metabolism of methyl tert-butyl ether.

Table 1. Results of gallstone dissolution (gallbladder stones) with methyl tert-butyl ether in 803 patients[12]

Number of patients	803
Placement of catheter successful	95%
Mean stone number per patient	7
Mean stone size	1.6 cm
Patients with solitary stones	26%
Patients with multiple stones	74%
Stone dissolution (> 90% of stone burden)	95%
Residual sludge in the gallbladder	43%

was necessary in only 1.6% (Table 2). There was no procedure-related death and the 30-day mortality was 0.4%.

Staffing was a major problem: after gallbladder puncture, each patient had to be treated by a nurse who had to instill 3–5 ml MTBE with a syringe and aspirate it immediately. Automatic pumps supplied by Baxter Co., USA, made it possible for one nurse to treat three patients simultaneously (Table 3), but unfortunately these are not available in most hospitals.

The recurrence rate after complete stone dissolution with MTBE was high (Figure 2), as with oral gallstone dissolution and shock wave lithotripsy. The

Table 2. Complications of contact litholysis with methyl tert-butyl ether in 803 patients[12]

Minor complications	16.1%
Leucocytosis	7.8%
Fever	5.6%
Increase in transaminases	8.0%
Haematobilia	0.7%
Bile leak after catheter removal	5.1%
Cholecystectomy due to bile leakage	1.6%
Procedure-related mortality	0.0%
30-day mortality	0.4%

Table 3. Comparison of treatment times of manual and automatic litholysis

	Manual	Automatic	Change (%)
Patients	42	42	
Stone number	11.1	11.4	
Stone size	1.9	1.9	
Treatment time (h)	9.2	12.9	
Time for patient care (h)	2.8	1.4	−50
Nurse's working time (h)	9.2	2.8	−78.3

Times are given as mean values.

recurrence rate after 5 years was 40% in patients with solitary stones, and 70–80% in patients with multiple concrements (Figure 3). There was no statistically significant difference in recurrence rate between patients with residual sludge in the gallbladder after catheter removal and patients without. Northfield's group have recommended that all patients be treated orally with chenodeoxycholic acid and ursodeoxycholic acid immediately after stone recurrence and not, as previously recommended, only after symptoms have recurred. Immediate treatment of patients with recurrent stones should reduce stone recurrence after 5 years to 20–30%[13].

ETHYL PROPIONATE (EP)

Ethyl propionate is a C5-ester. Esters have stronger internal hydrogen bonding and polarity than ethers. The binding of the hydrogen of the C_3-hydroxy-group of cholesterol is stronger to the oxygen of the carbonyl group of EP than to the etheric oxygen of MTBE. Its solubilizing capacity for cholesterol is comparable to that of MTBE. Its boiling point is 99°C, whilst its vapour pressure is 40 mmHg at 27°C – much lower than that of MTBE, and it is therefore less flammable. EP is not detectable in the blood after treatment, and is metabolized

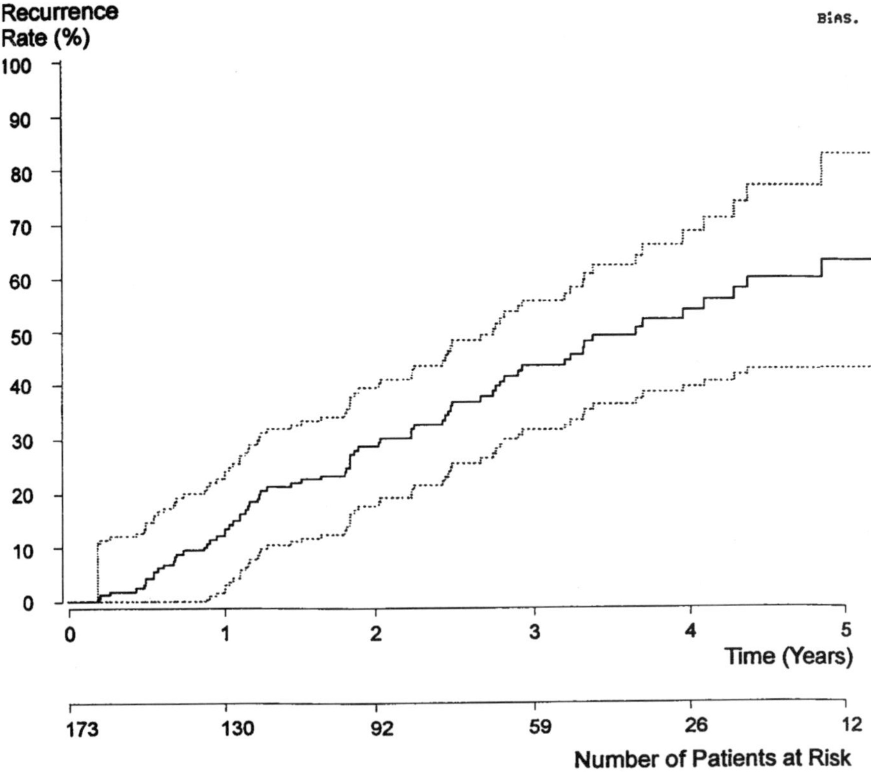

Figure 2. Probability of stone recurrence in patients after stone dissolution (Kaplan-Meier estimator with Hall-Wellner confidence bonds of 95% confidence)[12].

to ethanol and propionic acid, both of which are non-toxic. It is approved as a flavouring agent. Unwanted effects with EP therapy seem to be less frequent and severe than with MTBE[14].

In 1997 Zakko reported dissolution rate, treatment time and costs to be comparable with MTBE[7,14], whilst EP is easier to handle for nurses and more comfortable for patients.

CONCLUSIONS

Contact dissolution of cholesterol gallbladder and bile duct stones has a high success rate, is easy to perform, has a low complication rate and is relatively cheap. Contact dissolution has lost its importance since laparoscopic cholecystectomy and endoscopic extraction of bile duct stones came into fashion. It is indicated only in high risk patients and in patients with multiple intrahepatic stones.

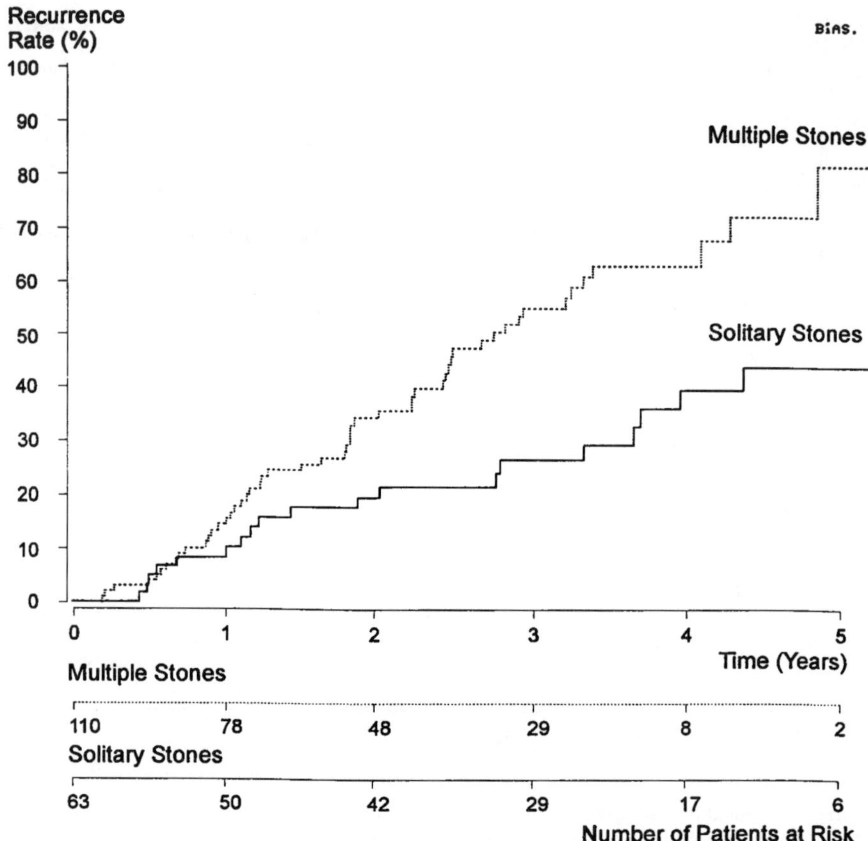

Figure 3. Probability of stone recurrence in patients with stolitary or multiple gallbladder stones $(p < 0.001)$[12].

REFERENCES

1. Pribram BOC. Ether treatment of gallstones impacted in the common duct. Lancet. 1939;1:1311–1313.
2. Torresyap FC. Chloroform instillation of common bile duct. AMA Arch Surg. 1958;77:903–907.
3. Thistle JL, Carlson GL, Hofmann AF et al. Monooctanoin, a dissolution agent for retained cholesterol bile duct stones: Physical properties and clinical application. Gastroenterology. 1980;78:1016–1022.
4. Leuschner U, Baumgärtel H. Gallstone dissolution in the biliary tract: in vitro investigations on inhibiting factors and special dissolution agents. Am J Gastroenterol. 1982;77:222–226.
5. Leuschner U, Baumgärtel H, David R et al. Biochemical and morphological investigations of the toxicity of a Capmul preparation and a bile salt-EDTA solution in patients with bile duct stones. Am J Gastroenterol. 1984;79:291–298.
6. Allen MJ, Borody TJ, Bugliosi TF, May GR, LaRusso NF, Thistle JL. Rapid dissolution of gallstones by methyl tert-butyl ether. Preliminary observations. N Engl J Med. 1985;312:217–220.
7. Zakko SF, Scirica JC, Guttermuth MC, Dodge J, Hajjar J-J. Ethyl propionate is more effective and less toxic than methyl tert-butyl ether for topical gallstone dissolution. Gastroenterology. 1997;113:232–237.

8. Palmer KR, Hofmann AF. Intraductal mono-octanoin for the direct dissolution of bile duct stones: experience in 343 patients. Gut. 1986;27:196–202.
9. Robinson GP. Monooctanoin (Moctanin®) – A new agent for the dissolution of retained cholesterol bile duct stones. Drugs Today. 1986;22:443–447.
10. Wosiewitz U, Sabinski F, Haus C, Güldütuna S, Leuschner U. Experimental dissolution of pigment gallstone material using alkaline EDTA and adjuvant bile salts/non-bile salt detergents, thiols and urea, with respect to local chemolitholysis. J Hepatol. 1992;14:7–15.
11. Leuschner U, Hellstern A, Schmidt K et al. Gallstone dissolution with methyl tert-butyl ether in 120 patients – Efficacy and safety. Dig Dis Sci. 1991;36:193–199.
12. Hellstern A, Leuschner U, Benjaminov A et al. Dissolution of gallbladder stones with methyl tert-butyl ether and stone recurrence. A European survey. Dig Dis Sci. 1998;43:911–920.
13. Petroni M, Jazrawi RP, Lanzini A et al. Repeated bile acid therapy for the long-term management of cholesterol gallstones. J Hepatol. 1996;25:719–724.
14. Hofmann AF, Amelsberg A, Esch O et al. Successful topical dissolution of cholesterol gallbladder stones using ethyl propionate. Dig Dis Sci. 1997;42:1274–1282.

26
Mechanisms of dissolution of cholesterol gallstones

H.A. AHMED, R.P. JAZRAWI, G. LAUFFER and T.C. NORTHFIELD

Cholesterol gallstones tend to dissolve within hours when exposed to a contact solvent like mono-octanoin (MO)[1], methyl tertiary butyl ether (MTBE)[2,3], ethyl propionate (EP)[4] and isopropyl acetate (IA)[5]. Gallstone dissolution takes months or years, in contrast, when bile is rendered unsaturated with cholesterol using oral bile acid therapy with chenodeoxycholic acid (CDCA)[6] or ursodeoxycholic acid (UDCA)[7]. The mechanisms of dissolution in both approaches are different.

CONTACT DISSOLUTION

During dissolution with MTBE, we have noticed that the gallbladder aspirates separate into three layers in storage cylinders[8,9] (Figure 1). MTBE constitutes the top layer and bile forms the bottom layer, with a third intermediate creamy layer in between. This layer is not a mixture of the other two layers for the following reasons. First, its chemical composition (Table 1) is not an average of the two

Table 1. Physical and chemical properties

	MTBE	Intermediate layer	Bile
Colour	colourless	yellow	dark green
Specific gravity	0.80	0.85	0.95
Cholesterol*	5.8 ± 3.3	8.9 ± 2.7	3.7 ± 1.5
Phospholipid*	0	7.1 ± 2.4	13.4 ± 3.0
Bile acids*	0	5.3 ± 2.1	40.6 ± 14.3
Protein*	0	4.1 ± 1.7	7.8 ± 2.3
Bilirubin*	0	2.16 ± 0.53	51.7 ± 24.3
Calcium*	0	0.04 + 0.02	0.09 ± 0.03

*results expressed in g/l, as mean + SD ($n = 6$).

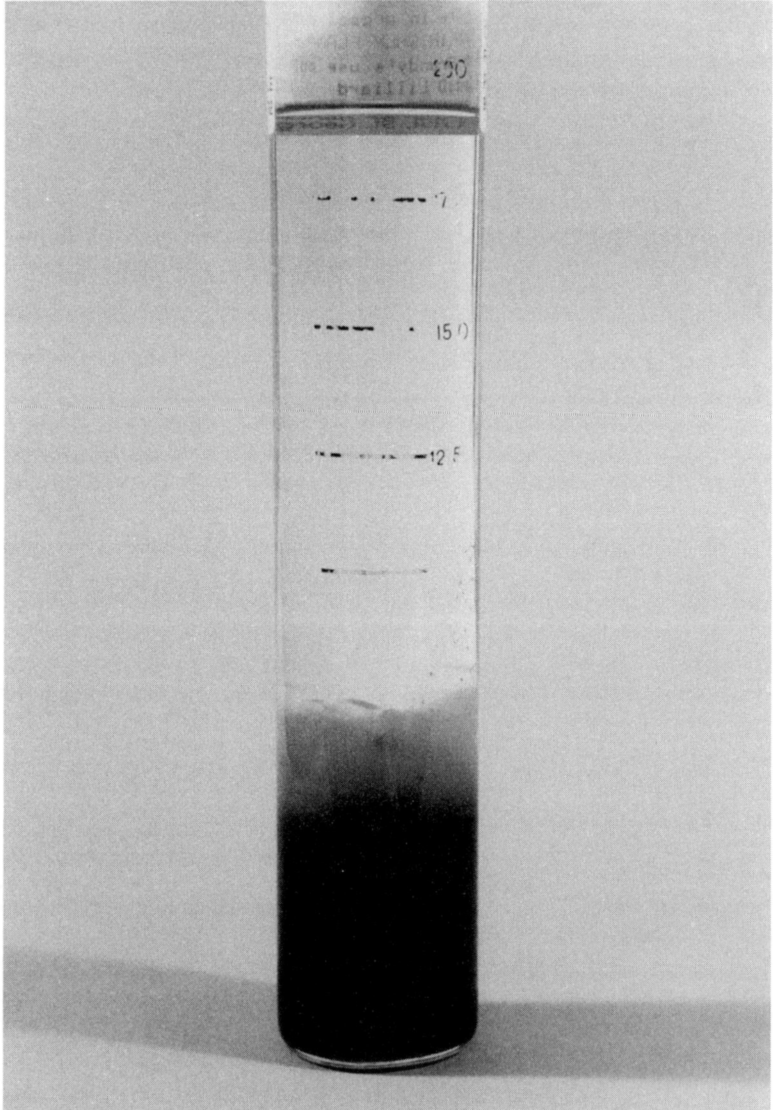

Figure 1. A glass cylinder containing the efflux from a patient's gallbladder during gallstone dissolution with MTBE. The contents separate into a colourless transparent MTBE layer at the top, dark green bile layer at the bottom and a third intermediate yellowish green layer in between.

other layers, since cholesterol concentration was higher in the intermediate layer (8.9 ± 2.7 g/l) than in the bile (3.7 ± 1.5) and MTBE (5.8 ± 3.3) layers. There was a direct correlation (Figure 2, r = 0.81, p = 0.001) between the concentrations of cholesterol in the intermediate layer and in the MTBE layer, but not

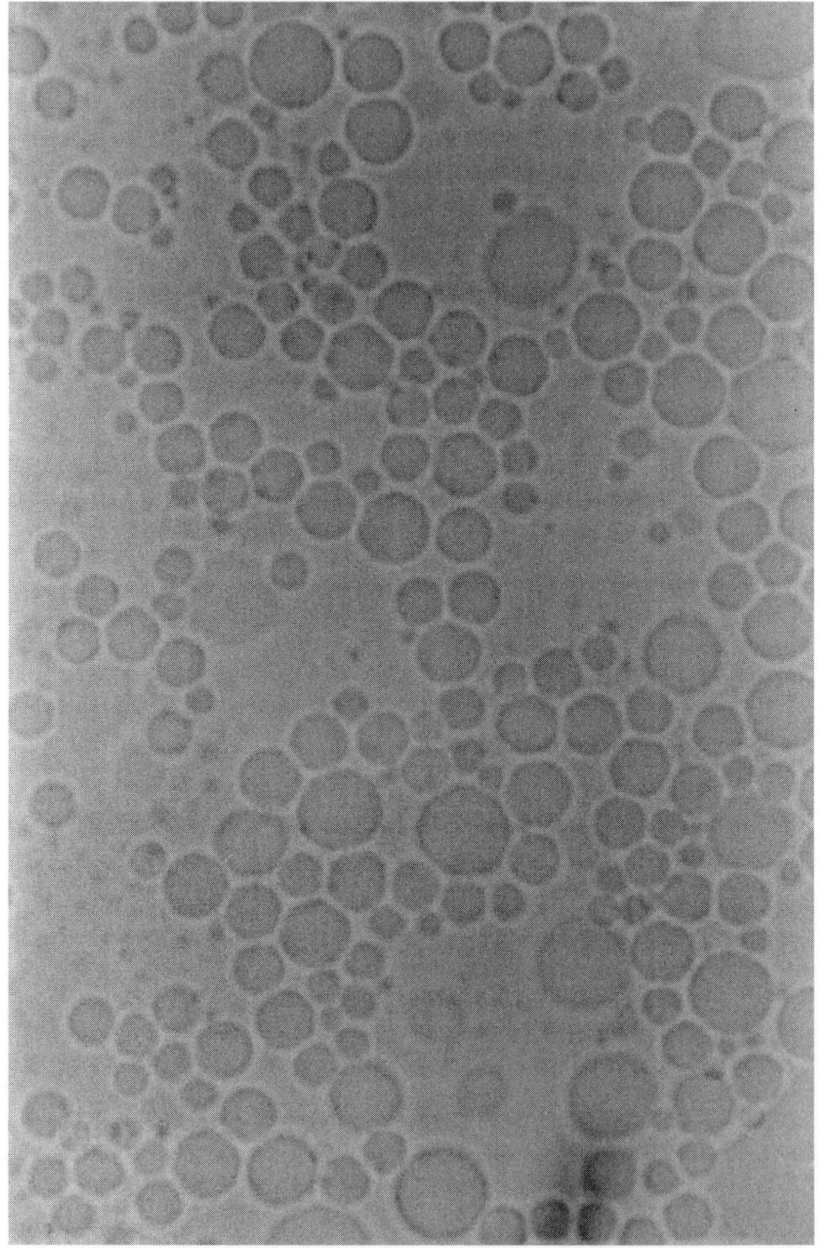

Figure 2. Direct light microscopic examination of a drop of the intermediate layer (× 400) shows globular structures with variable sizes (5–100 μm).

with that in the bile layer. This suggests that the intermediate layer may act as the direct supplier of cholesterol to the MTBE layer, i.e. it is intermediate in the transport of cholesterol from the stone to MTBE. In addition, the bile acid concentration in the intermediate layer (5.3 ± 2.1) was about 1/5th that in bile

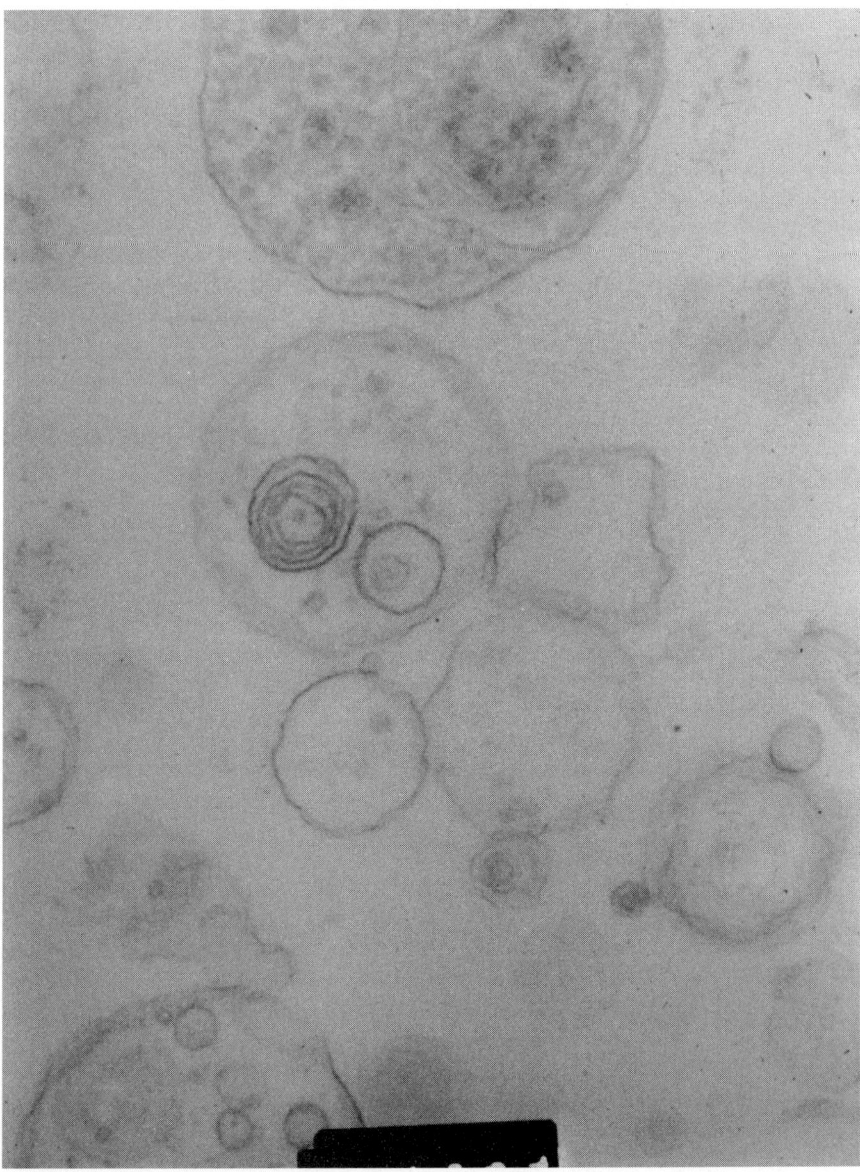

Figure 3. A transmission electron micrograph ($\times$ 20 000) of the intermediate layer showing the globular structures in Figure 2 as multilamellar vesicles.

(40.6 ± 14.3), and the bilirubin concentration (2.16 ± 0.53) was about 1/25th that in bile (51.7 ± 24.3). Second, the intermediate layer was resistant to separation by centrifugation up to 20 000 g even after saturation with solid sodium chloride. Light microscopic examination of this layer (Figure 3) has shown multiple globular bodies, with considerable size variability, while electron microscopy (Figure 4) has shown different sized multilamellar vesicular formations.

We have performed a series of experiments in vitro[10] to compare the dissolution of matched gallstones in an artificially prepared intermediate layer and in MTBE (Figure 5). In both conditions there was a curvilinear relationship between the time to dissolution and the initial stone size. Although there was no statistically significant difference between the two solvents taking into account all the stones studied, the artificial intermediate layer showed a shorter dissolution time for matched stones with an initial weight over 150 mg ($p = 0.005$). For an average stone of 700 mg, dissolution time was about 20% shorter using the intermediate layer. We also found a significantly shorter dissolution time for matched stones when MTBE was prewarmed to 35°C rather than instilled at room temperature of 18°C (Figure 6) ($p = 0.02$). With calcified stones (attenuation values > 50 Hounsfield units) the addition of the calcium chelator EDTA (1%) shortened the dissolution time compared to MTBE alone ($p = 0.05$, Figure 7).

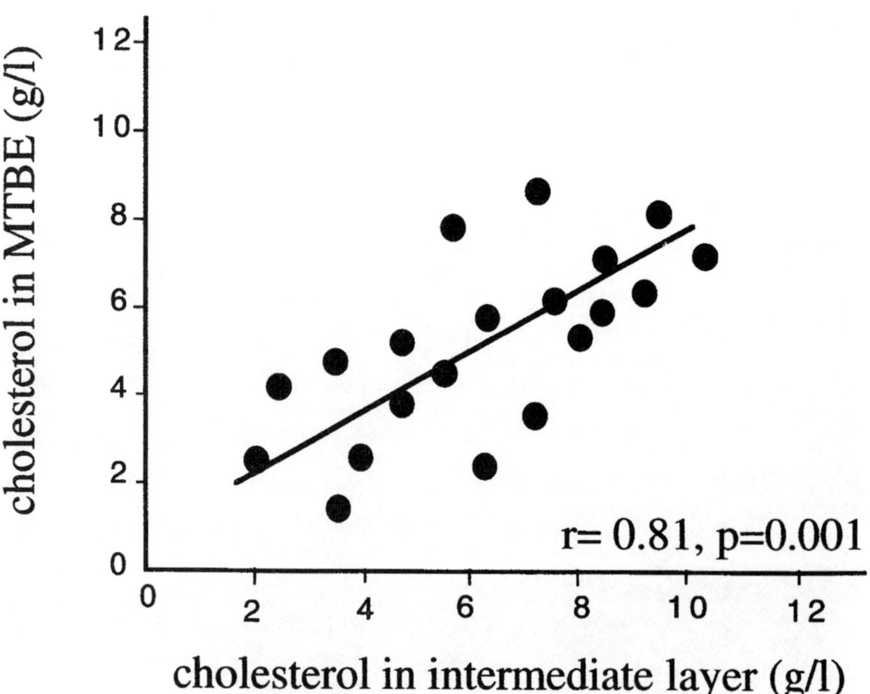

Figure 4. Cholesterol concentration in the intermediate layer is directly correlated to the concentration in the MTBE layer, but not in bile.

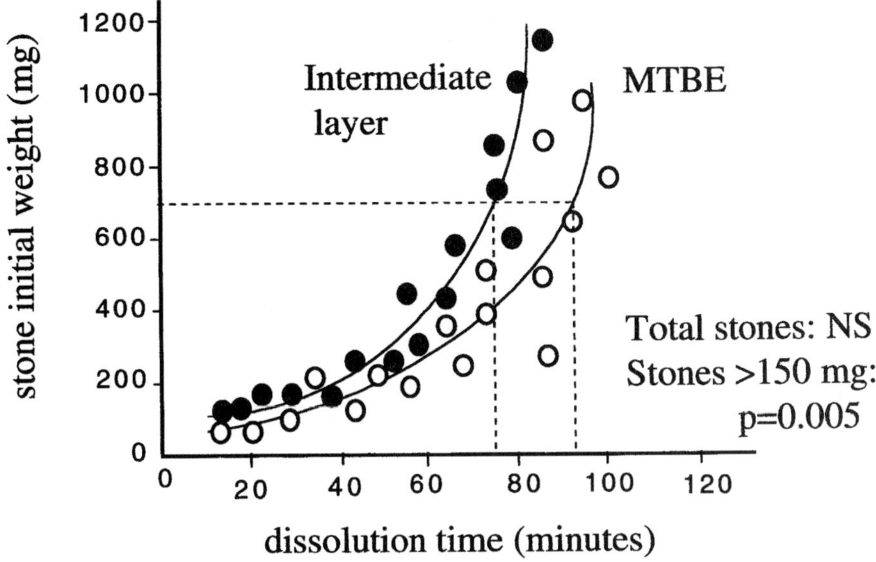

Figure 5. There is a curvilinear relationship between the time to dissolution and the stone initial weight, when using MTBE or artificially prepared intermediate layer. The time to dissolution was significantly shorter for the stones with initial weight of more than 150 mg when dissolved in artificially prepared intermediate layer.

Bergman and colleagues[11] have shown that the addition of the bilirubin solvent dimethylsulphoxide (DMS) to MTBE or ethyl propionate significantly shortens the time to dissolution. The reduction in the dissolution time with MTBE/DMS was about 40% compared to MTBE alone. They have also reported that DMS overcame the inhibitory effect of bile on cholesterol dissolution with MTBE and EP.

Zakko and colleagues[12] have shown that EP tends to dissolve more stones than MTBE (88% vs. 79%, NS), and dissolves matched stones more rapidly than MTBE (38 ± 8 vs. 60 ± 13 min, $p < 0.03$) or isopropyl acetate (55 ± 12 min, $p < 0.001$). These authors also reported that EP and IA were less toxic to the intestinal mucosa than MTBE, which caused more inhibition of active absorption and a greater increase in passive permeation than the other two solvents. Earlier reports from Esch and colleagues[13], studying anaesthetized piglets under conditions simulating contact gallstone dissolution, have shown that the blood levels of MTBE increased steadily to 0.3–0.4 ml/l during infusion of MTBE, and declined to half the peak value within 90 min when MTBE was replaced by saline. By contrast, when EP was infused blood levels remained below the detection limit of gas chromatography, probably because of high first-pass hepatic extraction.

ORAL DISSOLUTION

Ursodeoxycholic (UDCA) and chenodeoxycholic (CDCA) acids act much more slowly by decreasing biliary cholesterol secretion and thus enhancing the secre-

Effect of Temperature

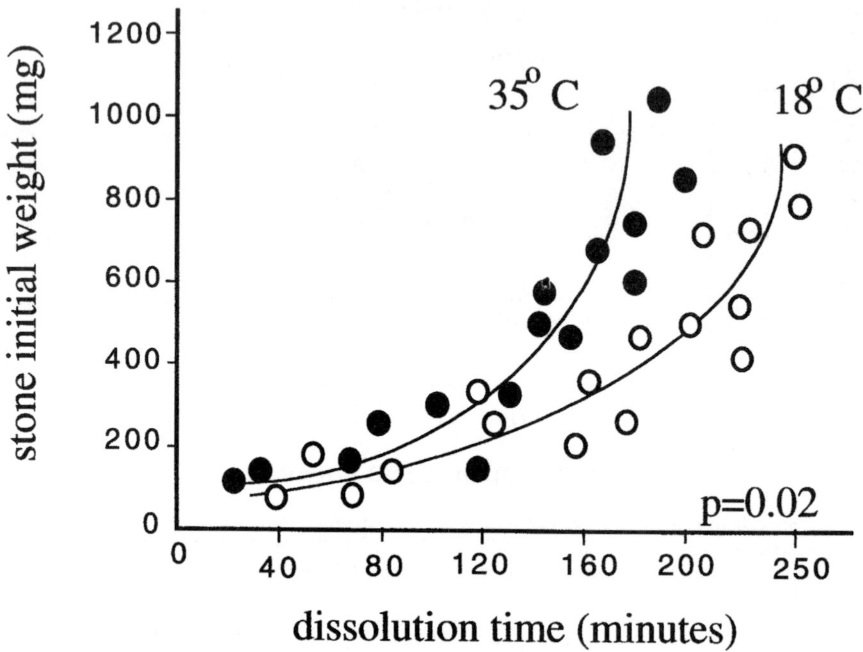

Figure 6. Time to dissolution of stones using MTBE is significantly shorter when the solvent is pre-warmed to 35°C before instillation than when used at room temperature.

tion of unsaturated bile. Northfield and colleagues[14] showed that chenodeoxycholic acid decreases biliary cholesterol secretion, and Ponz De Leon and colleagues[15] have shown that UDCA treatment reduces biliary cholesterol to nearly half the pre-treatment values, both in concentration and as a molar proportion of biliary lipids; although it marginally reduces the absolute bile acid concentration by 8–9%, it increases the molar proportion of bile acids by the same amount and enriches bile with UDCA to about 40% of total bile acids, at the expense of a reduction in cholate, chenodeoxycholate and deoxycholate. These changes all reduce cholesterol saturation in gallbladder bile, and this has also been shown for CDCA therapy in addition to UDCA therapy[16]. UDCA therapy also reduces intestinal cholesterol absorption, another major mechanism by which it reduces biliary cholesterol as shown by Ponz De Leon and colleagues, and later confirmed by many other groups[15]. Both UDCA and CDCA reduce the activity of the cholesterol esterifying enzyme acyl-CoA cholesterol acyltransferase (ACAT) in the microsomes of the gallbladder mucosal cells, by 60–65%[17]. The authors speculate that this might be because they decrease absorption of cholesterol from the bile.

Another effect of both UDCA and CDCA is to prolong the nucleation time in bile from treated gallstone subjects to levels found in gallstone-free subjects[18].

Calcified Stones

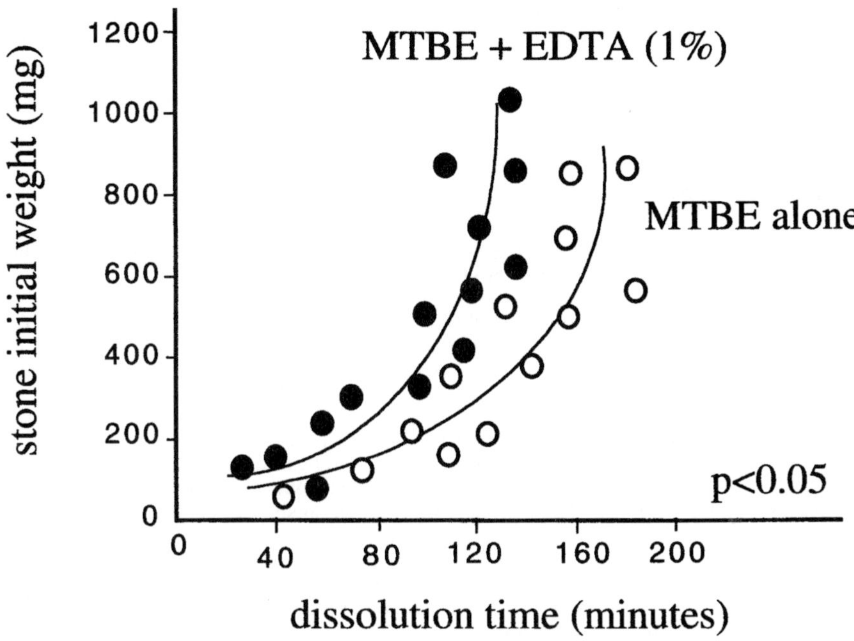

Figure 7. The addition of the calcium chelator EDTA to MTBE significantly shortens the time to dissolution of calcified stones (> 50 HU) compared to MTBE alone.

This may be simply because they reduce biliary cholesterol saturation, but might also reflect changes in gallbladder glycoproteins which are pronucleating proteins. O'Leary and colleagues[19] have shown that for a given bile acid concentration, UDCA and its taurine conjugate t-UDCA are much less effective in stimulating the release of biliary glycoproteins[20,21]. With UDCA therapy, the bile acid mixture in the gallbladder (with about 40% in the form of UDCA) releases less glycoproteins, and this can prolong the nucleation time in vitro. We have demonstrated in model bile[22] that pronucleators tend to be relatively more hydrophilic while antinucleators tend to be more hydrophobic, and that pronucleator proteins enhance the transfer of biliary cholesterol from the micellar to the vesicular phase. Mizuno and colleagues[23] have described discoid phospholipid lamellae separated between the micellar and vesicular phases obtained from bile by gel filtration and visualized by electron microscopy. They have shown that UDCA treatment stabilizes these discoid lamellae and inhibits their transformation into vesicular structures and cholesterol microcrystals, a process which occurs in the bile of untreated gallstone patients as part of the nucleation process.

The effects of bile acid therapy can be enhanced by concomitant administration of an HMG-CoA reductase inhibitor[24]. However, the statins alone have proved disappointing in studies of cholesterol gallstone dissolution[25].

Dissolution rate can also be accelerated by about two-fold by increasing the surface area via lithotriptic stone fragmentation[26].

Ursodeoxycholyl-diethylenetriamine-triacetic acid (UDCA-DTTA) is a synthetic compound that includes both UDCA and calcium chelating domains[27]. It has been shown in vitro to dissolve sliced human gallstones with a composition of more than 50% calcium bilirubinate. Further studies are required to examine the efficacy and safety of this interesting prodrug in vivo.

REFERENCES

1. Thistle JL, Carlson GL, Hofmann AF et al. Monooctanoin a dissolution agent for retained cholesterol bile duct stones: physical properties and clinical application. Gastroenterology. 1980;78:1016–1022.
2. Allen MJ, Borody TJ, Bugliosi TF et al. Rapid dissolution of gallstones by methyl tert-butyl ether. Preliminary observations. N Engl J Med. 1985;312:217–220.
3. Allen MJ, Borody TJ, Bugliosi TF et al. Cholelitholysis using methyl tertiary butyl ether. Gastroenterology. 1985;88:122–125.
4. Hofmann AF, Schteingart CD, van Sonnenberg E et al. Contact dissolution of cholesterol gallstones with organic solvents. Gastroenterol Clin North Am. 1991;20:183–199.
5. Long CA, Teplick SK, Baker MB et al. In vitro cholesterol gallstone dissolution: comparison of methyl tert-butyl ether with three new ester solvents. Radiology. 1991;180:47–49.
6. Danzinger RG, Hofmann AF, Schoenfield LJ et al. Dissolution of cholesterol gallstones by chenodeoxycholic acid. N Engl J Med. 1972;286:1–8.
7. Okumura M, Tanikawa K, Chuman Y. Clinical studies on dissolution of gallstones using ursodeoxycholic acid. Gastroenterol Jpn. 1977;12:469–475.
8. Lauffer GL, Ahmed HA, Jazrawi RP et al. Do biliary lipids and proteins enhance gallstone dissolution with methyl tert-butyl ether (MTBE)? Gut. 1992;33:S26.
9. Lauffer GL, Jazrawi RP, Ahmed HA et al. In vivo comparison for gallstone dissolution (using MTBE) with a computerized pump and hand syringe at two temperatures. Gastroenterology. 1993;104:A368.
10. Lauffer GL, Jazrawi RP, Ahmed HA et al. In vitro gallstone dissolution characteristics with MTBE using a computerized pump: Methods of improving efficacy. Gastroenterology. 1992;102(Suppl):4A.
11. Bergman JJ, Groen AK, Huibregtse K et al. Addition of dimethylsulphoxide to methyl-tert-butyl ether and ethyl propionate increases cholesterol dissolving capacity and cholesterol gallstone dissolution in vitro. Gut. 1994;35(11):1653–1658.
12. Zakko SF, Scirica JC, Guttermuth MC et al. Ethyl propionate is more effective and less cytotoxic than methyl tert-butyl ether for topical gallstone dissolution. Gastroenterology. 1997;113:232–237.
13. Esch O, Schteingart CD, Pappert D et al. Increased blood levels of methyl tert-butyl ether but not of ethyl propionate during instillation with contact gallstone dissolution agents in the pig. Hepatology. 1993;18:373–379.
14. Northfield TC, LaRusso NF, Hofmann AF, Thistle JL. Biliary lipid output during three meals and an overnight fast. II. Effect of chenodeoxycholic acid treatment in gallstone subjects. Gut. 1975;16:1–11.
15. Ponz De Leon M, Carulli N, Loria P et al. Cholesterol absorption during bile acid feeding. Effect of ursodeoxycholic acid (UDCA) administration. Gastroenterology. 1980;78:214–219.
16. Sahlin S, Ahlberg J, Reihner E et al. Nucleation time of gallbladder bile in gallstone patients: influence of bile acid treatment. Gut. 1991;32:1554–1557.
17. Sahlin S, Ahlberg J, Reihner E et al. Cholesterol metabolism in human gallbladder mucosa: relationship to cholesterol gallstone disease and effects of chenodeoxycholic acid and ursodeoxycholic acid treatment. Hepatology. 1992;16:320–326.
18. Miettinen TE, Kiviluoto T, Taavitsainen M et al. Cholesterol metabolism and serum and biliary noncholesterol sterols in gallstone patients during simvastatin and ursodeoxycholic acid treatments. Hepatology. 1998;27:649–655.

19. O'Leary DP. Artificial bile inhibits bile salt-induced gallbladder glycoprotein release in vitro. Hepatology. 1994;19:771–774.
20. Smith BF. Human gallbladder mucin binds biliary lipids and promotes cholesterol nucleation in model bile. J Lipid Res. 1987;28:1088–1097.
21. Groen AK, Noordam CN, Drapers JAG et al. Isolation of a potent cholesterol nucleation-promoting activity from human gallbladder bile: role in the pathogenesis of gallstone disease. Hepatology. 1990;11:525–533.
22. Ahmed HA, Petroni ML, Abu-Hamdiyyah M et al. Hydrophobic/hydrophilic balance of proteins: a major determinant of cholesterol crystal formation in model bile. J Lipid Res. 1994;35:211–219.
23. Mizuno S, Tazuma S, Kajiyama G. Stabilization of biliary lipid particles by ursodeoxycholic acid. Prolonged nucleation time in human gallbladder bile. Dig Dis Sci. 1993;38:684–693.
24. Hanson DS, Duane WC. Effects of lovastatin and chenodiol on bile acid synthesis, bile lipid composition and biliary lipid secretion in healthy human subjects. J Lipid Res. 1994;35:1462–1468.
25. Chapman BA, Burt MJ, Chisholm RJ et al. Dissolution of gallstones with simvastatin, an HMG CoA reductase inhibitor. Dig Dis Sci. 1998;43:349–353.
26. Tint GS, Dyrska H, Sanghavi B et al. Lithotripsy plus ursodiol is superior to ursodiol alone for cholesterol gallstones. Gastroenterology. 1992;102:2042–2049.
27. Takahashi M, Konishi T, Maeda Y et al. Basic studies on N″-ursodeoxycholyldiethylene-triamine-N,N,N′-triacetic acid for the dissolution of calcified gallstones. Biol Pharm Bull. 1998;21:551–557.

27
Extracorporeal shock-wave lithotripsy of gallstones

G.H. SAUTER, M. SACKMANN and G. PAUMGARTNER

INTRODUCTION

There is general agreement that laparoscopic cholecystectomy is the standard treatment for symptomatic gallstone disease[1]. Many patients however, and especially those at increased operative risk, are reluctant to undergo surgery or general anaesthesia and ask for non-invasive treatment. Oral bile acid dissolution is non-invasive, but sufficiently effective only in patients with very small radiolucent stones[2]. To overcome this limitation, we have combined bile acid dissolution with fragmentation therapy.

In 1985, our group in Munich was the first to use shock-waves, generated by an electrohydraulic lithotripter, to fragment gallstones[3,4]. The fragments that remained were dissolved by combination therapy with ursodeoxycholic acid plus chenodeoxycholic acid. Today, we prefer adjuvant dissolution therapy with ursodeoxycholic acid alone, which has been shown to be as effective as combination therapy but with fewer unwanted effects[5]. We summarize here our 15 years experience with this non-invasive therapy for gallstones.

CLINICAL TRIALS OF EFFICACY

Our first study examined the influence of stone characteristics on the efficacy of ESWL in more than 900 patients[6]. Patients with single stones $\leq$ 20 mm in diameter, single stones 21–30 mm in diameter, 2–3 stones with a cumulative diameter $\leq$ 30 mm, and patients with single stones exhibiting a thin calcified rim were included. In the subgroup of patients with single radiolucent stones $\leq$ 20 mm in diameter, the percentage of stone-free patients at 6, 12, and 18 months was 69%, 81%, and 90%, respectively. The stone-free rate decreased with the number, the size, and calcification of the stones. In addition, when patients were grouped according to the size of the largest fragment observed 24 h after lithotripsy, stone clearance occurred at a higher rate in patients with fragments < 3 mm than in those with fragments 4–5 mm or > 5 mm. The degree of fragmentation therefore seems to be another important determinant for stone clearance after ESWL.

Our second study investigated the influence of gallbladder emptying on gallstone clearance after ESWL in patients with a single radiolucent gallbladder stone $\leq$ 20 mm in diameter[7]. Three months after lithotripsy, patients with an ejection fraction > 60% after a test meal achieved complete gallstone clearance at significantly higher rates than patients with an ejection fraction < 60% (66% vs. 29%, $p = 0.005$).

Our third study examined whether repeated treatment would allow ESWL to be used without subsequent oral bile acid dissolution therapy, and would extend the spectrum of gallbladder stones that could successfully be treated by ESWL[8]. We found that complete stone clearance rates at 6 months after lithotripsy were higher in patients with single stones < 20 mm in diameter than in patients with larger single stones or multiple stones (77% vs. 60%, $p < 0.05$, and 41%, $p < 0.0001$ respectively). Thus, in our hands, repeated ESWL improved gallstone fragmentation, but did not overcome the limitations imposed by the initial adverse characteristics of the stones. Other groups have reported similar findings[9]. In our group of patients oral bile acid dissolution therapy did not further improve clearance of fragments after repeated ESWL.

UNWANTED EFFECTS

Unwanted effects and complication directly related to ESWL have been minimal in nearly 1000 patients treated for gallstones over the last 15 years. Biliary colic was most common (32%), while complications such as mild pancreatitis (2%), cholestasis (2%), and liver haematoma (0.2%) were rare. Endoscopic sphincterotomy had to be performed in 1.1% of our patients and 0.2% underwent cholecystectomy because of acute cholecystitis.

GALLSTONE RECURRENCE

Patients who have cleared their stones are at risk of stone recurrence. The cumulative stone recurrence rates 4 years after successful bile acid dissolution therapy have been reported to be significantly lower in patients who initially had a single stone than in patients who had multiple stones (12% and 45%, respectively)[10]. In our patients with single stones, recurrence rates at 1 year and 4 years after successful treatment with ESWL combined with oral bile acid dissolution therapy were 7% and 19%, respectively[11]. In certain subgroups of patients, however, recurrence rates may differ considerably from these values. In our prospective follow-up study of patients with solitary stones, the recurrence rate in patients with good gallbladder function was significantly lower than in patients with an ejection fraction of < 60% after a test meal (53% vs. 13% respectively; $p = 0.002$)[12]. In another study, we found that patients with increased bacterial conversion of cholic acid to deoxycholic acid in the intestine were at a considerably increased risk of gallstone recurrence after successful ESWL[13].

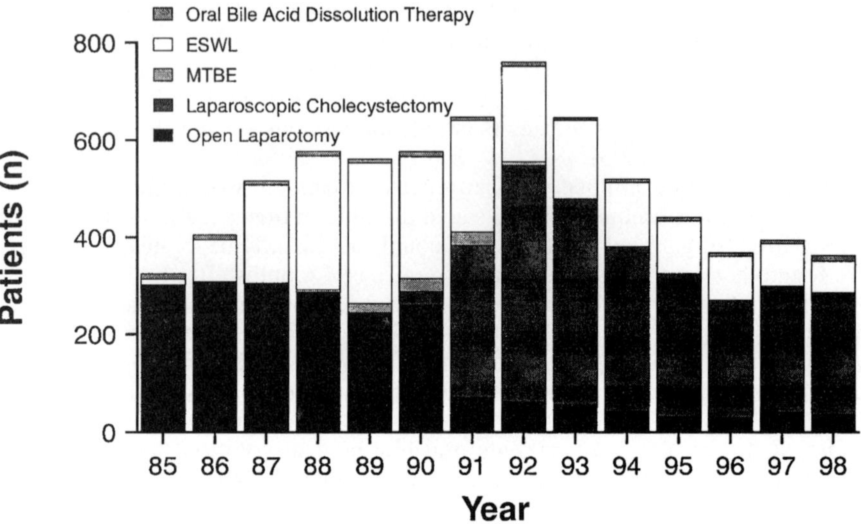

Figure 1. Treatment of gallbladder stones since 1985 in the University Hospital Grosshadern of the Ludwig-Maximilians-University in Munich, Germany.

TRENDS IN CLINICAL PRACTICE

Figure 1 shows the numbers of patients treated by each modality over the last 14 years in our hospital. In 1998, of nearly 400 patients treated for symptomatic gallstone disease, the majority underwent laparoscopic cholecystectomy (69%), and about 18% underwent ESWL.

CONCLUSION

ESWL continues to be a safe and effective non-surgical treatment for selected patients with symptomatic gallstone disease. It should be considered primarily in patients with solitary, radiolucent stones ≤ 20 mm in diameter and good gallbladder emptying, most of whom will become stone-free within 1 year after ESWL and suffer little stone recurrence.

REFERENCES

1. Paumgartner G, Carr-Locke DL, Dubois F, Roda E, Thistle JL. Strategies in the treatment of gallstone disease. Working team report. Gastroenterol Int. 1993;6:65–75.
2. May GR, Sutherland LR, Shaffer EA. Efficacy of bile acid therapy for gallstone dissolution: a meta-analysis of randomized trials. Aliment Pharmacol Ther. 1993;7:139–148.
3. Sauerbruch T, Delius M, Paumgartner G et al. Fragmentation of gallstones by extracorporeal shock waves. N Engl J Med. 1986;314:818–822.
4. Sackmann M, Delius M, Sauerbruch T et al. Shock-wave lithotripsy of gallbladder stones. The first 175 patients. N Engl J Med. 1988;318:393–397.

5. Sackmann M, Pauletzki J, Aydemir U et al. Efficacy and safety of ursodeoxycholic acid for dissolution of gallstone fragments: comparison with the combination of ursodeoxycholic acid and chenodeoxycholic acid. Hepatology. 1991;14:1136–1141.
6. Paumgartner G, Pauletzki J, Sackmann M. Ursodeoxycholic acid treatment of cholesterol gallstone disease. Scand J Gastroenterol. 1994;204(Suppl):27–31.
7. Pauletzki J, Sailer C, Kluppelberg U et al. Gallbladder emptying determines early gallstone clearance after shock-wave lithotripsy. Gastroenterology. 1994;107:1496–1502.
8. Sauter G, Kullak-Ublick G-A, Schumacher R et al. Safety and efficacy of repeated shockwave lithotripsy of gallstones with and without adjuvant bile acid therapy. Gastroenterology. 1997;112:1603–1609.
9. Tsuchiya Y, Ishihara F, Kajiyama G et al. Repeated piezoelectric lithotripsy for gallstones with and without ursodeoxycholic acid dissolution: A multicenter trial. J Gastroenterol. 1995;30:768–774.
10. Villanova N, Bazzoli F, Taroni F et al. Gallstone recurrence after successful oral bile acid treatment. A 12-year follow-up study and evaluation of long-term postdissolution treatment. Gastroenterology. 1989;97:726–731.
11. Sackmann M, Niller H, Kluppelberg U et al. Gallstone recurrence after shock-wave therapy. Gastroenterology. 1994;106:225–230.
12. Pauletzki J, Althaus R, Holl J, Sackmann M, Paumgartner G. Gallbladder emptying and gallstone formation: a prospective study on gallstone recurrence. Gastroenterology. 1996;111:765–771.
13. Berr F, Mayer M, Sackmann M, Sauerbruch T, Holl J, Paumgartner G. Pathogenetic factors in early recurrence of cholesterol gallstones. Gastroenterology. 1994;106:215–224.

28
Management of gallstone recurrence

T.C. NORTHFIELD, M.L. PETRONI and R.P. JAZRAWI

In the context of non-surgical treatment of gallstones, the main problem is that of gallstone recurrence. In discussing this problem, we plan to address the following questions:

(1) How frequent is gallstone recurrence?
(2) Can it be prevented?
(3) Can it be predicted?
(4) Can recurrent gallstones be retreated non-surgically?

FREQUENCY OF GALLSTONE RECURRENCE

The earliest study on this subject[1] used cumulative recurrence rate, and suggested that gallstone recurrence was inevitable in the long term. This was because, in assessing cumulative recurrence, all patients who have a recurrence are counted in the results, whereas patients who have not had a recurrence are not counted unless they have achieved the full period of follow up. A more realistic estimate can be obtained using actuarial methods[2], in accordance with those used for survival rates following surgical treatment for cancer. A prospective comparison by us of the two methods, and also of overall recurrence rate on 42 patients, is shown in Figure 1. Using actuarial analysis, recurrence rate reached a plateau of approximately 50% at 5 years. Actuarial analysis was also employed by the Bristol group[3] for their 40 patients, and in a more recent study[4] by us on 100 patients, giving similar results.

Different results have been obtained by the Bologna group[5], who also used actuarial analysis. Their recurrence rates failed to plateau off at 5 years, so that a higher recurrence rate was eventually obtained. The most recent results were those published by Leuschner and colleagues[6], based on patients from a large number of different centres who had been treated initially with direct installation of methyl-tert-butyl-ether. They found a higher actuarial recurrence rate in 110 patients with multiple gallstones, by comparison with that in 63 patients with solitary stones, a highly significant difference. The follow up period

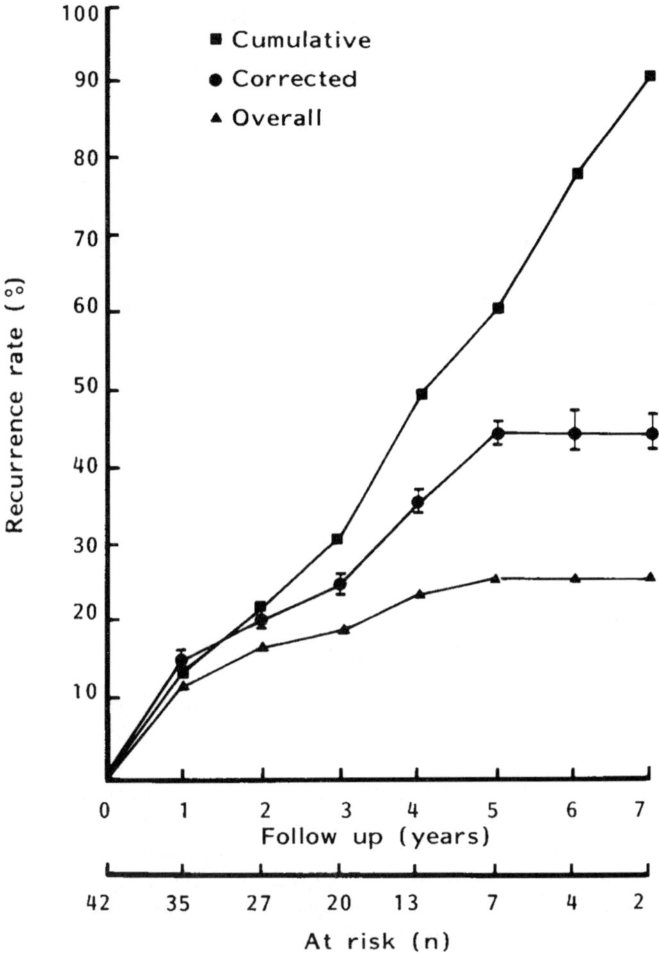

Figure 1. Different methods of expressing gallstone recurrence rate (the 95% confidence limits are shown for corrected or actuarial recurrence rate). (Reproduced by kind permission of the publishers of the Journal of Hepatology).

was only 5 years, so it is not clear whether or not a plateau was reached at this time.

The fact that the majority of studies have shown that only about 50% of the gallstone patients have recurrent stones following non-surgical treatment suggests that there are two gallstone populations. This in turn implies at least two types of defect leading to gallstone formation, one of which is permanent, whereas the other is only transitory, for instance pregnancy, the oral contraceptive pill or a period of rapid weight loss.

PREVENTION OF RECURRENT GALLSTONES

This question has been the subject of controlled trials from two different groups. One of these was the British/Belgian Gallstone Study[7], and the other was from the Bologna group[5]. Both studies compared a low dose of bedtime ursodeoxycholic acid (UCDA) with placebo treatment, and the British/Belgian study also had a group on a diet high in fibre and low in refined carbohydrate. The British/Belgian Gallstone Study showed no significant difference between the three groups at the end of 4 years. On retrospective questioning of the patients[8], it was found that those who were taking non-steroidal anti-inflammatory drugs (NSAIDs) regularly for some other reason had significantly lower recurrence rates than those who were not taking regular NSAIDs (Table 1). This finding has not, however, been subjected to a prospective controlled trial.

The results from the Bologna group were different in several respects[5] (Figure 2). First, there was no tendency for a plateau effect at 50% at 5 years, except in the one group (solitary stones having post-dissolution therapy, PDT). Second, PDT with UCDA did tend to reduce recurrence rate in most of the multiple and solitary stones, compared with no post-dissolution treatment (NPDT). In agreement with other groups, the authors found a higher recurrence rate for multiple stones than for solitary stones.

PREDICTION OF GALLSTONE RECURRENCE

This is important, because if prediction could be achieved reliably it would be possible to concentrate non-surgical treatment on those patients not liable to recurrence.

In the same group of patients, the characteristics of primary and recurrent gallstones[4] were compared. The results were limited to patients with primary radiolucent stones and gallbladder opacification, because it was not thought ethical to treat any other patients non-surgically. Ninety-five per cent of the recurrent gallstones in these patients were also radiolucent and showed gallbladder opacification. A similar figure was obtained for the proportion having multiple as opposed to single stones. On the other hand, the recurrent stones were smaller, 85% of them having a diameter < 6 mm, compared with 50% of the primary stones. This was because, following initial non-surgical treatment, the

Table 1. Effect of NSAIDs on gallstone recurrence rate. (Reproduced by kind permission of the publishers of Lancet)

| | | Recurrence | | |
		+	−	Total
NSAID use	+	0	12	12
	−	20	43	63
	Total	20	55	75

$p < 0.05$

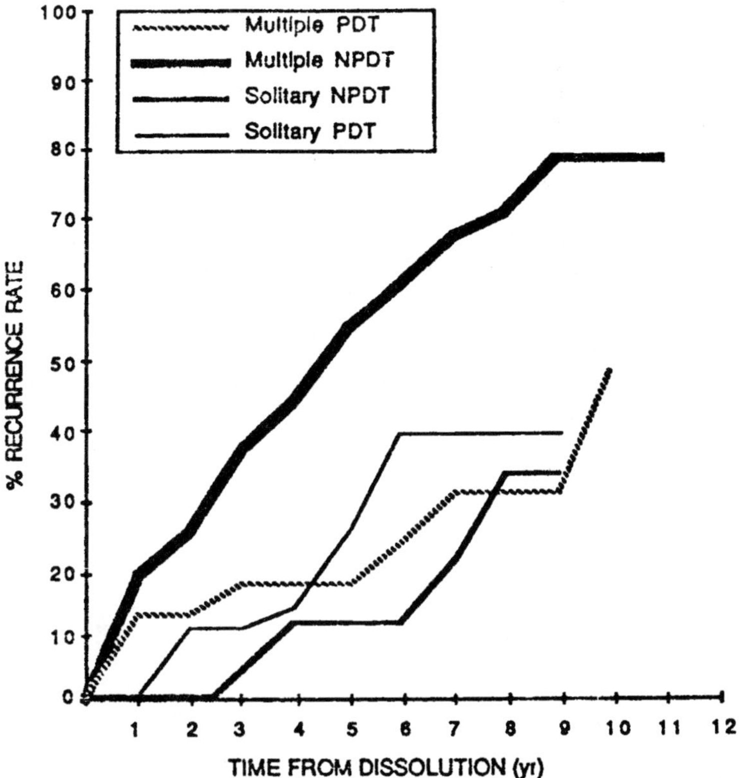

Figure 2. Cumulative recurrence rate for multiple and single gallstones with and without post-dissolution treatment with ursodeoxycholic acid (300 mg daily). (Reproduced by kind permission of the publishers of Gastroenterology).

patients were followed up with regular ultrasound monitoring, so that the stones were detected at an earlier stage. For all characteristics, the proportion in the primary and recurrent stones was higher than that in the general gallstone population. Those patients who had multiple primary stones tended to have multiple recurrent stones, and those who had single primary stones to have single recurrent stones, and this was a significant difference. A large proportion of patients having recurrence experienced biliary symptoms within a short interval after detection of their recurrence, despite the fact that they were retreated with bedtime ursodeoxycholic acid as soon as recurrent gallstones were detected on regular 6-monthly ultrasound monitoring (closed circles in Figure 3). All these patients had had biliary pain at the time when their primary gallstones were treated non-surgically.

Thus, all recurrent stones showed a strong tendency to breed true, with the same characteristics as the primary stones from the same individual. This suggests that the best candidates for non-surgical treatment are those with single stones. Not only are they suitable for extra-corporeal shock-wave lithotripsy

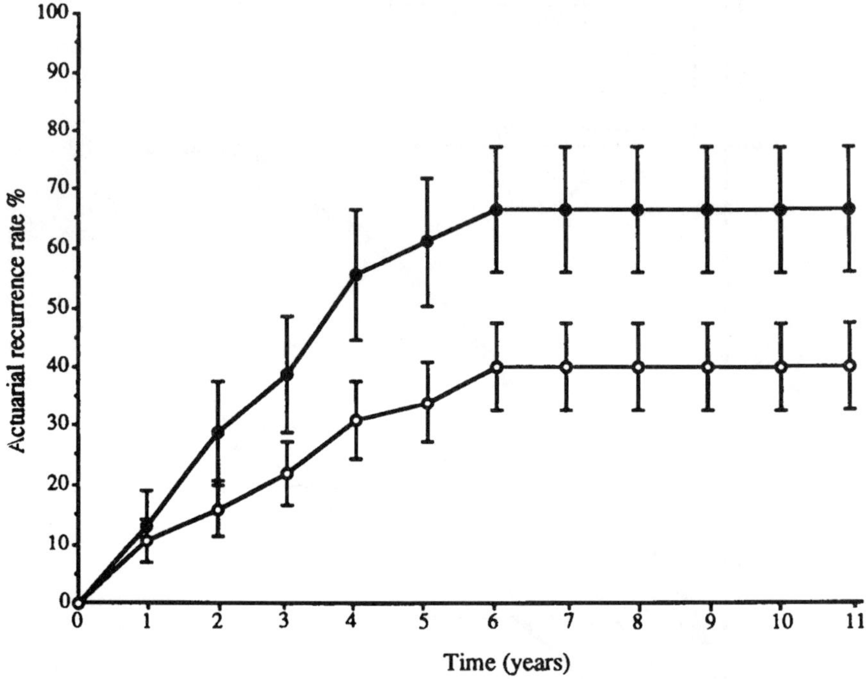

Figure 3. Actuarial recurrence rate in patients with post-dissolution biliary symptoms (upper curve) and in patients who remained asymptomatic during follow-up. Recurrence rate is significantly higher in the symptomatic patients ($p < 0.05$). Diagnosis of recurrence rate was based on regular annual ultrasound monitoring. (Reproduced by kind permission of the publishers of European Journal of Gastroenterology and Hepatology).

(ESWL) in addition to bile acid therapy, but also they are unlikely to have a recurrence.

TREATMENT OF RECURRENT GALLSTONES

The above section suggests that recurrent gallstones should be retreated early, because they develop symptoms early. They are suitable for non-surgical retreatment, because the patients develop radiolucent stones in a functioning gallbladder. They are suitable for bile acid therapy, without the need for ESWL because, with regular ultrasound monitoring, the stones are small as well as multiple at the time of detection.

Figure 4 shows a mathematical model[9] which we used to predict the results of retreatment with bile acid therapy in a cohort of 100 hypothetical gallstone free patients following non-surgical treatment. We assumed a gallstone recurrence rate of 20% and a redissolution rate of 40%. Using this model, a steady state situation was reached in patients remaining gallstone free, with only a small proportion undergoing gallstone recurrence and redissolution.

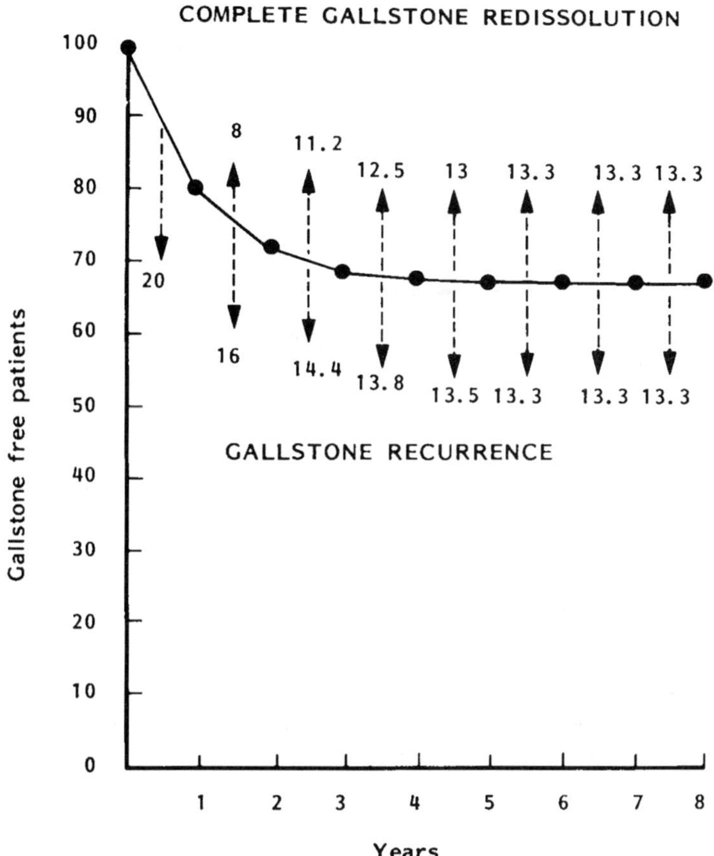

Figure 4. Application of a mathematical model for calculating the number of gallstone free patients, based on initial cohort of 100 patients, assuming a gallstone recurrence rate of 20% annually and a gallstone redissolution rate of 40% annually. (Reproduced by kind permission of Kluwer Academic Publishers Ltd.).

We have subjected this mathematical model to a controlled clinical trial[10] in a total of 172 patients from six centres in England and Italy (the British/Italian Gallstone (BIG) study). The observed gallstone recurrence rate was 12% per annum and the redissolution rate was 41% per annum. Figure 5 shows the predicted recurrence rate according to the mathematical model, using the real-life recurrence and redissolution rates observed in this group of patients. As can be seen, the proportion of gallstone free patients reached a reasonably steady state situation by 3 years, at which stage 61 patients were still being followed up. It can be seen that the observed figure for gallstone free patients in the trial lay reasonably close to the predicted curve, thus confirming the validity of the mathematical model. It was also found that in the long term the proportion of gallstone free patients was considerably higher for single gallstones than for multiple stones, with a plateau proportion of 90%. In accordance with this, there

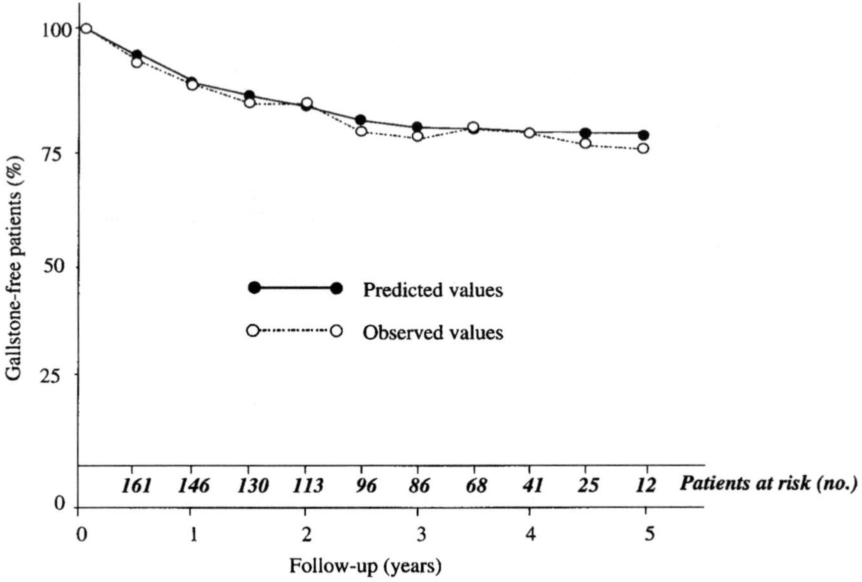

Figure 5. Proportion of gallstone free patients in the British/Italian Gallstone (BIG) study. (Reproduced by kind permission of the publishers of the Journal of Hepatology).

was a trend for a higher proportion of patients to remain gallstone free following ESWL than following bile acid therapy alone.

SUMMARY

In the majority of published trials, the proportion of gallstone patients having recurrence following non-surgical treatment reaches a plateau of 50% at 5 years. This plateau recurrence rate is considerably lower after single primary stones than after multiple primary stones. Gallstone recurrence cannot be prevented by diet or low-dose ursodeoxycholic acid. It may be prevented by NSAIDs, but this has not been the subject of a prospective trial. Small, radiolucent gallstones can be retreated with full-dose ursodeoxycholic acid, and this is a viable long-term strategy for these patients. Those with single stones are unlikely to suffer from gallstone recurrence, and are therefore worth treating non-surgically with lithotripsy and bile acid therapy, if they have biliary symptoms and other indications for non-surgical treatment.

REFERENCES

1. Ruppin DC, Dowling RH. Is recurrence inevitable after gallstone dissolution by bile acid treatment? Lancet. 1982;1:181–185.
2. Lanzini A, Jazrawi RP, Kupfer RM et al. Gallstone recurrence after medical dissolution: an over-estimated threat? J Hepatol. 1986;3:241–246.

3. O'Donnell LDJ, Heaton KW. Recurrence and re-recurrence of gallstones after medical dissolution: A long follow-up. Gut. 1988;29:655–658.
4. Petroni ML, Jazrawi RP, Goggin PM et al. Characteristics of recurrent gallstones following non-surgical treatment: Implications for retreatment. Eur J Gastroenterol Hepatol. 1991;3:473–478.
5. Villanova N, Bazzoli F, Taroni F et al. Gallstone recurrence after successful oral bile acid treatment: A 12-year follow up study and evaluation of long term post-dissolution treatment. Gastroenterology. 1989;97:726–731.
6. Hellstern A, Leuschner U, Benjaminov A et al. Dissolution of gallbladder stones with methyl-tert-butyl-ether and stone recurrence. A European Survey. Dig Dis Sci. 1998;43: 911–920.
7. Hood KA, Gleeson D, Ruppin RH and the British-Belgian Gallstone Study Group. Gallstone recurrence and its prevention: the British-Belgian Gallstone Study Group's post-dissolution trial. Gut. 1993;34:1277–1288.
8. Hood KA, Gleeson D, Ruppin DC and the British/Belgian Gallstone Study Group. Prevention of gallstone recurrence by non-steroidal anti-inflammatory drugs. Lancet. 1988;ii:1223–1225.
9. Northfield TC, Jazrawi RP. Patient selection for bile acid therapy. In: Paumgartner G, Stiehl A, Gerok W, eds. Bile Acid and the Liver. Lancaster: MTP Press Ltd., 1988.
10. Petroni ML, Jazrawi RP, Lanzini A et al. Repeated bile acid therapy for the long-term management of cholesterol gallstones. J Hepatol. 1996;25:719–724.

29
Laparoscopic cholecystectomy

A.G. JOHNSON

INTRODUCTION

Laparoscopic cholecystectomy was introduced at the end of the 1980s, with the hope that it would lead to a shorter hospital stay, quicker return to work, and would also save money. However, it swept the surgical world without any proper evaluation of safety or cost effectiveness and, during this time, hospital stay for all operations was rapidly diminishing and smaller incisions were being used for open surgery. On the one hand, the operation has been called 'the greatest advance in surgery since general anaesthesia' and on the other, 'the socio-economic tyranny of surgical technology'. It is, therefore, important, 10 years after it came into regular use, to evaluate its place in the management of gallstones.

LAPAROSCOPIC TECHNIQUES

The laparoscope is not new, and has been used in gynaecology for decades. In general surgery, it was used diagnostically in the past and for taking liver biopsies when there was not accurate imaging of discrete lesions. The invention of miniature television cameras that could be placed on the end of the laparo-scope widened the surgical possibilities dramatically. However, it is only the access to the abdomen that differs from open surgery, and the procedure of cholecystectomy is exactly the same; therefore, the term 'minimally invasive' was rapidly changed to 'minimal access surgery'. From the first principles, it is obvious that the smaller the incision is the less impact the laparoscopic access will have. Large mid-line paramedian or subcostal incisions had been the norm for cholecystectomy and, surprisingly, the surface marking of the fundus of the gallbladder was often thought to be important, whereas it is the ducts that are the difficult area. Large incisions were justified before the days of good imaging and good muscle relaxation with anaesthesia, but small high transverse or mid-line incisions had been used well before laparoscopic surgery was introduced. The question, therefore, is whether a laparoscopic approach is quicker, safer, leads to more rapid recovery and shorter time off work, is cheaper or more cosmetic, than an accurately placed small incision.

THE EVIDENCE

Unfortunately, of well over 1000 publications, only three have reported prospective randomized trials[1-3] with more than 50 patients in each group, and these three compare 'mini' or small incision with laparoscopic cholecystectomy. One of the trials was blinded so that the carers and patients did not know which operation was to be performed or which had been performed. All three trials showed that the laparoscopic took longer to perform than the small incision operation. In two of the trials, the hospital stay was reduced after laparoscopic surgery, but in the one that was blinded there was no difference in hospital stay, nor in the time back to work or full activity.

METABOLIC RESPONSE TO SURGERY

The hope of minimal access surgery is that the surgical trauma and the metabolic response would be reduced. Pain scores were low in both groups, but less after laparoscopic cholecystectomy, whereas antiemetic requirements were higher[4]. The difference in metabolic response, e.g. cortisol and glucose levels and respiratory function, was minimal[5] (Figure 1). Indeed, the variation within the groups was greater than those between the groups. A detailed metabolic analysis by Ortega and colleagues[6] showed a different pattern between the two groups, but no overall differences. They particularly noted a surge of noradrenaline and antidiuretic hormone at the time that the pneumoperitoneum was being put in (Figure 2).

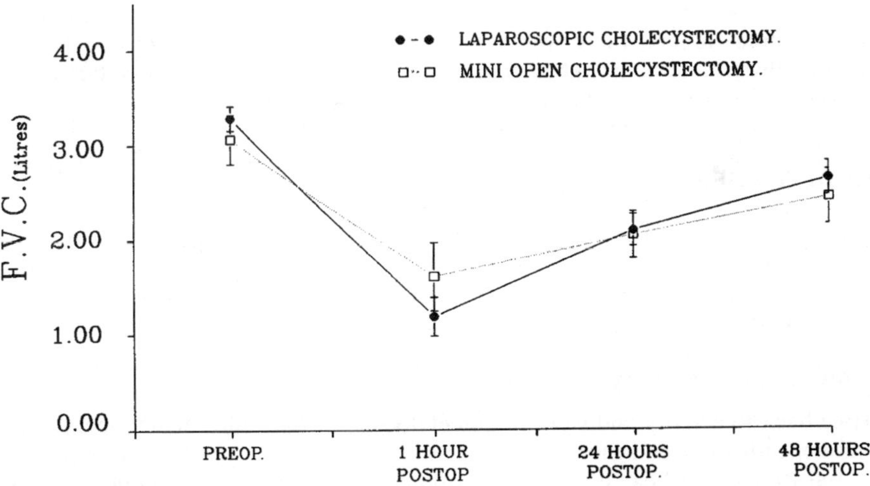

Figure 1. Respiratory changes after laparoscopic and mini cholecystectomy[5]. (Reproduced by permission of Dr DM Squirrell).

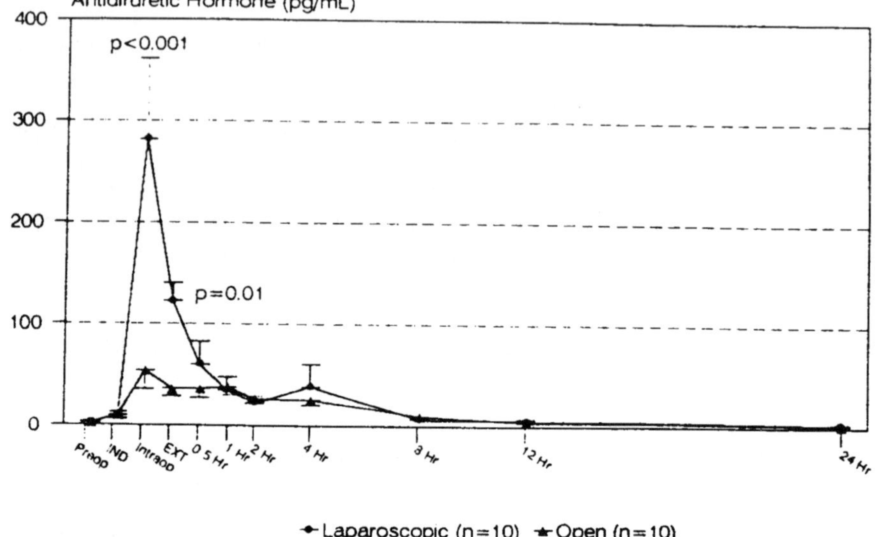

Figure 2. Changes in levels of antidiuretic hormone after laparoscopic and open cholecystectomy. (Reproduced from ref. 6 by permission of the Editor of the Journal of the American College of Surgeons).

COSTS

Two trials have done a cost analysis and both found that laparoscopic cholecystectomy was about £400 more expensive than 'mini' cholecystectomy, and this was largely accounted for by the increased theatre time and the more expensive instruments. If more disposable instruments are used, then the cost goes up considerably more. Even in the Glasgow trial, when the length of stay was less after laparoscopic surgery, there was still a cost difference. Both laparoscopic and mini-cholecystectomy have been performed with stays of 24 h or less, but as the main cost difference is in the operating theatre, this will still be present.

QUALITY OF LIFE

Quality of life analysis shows no overall differences between laparoscopic and mini cholecystectomy pre-operatively, at 3 weeks, or up to 12 weeks post-operatively[1,3] (Table 1). The end result – removing the gallbladder – is exactly the same in each.

Time back to activity and work

Time back to activity and work is tremendously variable after many operations, and depends on social factors, whether a patient is employed or self-employed and attitudes that bear no relation to the actual operative technique used. In Britain, the general practitioner who signs the patient back to work has a major influence on this time. However, in controlled trials there has been no difference

Table 1. Quality of life after cholecystectomy

	Laparoscopic (%)	Mini (%)
Excellent or good		
1 week	86*	86
4 weeks	91	90
12 weeks	92	93

*There was a slightly higher proportion of excellent results after 1 week with laparoscopic cholecystectomy.

in median time back to paid work, being 5–6 weeks after both operations in one study and 5 weeks for laparoscopic and 4 weeks for mini in another. Mean time back to sexual activity was 21 days after both operations.

OTHER EFFECTS OF LAPAROSCOPIC CHOLECYSTECTOMY

Threshold for elective cholecystectomy

Throughout the world there has been an increase in the operation rate, varying from about 20% to as high as 70%[7,8] since the introduction of the laparoscopic operation. This highlights the very soft nature of the indications for elective cholecystectomy and the very variable threshold. Scott and Black in 1992[9] assessed the appropriateness of cholecystectomy by giving the case notes of over 200 patients to a panel of nine doctors of varying specialties and a panel of nine surgeons. There was very poor agreement on whether the operation should have been performed at all (Table 2). This, again, has considerable implications for the overall cost of treating gallstones.

Complications

In no country in the world has there been a detailed prospective record of bile duct damage or other complications before and since the introduction of laparoscopic cholecystectomy. Estimates from various countries, e.g. Holland[10], Canada[7], USA[11], show a range from a 2- to 5-fold increase. Certainly, there has been a considerable increase in litigation for this damage, so much so that it has been estimated that in Britain, £500 should be added to every cholecystectomy

Table 2. Appropriateness of cholecystectomy

	Mixed specialists (%)	Surgeons (%)
Appropriate	41	52
Inappropriate	30	2
Could not agree	29	44
Total	100	98*

*2% were equivocal.

for the cost of litigation and treatment of complications (which, under the National Health system, are borne by the Institution). Whether this increase in litigation would have occurred if laparoscopic surgery had not been introduced is impossible to tell. Surprisingly, one of the other effects of laparoscopic surgery has been that most surgeons who previously performed an intraoperative cholangiogram no longer do so, under the mistaken impression that it is difficult to do laparoscopically. However, it still has a very important role in delineating anatomy, provided there is real time screening, whether or not it is important in detecting stones in the duct. However, this has had the effect of increasing the number of pre-operative and post-operative ERCPs, which has also added to the cost. Fletcher[12] has calculated that, with the additional investigations, the increased operation rates and complications, the introduction of laparoscopic surgery has actually increased, not decreased, the number of bed-days occupied in the treatment of gallstones in Western Australia.

ALTERNATIVES

The three major trials have compared laparoscopic surgery, not with the traditional large incision, but with a small transverse upper-abdominal incision (Figure 3). Many surgeons still make the small incision over the gallbladder fundus, rather than high up over the cystic duct/common duct junction, and therefore find it an unnecessarily difficult procedure. When properly placed, even for a fat patient, the operation is straightforward and the vision is good. We await with eager anticipation the results of the multicentre Swedish trial of

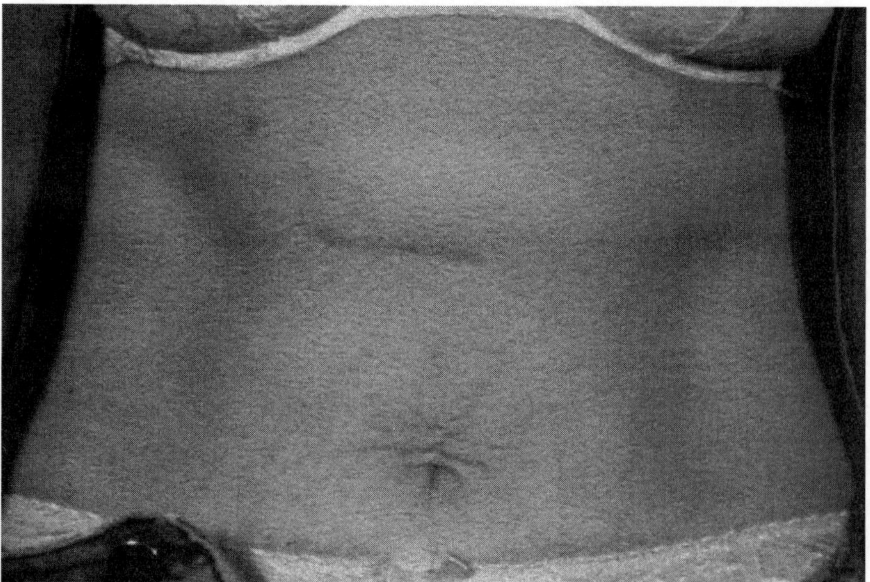

Figure 3.   Recent incision for mini cholecystectomy (Medical Illustration Dept., Royal Hallamshire Hospital).

laparoscopic versus mini cholecystectomy performed by Residents as well as Consultants, which includes many hundreds of patients.

CONCLUSION

The evidence, so far, suggests that laparoscopic cholecystectomy has had little beneficial impact on the management of gallstones. It is not safer or quicker to perform, although there may be a slightly shorter stay in hospital. It is, overall, significantly more expensive, and with the lowering of the threshold, the cost of treating gallstones as a whole has increased considerably. It is slightly more cosmetic, but not very much so, compared with the small high 'mini' incision. The serious complication rate is certainly not less, and all the evidence points to it being greater. The main influence on length of hospital stay and getting back to work is the attitude of doctors, nurses and patients, rather than a slight variation in technique. If even half the operations which are now performed laparoscopically were done by a small incision technique, tens of millions of pounds would be saved each year. The millions of pounds that have been put into designing and making new instruments for what is really just a minor alteration in access for cholecystectomy could have been far better employed researching into the cause and prevention of gallstones, which is a metabolic rather than a structural disease.

REFERENCES

1. McMahon AJ, Russell IT, Baxter JN et al. Laparoscopic vs. mini-laparotomy cholecystectomy: A randomized trial. Lancet. 1994;343:135–138.
2. McGinn FP, Miles AJG, Uglow M et al. Randomized trial of laparoscopic cholecystectomy and mini-cholecystectomy. Br J Surg. 1995;82:1374–1377.
3. Majeed AW, Troy G, Nicholl JP et al. Randomized, prospective, single blind comparison of laparoscopic vs. small-incision cholecystectomy. Lancet. 1996;347:989–994.
4. Squirrell DM, Majeed AW, Troy G et al. A randomized, prospective, blinded comparison of postoperative pain, metabolic response, and perceived health after laparoscopic and small incision cholecystectomy. Surgery. 1998;123:485–495.
5. Squirrell DM. B Med Sci Thesis, University of Sheffield.
6. Ortega AE, Peters JH, Incarborne R et al. A prospective randomized comparison of the metabolic and stress hormone responses of laparoscopic and open cholecystectomy. J Am Coll Surg. 1996;183:249–256.
7. Cohen MM, Young W, Thériault M-E et al. Has laparoscopic cholecystectomy changed patterns of practice and patient outcome in Ontario? Can Med Assoc J. 1996;154:491–500.
8. Lothian Surgical Audit 1995. Department of Surgery, Royal Infirmary, Edinburgh.
9. Scott EA, Black N. Appropriateness of cholecystectomy. Ann R Coll Surg. 1992;74(suppl): 97–101.
10. Gouma DJ, Go PMNYH. Bile duct injury during laparoscopic and conventional cholecystectomy. J Am Coll Surg. 1994;178:229–233.
11. Strasberg SM, Hertl M, Soper NJ. An analysis of the problem of biliary injury during laparoscopic cholecystectomy. J Am Coll Surg. 1995;180:101–125.
12. Fletcher DR. Laparoscopic cholecystectomy: what national benefits have been achieved and at what cost? Med J Austr. 1995;163:535–538.

30
Combination of ursodeoxycholic acid and chenodeoxycholic acid for dissolution of cholesterol gallstones

M.L. PETRONI, R.P. JAZRAWI, A. LANZINI, P. PAZZI,
H.A. AHMED and T.C. NORTHFIELD

INTRODUCTION

Over the past 25 years, bile acids have provided an alternative therapeutic strategy to cholecystectomy for treating cholesterol gallstones. Bile acid therapy can be used as sole treatment for small stones or as adjuvant to extracorporeal shock-wave lithotripsy for large stones[1,2].

Two naturally occurring bile acids, chenodeoxycholic acid (CDCA) and ursodeoxycholic acid (UDCA), have been used for the pharmacological treatment of cholesterol gallstones. Oral administration of these bile acids has been shown to reduce cholesterol secretion and cholesterol saturation of gallbladder bile[3-7]. Clinical trials comparing the two bile acids have shown that, at equimolar doses and similar dose timing, UDCA is superior to CDCA in inducing gallstone dissolution[7,8]. The standard medical treatment for cholesterol gallstones has become UDCA 8–12 mg/kg/day. The combination of UDCA and CDCA was, however, advocated in the early 1980s as a cheaper and more effective alternative to standard treatment[9].

RATIONALE FOR THE COMBINED ADMINISTRATION OF UDCA AND CDCA

UDCA and CDCA have different and, in some respects, complementary metabolic and pharmacological effects. Their combined administration might, therefore, create more favourable conditions for cholesterol gallstones dissolution.

Cholesterol solubilization

The mechanism of cholesterol solubilization in bile is different for the two bile acids. CDCA acts only via micellar dissolution[10], the amount of cholesterol solubilized depending on micellar saturation. In contrast, UDCA, which has a lower micellar cholesterol solubilizing capacity than CDCA, promotes dissolution mainly by liquid crystalline dispersion of cholesterol[10,11]. The consequent development of a two-phase system (micelles and liquid crystals) allows solubilization of cholesterol in amounts exceeding micellar saturation. It is likely that the combined administration of the two bile acids allows both mechanisms to be active at the same time.

Cholesterol secretion

Oral bile acid therapy enriches the bile acid pool with the administered bile acid. The relative biliary enrichment is greater following CDCA than UDCA administration because, unlike UDCA, CDCA inhibits de novo bile acid synthesis by acting on the rate-limiting enzyme, cholesterol 7α-hydroxylase[12]. Furthermore, the two bile acids affect biliary cholesterol secretion by different mechanisms. CDCA reduces hepatic cholesterogenesis by acting on the rate-limiting enzyme, HMG CoA reductase[13]. UDCA does not influence hepatic cholesterogenesis, but nevertheless reduces cholesterol secretion into bile even more than CDCA[3,4] by reducing intestinal cholesterol absorption[14], and by increasing the conversion of hepatic cholesterol to bile acids, so that less cholesterol is available to be secreted in bile[15]. In addition, chronic treatment with UDCA is associated with a significant reduction in both bile acid–cholesterol, and bile acid–phospholipid coupling[14]. This effect on biliary lipids is likely to be due to the lower detergency of the UDCA-enriched bile acid pool.

Side effects of monotherapy

CDCA therapy causes dose-related diarrhoea and hypertransaminasaemia[5,6], due to its secretory effect on the colonic mucosa and its hepatotoxicity respectively. UDCA causes less or no inhibition of colonic absorption of sodium and water[16] and has been shown to have a specific protective effect against CDCA-induced hepatocyte damage[17,18]. Thus, both unwanted effects could theoretically be reduced by using a lower dose of CDCA in combination with UDCA.

Radiolucent gallstones become calcified in up to 10% of patients during therapy with UDCA[19–21], probably because calcium becomes less soluble in an aqueous bile salt–lecithin mixture with increasing concentrations of UDCA[19]. This unwanted effect could also be reduced by using a smaller dose of UDCA in combination therapy.

EFFECT OF COMBINATION THERAPY ON BILIARY LIPID COMPOSITION

The equimolar combination of UDCA plus CDCA at the total dose of 10 mg/kg/day has been shown to be as effective as UDCA monotherapy at the same total dose, and both regimens are more effective than CDCA monotherapy in reducing biliary cholesterol in non-obese subjects[9,22]. Combination therapy reduced cholesterol saturation index significantly more than did monotherapy with either bile acid[9]. Furthermore, 10 mg/kg/day of CDCA plus 5 mg/kg/day

UDCA caused gallstone dissolution even in the presence of bile supersaturated with cholesterol[23]. This finding is in agreement with the suggestion that both micellation and liquid crystal formation contribute to cholesterol solubilization with combination therapy. These favourable changes in biliary lipids were more marked in obese patients at the total dose of 15 mg/kg/day[23], and produced desaturated bile in over 80% of patients on combination therapy, compared with one-third or less of patients on monotherapy with either bile acid. Total bile acid pool size increased in non-obese subjects on combination therapy at standard dose, but not on UDCA monotherapy[9], nor in obese subjects whether on high dose UDCA monotherapy or on combination therapy[24].

CLINICAL EFFICACY OF COMBINATION THERAPY IN GALLSTONE DISSOLUTION

Bile acid therapy alone

The largest published study on the clinical efficacy of combination therapy was that of Podda and colleagues[22]. They compared combination therapy with equimolar UDCA and CDCA (5 mg/kg/day each) at mealtimes with UDCA monotherapy (10 mg/kg/day), in a randomized single-blind study in 120 patients. They used strict admission criteria (non-obese patients, with gallstones < 15 mm in diameter of which most were floating, i.e. cholesterol-rich). A significantly higher proportion of patients with small stone (≤ 5 mm in diameter) achieved complete dissolution at 6 months with combination therapy than with UDCA alone (52% vs 24%); this was also true for larger stones when complete plus partial dissolution results were pooled together. There was no difference in efficacy between the two treatments after 12 months. They concluded that combination therapy caused faster gallstone dissolution than UDCA monotherapy.

The main difficulty in conducting studies of gallstone dissolution is that the use of complete gallstone dissolution as an end-point requires a large number of patients to be enrolled for a long follow-up period in order to detect significant differences between treatment groups. Our group has developed a different approach to compare the efficacy of different bile acid regimens[8]. We have used a standardized oral cholecystographic technique to measure changes in gallstone volume over time, and thus to define gallstone dissolution rate: the percentage reduction in gallstone volume at different time intervals after the start of treatment. We found gallstone dissolution rate to be higher on combination therapy at the dose of 12 mg/kg/day (6 mg/kg/day of each bile acid) than on CDCA alone at the dose of 12 mg/kg/day. However, no difference was found between combination therapy and UDCA monotherapy after 6 and after 12 months of treatment.

Bile acid plus lithotripsy treatment

Combination therapy with CDCA and UDCA has also been evaluated as an adjuvant therapy to extracorporeal shock-wave lithotripsy (ESWL), and compared with either CDCA[25] or UDCA monotherapy[26]. Uribe and colleagues[25] randomized 40 patients with a single cholesterol stone treated by ESWL until stone fragments were 5 mm in diameter to receive either CDCA 750 mg/day (equivalent to 10–14 mg/kg/day) or CDCA 500 mg/day plus UDCA 500 mg/day (equivalent to a total dose of 14–18 mg/kg/day). Combination therapy resulted in significantly faster dissolution than CDCA treatment, with 90% of patients achieving complete stone dissolution by 6 months compared with only 20% in the CDCA group. Both treatments showed a similar overall efficacy at 9 months with 85% of patients achieving complete dissolution.

Sackmann and colleagues[26] compared UDCA monotherapy at a dose of 750 mg/day (9–13 mg/kg/day) with combination therapy using UDCA 500 mg/day plus CDCA 500 mg/day (12–18 mg/kg/day) in 282 post ESWL patients (82% having a single stone). They found UDCA monotherapy to be as effective as combination therapy for complete fragment dissolution at all follow-up intervals: the rate of clearance at 12 months was 46% and 49% respectively.

Safety

Data from earlier small series[23,27,28] suggested that the combination of UDCA plus CDCA is well tolerated. Occasional diarrhoea and a transient rise in amino-transferases have been reported in a small proportion of patients. Podda and colleagues[22] reported that only one patient had to reduce the dose of bile acids because of diarrhoea, and there was no difference in transminase levels between the two treatment groups over the whole study period. In contrast, Sackmann and colleagues[26] reported that combination therapy caused more adverse effects (diarrhoea) and treatment withdrawals than monotherapy with UDCA, possibly because of the higher dosage of CDCA used. No deleterious changes in plasma lipids have been reported in any of the studies. Thus, although the results of Podda and colleagues[22] strongly suggested that combination therapy was more efficacious than UDCA monotherapy in achieving complete gallstone dissolution, this was not confirmed by studies using dissolution rate[8] or studies on post ESWL patients[26].

THE BRITISH–ITALIAN STUDY ON GALLSTONE DISSOLUTION

The British–Italian Gallstone Study Group was established in order to compare, in a randomized double-blind fashion, the efficacy of the equimolar combination of UDCA and CDCA (5 mg/kg/day each) with UDCA monotherapy (10 mg/kg/day) in terms of complete gallstone dissolution and dissolution rate.

One-hundred and fifty-four patients (44 males and 110 females) fulfilling the standard criteria for medical treatment of gallstones (symptomatic gallstones ≤ 15 mm in diameter radiolucent on plain X-ray and functioning gallbladder at oral cholecystography) were enrolled. They were randomized to either of the two treatment regimens mentioned above. The study period was 24 months, with follow-up assessments carried out at 6-monthly intervals.

The two treatment groups were matched for sex, age, body mass index, gall-stone size and number (Table 1). During the study period, 61 patients (39%) dropped out (32 in the UDCA group and 29 in the combination group). Most dropouts occurred because patients decided to switch to surgical treatment, as

Table 1. Demographic and clinical characteristics of the British–Italian trial patients

		UDCA	Combination	Total
gender	male	22	22	44
	female	55	55	110
age (years) median, range		48 (18–89)	48 (21–78)	48 (18–89)
BMI (kg/m^2) median, range		24 (17–34)	25 (18–35)	25 (19–42)
stone no. Single Multiple		20 57	18 59	38 116
stone size (mm) median, range		8 (2–15)	10 (2–15)	9 (2–15)

laparoscopic cholecystectomy became available practice during the trial. Eight patients withdrew due to persistent diarrhoea (two in the UDCA group and six in the combination group). Gallstone calcification on plain abdominal X-ray developed in one patient in the UDCA group and in two patients in the combination group.

The mean gallstone dissolution rate at 6 months was 47% in the UDCA group and 44% in the combination group (NS), and was 60% and 53% (NS) respectively, at 12 months.

Complete gallstone dissolution on an intention-to-treat basis also showed no difference between the two regimens at any time interval. At 24 months, complete gallstone dissolution was 28% in the UDCA group vs 30% in the combination group.

A separate analysis was also carried out in a subgroup of patients with small stones ($\leq$ 5 mm): complete gallstone dissolution at 6 months was reported in 29% of patients on UDCA and 42% on combination therapy, a nonsignificant difference contrasting with the findings of Podda and colleagues[22].

COST-EFFECTIVENESS OF COMBINATION THERAPY

Combination therapy is 15–20% cheaper than the equivalent dose of UDCA alone, a definite advantage in terms of cost-effectiveness for cholesterol gallstone dissolution.

SUMMARY

The different metabolic and pharmacological effects of CDCA and UDCA on biliary lipids and on cholesterol solubilization provide a rationale for their use in combination. Unwanted effects with the combination are mild (mainly diarrhoea) and only slightly more frequent than those observed with UDCA treatment alone. Initial results suggested that combination therapy is more effective in achieving complete dissolution than UDCA alone, but this has not been confirmed by subsequent trials using bile acids as sole therapy or as adjuvant therapy to ESWL. Combination therapy has the advantage that it is cheaper and equally efficacious, and therefore more cost-effective.

REFERENCES

1. Northfield TC, Jazrawi RP. Patients selection for bile acid therapy. In Paumgartner G et al. (eds) Bile Acids and the Liver. Lancaster: MTP Press, 1987;329–342.
2. Petroni ML, Jazrawi RP, Grundy A et al. Prospective, multicenter study on value of computerized tomography (CT) in gallstone disease in predicting response to bile acid therapy. Dig Dis Sci. 1995;40:1956–1962.
3. Nilsell K, Angelin B, Leijd B, Einarsson K. Comparative effect of ursodeoxycholic acid and chenodeoxycholic acid on bile acid kinetics and biliary lipid secretion in man. Evidence for different modes of action on bile acid synthesis. Gastroenterology. 1983;85:1248–1256.
4. Von Bergmann K, Epple-Gutsfeld M, Leiss O. Differences in the effects of chenodcoxycholic and ursodeoxycholic acid in biliary lipid secretion and bile acid synthesis in patients with gallstones. Gastroenterology. 1984;87:136–143.
5. Mok HYI, Bell GD, Dowling RH. Effect of different doses of chenodeoxycholic acid on bile lipid composition and on frequency of side effects of patients with gallstones. Lancet. 1974;2:253–257.
6. Thistle JL, Hofmann AF, Ott BJ, Stephens DH. Chenotherapy for gallstone dissolution: I. Efficacy and safety. JAMA. 1978;239:1041–1046.
7. Bachrach WH, Hofmann AF. Ursodeoxycholic acid in the treatment of cholesterol cholelithiasis. Dig Dis Sci. 1982;27:737–761.
8. Jazrawi RP, Pigozzi MG, Galatola G, Lanzini A, Northfield TC. Optimum bile acid therapy for rapid gallstone dissolution. Gut. 1992;33:381–386.
9. Podda M, Zuin M, Dioguardi ML, Festorazzi S, Dioguardi N. A combination of ursodeoxycholic acid and chenodeoxycholic acid is more effective than either alone in reducing biliary cholesterol saturation. Hepatology. 1982;2:334–339.
10. Park YH, Igimi H, Carey MC. Dissolution of human cholesterol gallstones in stimulated chenodeoxycholate-rich and ursodeoxycholate-rich biles. An in vitro study of dissolution rates and mechanisms. Gastroenterology. 1984;87:150–158.
11. Corrigan OI, Su CC, Higuchi WI, Hofmann AF. Mesophase formation during cholesterol dissolution in ursodeoxycholic-lecithin solutions: new mechanisms for cholesterol dissolution in humans. J Pharmacol Sci. 1980;69:869–870.
12. Reihner E, Bjorkhem I, Angelin B, Ewerth S, Einarsson K. Bile acid synthesis in humans: regulation of hepatic microsomal cholesterol 7-alpha-hydroxylase activity. Gastroenterology. 1989;97:1498–1505.
13. Coyne MJ, Bonorris GG, Goldstein LI, Schoenfield LJ. Effect of chenodeoxycholic acid and phenobarbital on the rate-limiting enzymes of hepatic cholesterol and bile acid synthesis in patients with gallstones. J Lab Clin Med. 1976;87:281–291.
14. Lanzini A, Northfield TC. Effect of ursodeoxycholic acid on biliary lipid coupling and on cholesterol absorption during fasting and eating in subjects with cholesterol gallstones. Gastroenterology. 1988;95:408–416.
15. Angelin B, Ewerth S, Einarsson K. Ursodeoxycholic acid treatment in cholesterol gallstone disease: effects on hepatic 3-hydroxy-3-methylglutaryl coenzyme A reductase activity. biliary lipid composition, and plasma lipid levels. J Lipid Res. 1983;24:461–468.
16. Chadwick VS, Gaginella TS, Carlson GL, Debongnie JC, Phillips SF, Hofmann AF. Effect of molecular structure on bile acid-induced alterations in absorptive function, permeability, and morphology in the perfused rabbit colon. J Lab Clin Med. 1979;94:661–674.
17. Galle PR, Theilmann L, Raedsch R, Otto G, Stiehl A. Ursodeoxycholate reduces hepatotoxicity of bile salts in primary human hepatocytes. Hepatology. 1990;12:486–491.
18. Lim AG, Ahmed HA, Jazrawi RP, Levy JH, Northfield TC. Effects of bile acids on human hepatic mitochondria. Eur J Gastroenterol Hepatol. 1994;6:1157–1163.
19. Raedsch R, Stiehl A, Czygan P. Ursodeoxycholic acid and gallstone calcification. Lancet. 1981;2:1296.

20. Bateson MC. Calcification of radiolucent gallstones during treatment with ursodeoxycholic acid. Br Med J. 1981;283:645–646.
21. Meredith TJ, Williams GV, Murphy GM, Dowling RH. Retrospective comparison of cheno and urso in the medical treatment of gallstones. Gut. 1982;23:382–389.
22. Podda M, Zuin M, Battezzati PM, Ghezzi C, De Fazio C, Dioguardi ML. Efficacy and safety of a combination of chenodeoxycholic and ursodeoxycholic acid for gallstone dissolution: a comparison with ursodeoxycholic acid alone. Gastroenterology. 1989;96:222–229.
23. Thistle JL. Dissolution of gallstones using ursodeoxycholic acid with or without chenodeoxycholic acid or taurine. In Paumgartner G, Stiehl A, Gerok W (eds). Biological Effects of Bile Acids. Lancaster: MTP Press, 1987;353–354.
24. Zuin M, Petroni ML, Granddinetti G et al. Comparison of effects of chenodeoxycholic and ursodeoxycholic acid and their combination on biliary lipids in obese patients with gallstones. Scand J Gastroenterol. 1991;26:257–262.
25. Uribe M, Sanchez JM, Davila B, Mendez N, Merikanski A, Bosquez F. Rapid dissolution of gallstone fragments after high doses of the combination of ursodeoxycholic acid and chenodeoxycholic acid plus early shock-wave retreatment: a comparison with chenodeoxycholic acid. In Paumgartner G et al. (eds) Lithotripsy and Related Techniques for Gallstone Treatment. St. Louis: Mosby Year Book, 1991;119–124.
26. Sackmann M, Pauletzki J, Aydemir U et al. Efficacy and safety of ursodeoxycholic acid for dissolution of gallstone fragments: comparison with the combination of ursodeoxycholic acid and chenodeoxycholic acid. Hepatology. 1991;14:1136–1141.
27. Roehrkasse R, Fromme H, Malavolti M, Tunuguntla AK, Ceriak S. Gallstone dissolution treatment with a combination of chenodeoxycholic and ursodeoxycholic acid. Studies of safety, efficacy and effects on bile lithogenicity, bile acid pool and serum lipids. Dig Dis Sci. 1986;31:1032–1040.
28. Czygan P. Efficacy of combined ursodeoxycholic and chenodeoxycholic acid treatment. In Paumgartner G, Stiehl A, Gerok W. (eds), Biological Effects of Bile Acids. Lancaster: MTP Press, 1987;343–344.

Section IX
Other conditions

31
Role of bile acids in colonic neoplasia: experimental animal studies

C. EINARSSON

BILE ACIDS IN THE INTESTINE

The primary bile acids cholic acid and chenodeoxycholic acid are synthesized in the liver from cholesterol. After conjugation with glycine or taurine they are secreted into bile and thereafter pass into the intestine[1], whence more than 95% are reabsorbed partly by passive absorption throughout the small intestine but mainly by active absorption in the distal ileum. Bile acids which are not reabsorbed enter the colon where bacterial 7α-dehydroxylase metabolizes them, after deconjugation, to the secondary bile acids deoxycholic acid and lithocholic acid respectively[2]. Deoxycholic acid may partly be reabsorbed from the proximal colon, but lithocholic acid is almost entirely insoluble in water: very little is absorbed and is mostly excreted in faeces together with a complex mixture of other bile acid metabolites.

BILE ACID CARCINOGENESIS

Several lines of evidence suggest that bile acids may promote colonic carcinogenesis, and the secondary bile acids much more so than the primary bile acids. It has been suggested that it is the aqueous, rather than the total, concentration of bile acids which determines this effect in the colon. The solubility of a particular bile acid is determined by its pKa and by the luminal pH intestine; the lower the pH the less the solubility.

Most of the evidence comes from animal experiments showing that the secondary bile acids can be co-mutagenic and co-carcinogenic, that they can enhance colonic epithelial proliferation[3-7], and that this increases the risk of cancer development. Mucosal proliferation normally occurs in the lower and middle regions of the colonic crypts, but during enhanced proliferative activity, epithelial cells proliferate and accumulate in the upper parts of the mucosa.

Since spontaneous colorectal cancer is rare in laboratory animals, powerful organic carcinogens such as azoxymethane, 1,2-dimethylhydrazine, N-methyl-N-nitrosurea and N-methyl-N-nitro-N-nitrosoguanidine have been used for initiating neoplasia, mostly in rodent models. Bile acids have been added to the diet or administered to the animals by rectal installation to study their co-carcinogenic effect. Microbial mutagenicity tests such as the Ames test have demonstrated that deoxycholic acid and lithocholic acid (but not the primary bile acids) have a co-mutagenic activity but are not mutagenic themselves.

Animal models have several potential advantages and have expanded our knowledge of the fundamental biology of colonic neoplasia. They provide the opportunity to study the evolution of colon cancer from the initial damage to epithelial cell DNA in the target tissue to the development of an invasive adeno-carcinoma. They also provide an excellent test system in which to manipulate diet and colonic flora in order to study the complex rôles of dietary fat, endogenous steroids, bile acids and gut bacteria in tumour formation. Animal studies in this area should, however, be extrapolated to humans only with great caution.

CHEMOPROPHYLAXIS BY URSODEOXYCHOLIC ACID

To my knowledge, the first report on the effect of ursodeoxycholic acid on chemically induced colon cancer in rats was by Czygan et al.[8], who found that a diet supplemented with 1% chenodeoxycholic acid but not ursodeoxycholic acid enhanced dimethylhydrazine-induced colonic carcinogenesis in the rat.

Ten years later Earnest et al.[9] reported for the first time that dietary ursodeoxycholic acid decreased the incidence of experimental colonic carcinogenesis in rats. The animals were divided into groups and given either 0.2% or 0.4% cholic acid, 0.2% or 0.4% ursodeoxycholic acid, or 0.2% cholic acid plus 0.2% ursodeoxycholic acid in the diet. After 2 weeks half of the rats in each group were given weekly s.c. injections of azoxymethane for 2 weeks, and the others azoxymethane vehicle. The rats were maintained on bile acid treatment for a further 28 weeks and then sacrificed. About 50% of the rats developed tumours. Treatment with cholic acid increased the incidence of tumours, whereas 0.2% ursodeoxycholic acid did not, whilst 0.4% ursodeoxycholic acid decreased tumour development by about 50%. Moreover, the addition of 0.2% ursodeoxycholic acid to 0.2% cholic acid prevented the expected enhancement of tumour formation. In the rats receiving 0.4% cholic acid about 40% of the tumours were malignant whereas in those receiving 0.4% ursodeoxycholic acid no malignant tumour was found. Thus, ursodeoxycholic acid reduces the incidence of induced polyps and especially cancers, and their size.

Faecal bile acid excretion increased about five-fold during treatment with ursodeoxycholic acid[10]: the proportion of deoxycholic acid and hyodeoxycholic acid in faecal solids decreased, whereas those of ursodeoxycholic acid and lithocholic acid increased markedly. It seems strange that ursodeoxycholic acid-treated rats did not develop any malignant tumours, as they had a high level of lithocholic acid in the faeces. However, only a small proportion (2–7%) of the faecal bile acids was in the aqueous phase, even less for lithocholic acid, whilst hydrophilic bile acids including ursodeoxycholic acid and 5β muricholic acids dominated the aqueous phase, particularly on treatment with ursodeoxycholic acid. Treatment with ursodeoxycholic acid increased the ratio of hydrophilic to hydrophobic bile acids from 4 to 27, suggesting that ursodeoxycholic acid may prevent colonic carcinogenesis by diminishing the concentration of deoxycholic acid and enhancing the amounts of hydrophilic bile acids in the faecal aqueous phase.

MECHANISMS OF THE ANTICARCINOGENIC EFFECT OF URSODEOXYCHOLIC ACID

Cytoprotection

Several bile acids are cytotoxic against different cell types such as hepatocytes, erythrocytes and colonocytes. They probably act by disrupting membrane integrity. The degree of cytotoxicity parallels the relative hydrophobicity of each bile acid. Ursodeoxycholic acid, on the other hand, has a direct cytoprotective effect: it has been shown to stabilize the cell membranes of cultured hepatocytes and erythrocytes against other bile acids[11–13]. Tauroursodeoxycholic acid reverses the cytotoxicity of taurodeoxycholic acid and taurochenodeoxycholic acid on colonocytes[14]. The cytoprotective properties of ursodeoxycholic acid may contribute to its anticarcinogenic effect.

Ursodeoxycholic acid also increases the expression of class I and II major histocompatibility (MHC) antigens in premalignant colonocytes of rats treated with azoxymethane[15], suggesting that it may enhance the tumour immune surveillance system.

Protein kinase C constitutes a gene family of isoenzymes that are important in cellular proliferation and differentiation[16]. Azoxymethane changes the subcellular distribution and expression of protein kinase C isoforms[17], but cholic acid does not increase these changes when it enhances azoxymethane-induced colonic carcinogenesis in the rat model. Ursodeoxycholic acid, on the other hand, prevents most of the changes in protein kinase C isoform expression and distribution induced by azoxymethane[18]. This may contribute to its chemoprophylactic effect.

Alkaline sphingomyelinase is found in the intestinal mucosa, where it hydrolyses sphingomyelin to form ceramide, which is believed to inhibit cell proliferation and induce apoptosis. The colonic carcinogen dimethylhydrazine inhibits sphingomyelin hydrolysis in the colonic mucosa[19]. Alkaline sphingomyelinase may therefore be an important inhibitor of tumour genesis in the intestine. Duan et al.[20] have recently reported that some bile acids may dissociate alkaline sphingomyelinase from the intestinal mucosa in rats. Ursodeoxycholic acid, however, prevents the dissociation caused by other detergents and increases the level of mucosal sphingomyelinase in the colon. This may contribute to its inhibitory effect on azoxymethane-induced carcinogenesis.

URSODEOXYCHOLIC ACID AS CHEMOPROPHYLACTIC AGENT IN HUMANS

It is tempting to speculate that ursodeoxycholic acid might be a useful, potential cancer chemoprophylactic agent in patients at increased risk of colon cancer.

Earnest et al.[21] have recently reported that treatment of healthy volunteers with ursodeoxycholic acid 8–10 mg/kg daily reduces faecal aqueous phase deoxycholic acid to a potentially useful extent. Studies are now in progress to evaluate whether ursodeoxycholic acid reduces the incidence of colon cancer in patients with longstanding extensive ulcerative colitis or resected colorectal adenomatous polyps.

REFERENCES

1. Hofmann AF. Bile acids. In: Arias IM, Boyer JL, Fausto N, Jakoby WB, Schachter D, Shafritz D (eds) The Liver: Biology and Pathology. New York: Raven Press, 1994;677–718.
2. Hylemon PB. Metabolism of bile acids in intestinal microflora. In: Danielsson H, Sjovall J (eds). Sterols and Bile Acids. Amsterdam: Elsevier Publishing Co., 1985;331–343.
3. Reddy BS, Watanabe K, Weisburger JH, Wynder EL. Promoting effects of bile acids in colon carcinogenesis in germ-free and conventional F344 rats. Cancer Res. 1977;37:3238–3242.
4. Cohen BI, Raicht RF, Deschner EE, Takahashi M, Sarwal AN, Fazzini E. Effect of cholic acid feeding on N-methyl-N-nitrosurea-induced colon tumors and cell kinetics in rats. J Natl Cancer Inst. 1980;64:573–578.
5. Koga S, Kaibara N, Takeda R. Effect of bile acids on 1,2-dimethylhydrazine-induced colon cancer in rats. Cancer. 1982;50:543–547.
6. Wargovich MJ. Dietary promoters and antipromoters. In: Shankel DM, Hartman PE, Kaba T, Hollander A (eds). Antimutagenesis and Anticarcinogenesis Mechanisms. New York: Plenum Publishing Corp. 1986;409–420.
7. McSheery CK, Cohen BI, Bokkenheuser VD et al. Effect of calcium and bile acid feeding on colon tumors in the rat. Cancer Res. 1989;49:6039–6043.
8. Czygan P, Seitz H, Waldherr R, Stiehl A, Raedsch R, Kommerell B. Chenodeoxycholic acid but not ursodeoxycholic acid enhances colonic carcinogenesis in the rat. In: Paumgartner G, Stiehl A, Gerok W (eds). Bile Acids and Cholesterol in Health and Disease. Lancaster: MTP Press Ltd., 1984;383–385.
9. Earnest DL, Halubec H, Wali RK et al. Chemoprevention of azoxymethane-induced colonic carcinogenesis by supplemental dietary ursodeoxycholic acid. Cancer Res. 1994;54:5071–5074.
10. Batta AK, Salen G, Holubec H, Brasitus TA, Alberts D, Earnest DL. Enrichment of the more hydrophilic bile acid ursodeoxycholic acid in the fecal water-soluble fraction after feeding to rats with colon polyps. Cancer Res. 1998;58:1684–1687.
11. Galle P, Theilmann L, Raedsch R, Otto G, Stiehl A. Ursodeoxycholate reduces hepatotoxicity of bile salts in primary human hepatocytes. Hepatology. 1990;12:486–491.
12. Heuman DM, Pandak WMJ, Hylemon PB, Vlaheevik ZR. Conjugates of ursodeoxycholate protect against cytotoxicity of more hydrophobic bile salts: in vitro studies in rat hepatocytes and human erythyrocytes. Hepatology. 1991;14:920–926.
13. Guldutuna S, Zimmer G, Imhof M, Bhatti S, Yon T, Leuschner U. Molecular aspects of membrane stabilization by ursodeoxycholate. Gastroenterology. 1993;104:1736–1744.
14. Shekels LL, Beste JE, Ho SB. Tauroursodeoxycholic acid protects in vitro models of human colonic cancer cells from cytotoxic effects of hydrophobic bile acids. J Lab Clin Med. 1996;127:57–66.
15. Rigas B, Tsioulias GJ, Allan C, Wali RK, Brasitus TA. The effect of bile acids and piroxicam on HMC antigen expression in rat colonocytes during colon cancer development. Immunology. 1994;83:319–323.
16. Nishizuka Y. Intracellular signaling by hydrolysis of phospholipids and activation of protein kinase C. Science. 1992;258:607–614.
17. Craven PA, DeRubertis FR. Alterations in protein kinase C in 1,2-dimethylhydrazine induced colonic carcinogenesis. Cancer Res. 1992;52:2216–2221.
18. Wali RK, Frawley BP Jr, Hartmann S et al. Mechanisms of action of chemoprotective ursodeoxycholate in the azoxymethane model of rat colonic carcinogenesis: potential roles of protein kinase C-α, -β II and -ζ. Cancer Res. 1995;55:5257–5264.

19. Dudeja PK, Dahiya R, Brasitus TA. The role of sphingomyelin and sphingomyelinase in 1,2-dimethylhydrazine-induced lipid alterations of rat colonic plasma membrane. Biochim Biophys Acta. 1986;863:309–312.
20. Duan RD, Cheng Y, Tauschel HD, Nilsson A. Effects of ursodeoxycholate and other bile salts on levels of rat intestinal alkaline sphingomyelinase. A potential implication in tumorigenesis. Dig Dis Sci. 1998;43:26–32.
21. Earnest DL, Reid M, Heddens D et al. Treatment with 600 mg/day of ursodeoxycholic acid maximally supresses the proportion of deoxycholic acid in fecal water. Gastroenterology. 1998;114:A1120.

32
Role of bile acids in colonic neoplasia – human studies

M. STELLINI, M.J. VEYSEY, L.A. THOMAS, V. MILOVIC,
P.J. JENKINS, P. FAIRCLOUGH, G.M. MURPHY and
R.H. DOWLING

INTRODUCTION

The role of bile acids in colonic neoplasia is a large topic. Indeed, in the past, entire meetings, lasting two or three days, have been devoted to this subject. At this International Workshop, however, there were only two presentations of bile acids and colorectal cancer. The first (Chapter 31) dealt with studies in experimental animals. The second (the present chapter) discusses human studies in this field. We chose to study not bile acids in general, but one bile acid in particular, deoxycholic acid (DCA) and its role in the pathogenesis of large bowel cancer. Furthermore, we will discuss this subject mainly in relation to one disease, acromegaly, in which there is a high prevalence of colorectal neoplasia.

RATIONALE FOR STUDYING PATIENTS WITH ACROMEGALY

There were several reasons for concentrating on patients with acromegaly. First, patients with untreated acromegaly have abnormal DCA metabolism. For example, the proportion of DCA in fasting serum (expressed as a percentage of total serum bile acids) is increased in patients with acromegaly[1]. This is probably due to prolongation of large bowel transit times (LBTT)[2], since the percentage of DCA in fasting serum (Figure 1), the DCA input rate into the enterohepatic circulation and the DCA pool size[3] are each linearly related to LBTT.

Second, as noted above, patients with acromegaly have a high prevalence and incidence of colonic adenomatous polyps and cancers: in 11 prospective colonoscopic studies[4–15], the mean prevalence of neoplastic lesions (adenomas and carcinomas) in patients with acromegaly was 27%, compared with a mean of only 7% in matched controls[6] (Figure 2). The largest of these 11 surveys was that by Jenkins et al.[9] and at the time of publication (1997), these authors had examined 129 patients. They have now colonoscoped more than 200 patients, in whom

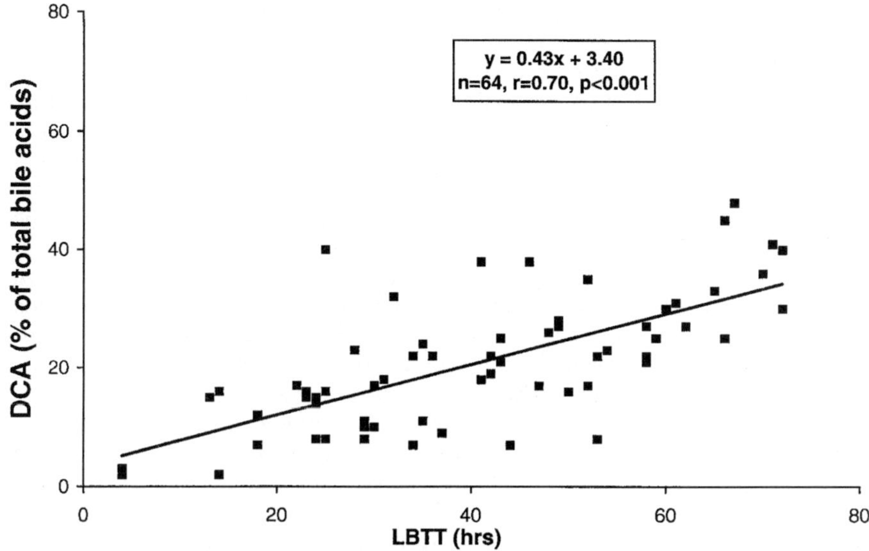

Figure 1. Relationship between large bowel transit time (LBTT measured in hours) and the proportion of deoxycholic acid (DCA) in fasting serum, expressed as a percentage of the total serum bile acids. (Reproduced with kind permission of BMJ Publishing Group (Gut. 1999;44:675–681).

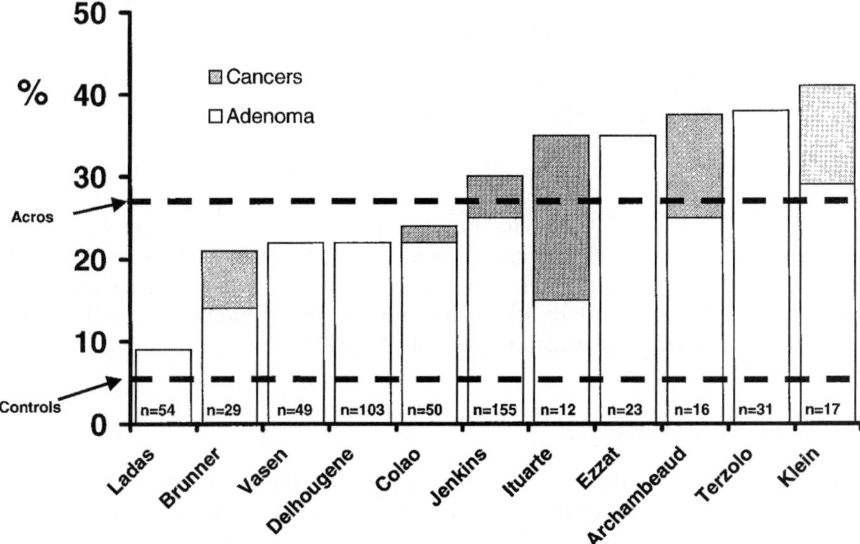

Figure 2. Results of 11 prospective colonoscopic studies of the prevalence of colorectal neoplasia in patients with acromegaly. The vertical axis refers to the percentage (%) of patients with endoscopically detected cancers (shaded bars) or adenomas (open bars). The numbers of patients examined is shown at the bottom of each histogram bar. The names listed on the vertical axis are the first authors of the relevant publication[4–15]. The upper broken horizontal line indicates the mean prevalence of colonoscopic lesions (cancers and adenomatous polyps) in acromegalic patients (acros), from all 11 studies. The lower broken horizontal line indicates the corresponding mean value in age-matched controls from the study by Vasen and colleagues[6].

they found 10 colorectal cancers, three of which were in the caecum (Jenkins and Fairclough, personal communication).

Third, acromegalic patients with colonoscopic lesions (adenomas and/or carcinomas) have higher concentrations of deoxycholic acid in fasting serum than acromegalics with normal colonoscopy, and 'controls' – patients undergoing clinically indicated colonoscopy who were found, in retrospect, to have a normal colon[16]. The pattern of serum DCA results in Jenkins' acromegalic population[14] was similar to that described by Bayerdorfer et al. in non-acromegalic patients with colonoscopic lesions[17,18].

Fourth, as well as having large peripheries (Greek: akron = extremity; megaly = great), acromegalic patients often have organomegaly of abdominal viscera including the gallbladder[2,19,20] and the colon ('colonomegaly')[21]. Thus, when Veysey et al.[21] measured colon size using an opsiometer (map measuring wheel) in barium enema radiographs of patients with acromegaly, they found that total colon length, and particularly the length of the sigmoid colon, were increased.

Fifth, patients with acromegaly have (by definition) increased circulating levels of growth hormone (GH) and insulin-like growth factor-1 (IGF-1). When Cats et al.[22] measured cell proliferation (using bromodeoxyuridine labelling) in mucosal biopsies of the sigmoid colon from acromegalic patients, they found that the labelling index was increased, and was linearly related to the serum levels of both GH and IGF-1.

RATIONALE FOR STUDYING DCA

Although bile acids in general have long been implicated in the pathogenesis of colorectal cancer[23–31], DCA is by far the greatest suspect. The evidence incriminating this hydrophobic secondary bile acid, both as an initiator and a promoter of colorectal neoplasia, has been summarized elsewhere in this book (Chapter 31). There is also a large body of evidence showing that in millimolar concentrations, DCA is 'toxic' to the colonic mucosa[32–39], causing epithelial damage ('epitheliolysis')[40] and inhibition of water and electrolyte transport[41]. In two human colon cancer cell lines (Caco-2 and HT 29), micromolar amounts (20–50 μM) of DCA stimulate cell proliferation as measured both by cell counts and by tritiated thymidine incorporation into DNA[42,43].

WORKING HYPOTHESIS

Based on the evidence discussed above, we postulated that in acromegaly, there are two potential 'colonotrophins', DCA and IGF-1, and that these two factors act in concert to stimulate cell proliferation, and a hyperplasia–adenoma–carcinoma sequence, in the large bowel mucosa.

STUDY DESIGN: PATIENTS AND METHODS

To test this hypothesis, we carried out a preliminary case-control study in two groups of patients recruited from the outpatient clinics at Guy's and

St. Bartholomew's Hospitals. There were nine acromegalic patients (mean age 57; range 38–72 years; four men and five women) undergoing surveillance colonoscopy to exclude colorectal neoplasia, and nine matched controls (mean age 58; range 43–73; four men and five women) selected from a total of 23 patients undergoing clinically indicated colonoscopy (for rectal bleeding in three and a change in bowel habit in six), all of whom had normal colonic mucosae both at endoscopy and by histology.

At colonoscopy, mucosal biopsies were taken from the caecum, transverse and sigmoid colon and, in addition to routine histology, the number of mitoses was counted using the technique described by Goodlad et al.[44]. In brief, the biopsies were stored in Carnoys solution for 2 h before being transferred into 70% alcohol. The tissue was then stained with the Fuelgen reaction, to facilitate counting of mitotic figures, in 20 microdissected crypts.

In the patients with acromegaly, fasting blood samples were obtained before colonoscopy for measurement of serum IGF-1 concentrations.

Ethical considerations

The protocol for these studies was approved by the Research Ethics Committees of Guy's Hospital, and the East London and the City Health Authority. Written consent was obtained from all patients.

Statistical methods

Unless otherwise stated, the results are given as means ± SEMs. The significance of differences between the means was tested using non-parametric methods. The relationship between mitotic counts and serum IGF-1 was examined using linear regression analysis.

RESULTS, INTERPRETATION AND DISCUSSION

Mitotic counts in colonic mucosal biopsies

There was a proximal-to-distal gradient in the number of mitoses per colonic crypt, particularly in the acromegalic patients. However at all three biopsy sites, the mitotic counts in the acromegalic patients were significantly greater than those in the controls (caecum: 12.2 ± 2.4 vs. 7.7 ± 1.4, $p < 0.005$; transverse: 10.1 ± 2.0 vs. 7.5 ± 1.5, $p < 0.01$; sigmoid: 8.8 ± 1.9 vs. 6.4 ± 1.0, $p < 0.01$). The difference in mean mitotic counts between the acromegalic patients and the 'controls' was greatest in the caecum. This may be relevant to the distribution of colorectal neoplasia in these two groups of individuals. In acromegalic patients, polyps and cancers occur relatively more often on the right than on the left, while in the non-acromegalic population, > 80% of lesions occur distal to the splenic flexure.

Relationship between serum IGF-1 and mitotic counts

Our initial results in the patients with acromegaly show that there was a significant linear relationship between the mitotic counts (at all three colonic biopsy sites), and the fasting, age-adjusted serum IGF-1 levels. For example, in the caecum the correlation coefficient (r) between these two variables was 0.69 ($p < 0.05$). This observation confirms and extends the results of Cats et al.[22], who showed a similar relationship, but only in the sigmoid colon. Taken together, these results suggest that growth hormone and insulin-like growth factor-1 may be trophic to the colon, a conclusion supported by the results of cell culture studies, which clearly show that IGF-1 promotes the growth of intestinal epithelial cells[45–48].

In our working hypothesis, we speculated that not only growth hormone/IGF-1 but also deoxycholic acid, might be trophic to the large bowel. The results of fasting serum DCA levels (measured by gas chromatography-mass spectrometry) in the patients studied here, are not yet available. In support of our hypothesis, however, Ochsenkuhn et al.[49] have shown a significant relationship between the percentage DCA in fasting serum and cell proliferation (measured by flow cytometry) in the colon. It remains to be seen whether the effects of IGF-1 and DCA are indeed *additive* in stimulating colonocyte proliferation thereby increasing the risk of colorectal neoplasia through the hyperplasia – adenoma – carcinoma sequence.

REFERENCES

1. Veysey MJ, Thomas LA, Mallet AI et al. Prolonged large bowel transit increases serum deoxycholic acid: a risk factor for octreotide induced gallstones. Gut. 1999;44:675–681.
2. Hussaini SH, Pereira SP, Veysey MJ et al. Roles of gall bladder emptying and intestinal transit in the pathogenesis of octreotide induced gall bladder stones. Gut. 1996;38:775–783.
3. Veysey MJ, Mallet A, Jenkins PJ, Besser GM, Dowling RH. Deoxycholic acid (DCA) and cholic acid (CA) kinetics in acromegalic patients treated with octreotide (OT). Gut. 1998;42:A11 (Abstr).
4. Ladas SD, Thalassinos NC, Ioannides G, Raptis SA. Does acromegaly really predispose to an increased prevalence of gastrointestinal tumours? Clin Endocrinol. 1994;41:597–601.
5. Brunner JE, Johnson CC, Zafar S, Peterson EL, Brunner JF, Mellinger RC. Colon cancer and polyps in acromegaly: increased risk associated with family history of colon cancer. Clin Endocrinol. 1990;32:65–71.
6. Vasen HF, van Erpecum KJ, Roelfsema F et al. Increased prevalence of colonic adenomas in patients with acromegaly. Eur J Endocrinol. 1994;131:235–237.
7. Delhougne B, Deneux C, Abs R et al. The prevalence of colonic polyps in acromegaly: a colonoscopic and pathological study in 103 patients (see comments). J Clin Endocrinol Metab. 1995;80:3223–3226.
8. Colao A, Balzano A, Ferone D et al. Increased prevalence of colonic polyps and altered lymphocyte subset pattern in the colonic lamina propria in acromegaly. Clin Endocrinol. 1997;47:23–28.
9. Jenkins PJ, Fairclough PD, Richards T et al. Acromegaly, colonic polyps and carcinoma (see comments). Clin Endocrinol. 1997;47:17–22.
10. Ituarte EM, Petrini J, Hershman JM. Acromegaly and colon cancer. Ann Intern Med. 1984;101:627–628.
11. Ezzat S. Hepatobiliary and gastrointestinal manifestations of acromegaly. Dig Dis. 1992;10:173–180.
12. Archambeaud-Mouveroux F, Geffray I, Teissar MP. Prevalence of colorectal carcinoma and polyps in acromegaly. 80th Annual meeting of The Endocrine Society; 1998 June 24–27, New Orleans, Bethesda 1998;504.
13. Terzolo M, Tappero G, Borretta G et al. High prevalence of colonic polyps in patients with acromegaly. Influence of sex and age (see comments). Arch Intern Med. 1994;154:1272–1276.
14. Klein I, Parveen G, Gavaler JS, Vanthiel DH. Colonic polyps in patients with acromegaly. Ann Intern Med. 1982;97:27–30.
15. Klein I. Acromegaly and cancer. Ann Intern Med. 1984;101:706–707.

16. Veysey MJ, Gathercole DJ, Jenkins PJ et al. Acromegalics with colorectal adenomas or carcinomas have increased serum deoxycholic acid (DCA) levels. Gut. 1997;41 (Suppl 3):A251 (Abstr).
17. Bayerdorffer E, Mannes GA, Ochsenkuhn T, Dirschedl P, Wiebecke B, Paumgartner G. Unconjugated secondary bile acids in the serum of patients with colorectal adenomas. Gut. 1995;36:268–273.
18. Bayerdorffer E, Mannes GA, Richter WO et al. Increased serum deoxycholic acid levels in men with colorectal adenomas (see comments). Gastroenterology. 1993;104:145–151.
19. Hopman WP, Van Liessum PA, Pieters GF et al. Postprandial gallbladder motility and plasma cholecystokinin at regular time intervals after injection of octreotide in acromegalics on long-term treatment. Dig Dis Sci. 1992;37:1685–1690.
20. Fuessl HS, Burrin JM, Williams G, Adrian TE, Bloom SR. The effect of a long-acting somatostatin analogue (SMS 201-995) on intermediary metabolism and gut hormones after a test meal in normal subjects. Aliment Pharmacol Ther. 1987;1:321–330.
21. Veysey MJ, Mills TD, Reynolds CR, Jenkins PJ, Besser GM, Dowling RH. 'Colonomegaly' in acromegaly – a link with colorectal neoplasia? Gut. 1997;41 (Suppl 3):A121 (Abstr).
22. Cats A, Dullaart RP, Kleibeuker JH et al. Increased epithelial cell proliferation in the colon of patients with acromegaly. Cancer Res. 1996;56:523–526.
23. Kanazawa K, Konishi F, Mitsuoka T et al. Factors influencing the development of sigmoid colon cancer. Bacteriologic and biochemical studies. Cancer. 1996;77:1701–1706.
24. Hill MJ, Aries VC. Faecal steroid composition and its relationship to cancer of the large bowel. J Pathol. 1971;104:129–139.
25. Reddy BS, Wynder EL. Large-bowel carcinogenesis: fecal constituents of populations with diverse incidence rates of colon cancer. J Natl Cancer Inst. 1973;501:1437–1442.
26. Reddy BS. Role of bile metabolites in colon carcinogenesis. Animal models. Cancer. 1975;36:2401–2406.
27. Reddy BS, Mastromarino A, Wynder EL. Further leads on metabolic epidemiology of large bowel cancer. Cancer Res. 1975;35:3403–3406.
28. Reddy BS, Mastromarino A, Gustafson C, Lipkin M, Wynder EL. Fecal bile acids and neutral sterols in patients with familial polyposis. Cancer. 1976;38:1694–1698.
29. Wynder EL, Reddy BS. The epidemiology of cancer of the large bowel. Am J Dig Dis. 1974;19:937–946.
30. Narisawa T, Magadia NE, Weisburger JH, Wynder EL. Promoting effect of bile acids on colon carcinogenesis after intrarectal instillation of N-methyl-N′-nitro-N-nitrosoguanidine in rats. J Natl Cancer Inst. 1974;53:1093–1097.
31. Crowther JS, Drasar BS, Hill MJ et al. Faecal steroids and bacteria and large bowel cancer in Hong Kong by socio-economic groups. Br J Cancer. 1976;34:191–198.
32. Marchetti C, Migliorati G, Moraca R et al. Deoxycholic acid and SFCA-induced apoptosis in the human tumor cell-line HT-29 and possible mechanisms. Cancer Lett. 1997;114:97–99.
33. Martinez JD, Stratagoules ED, LaRue JM et al. Different bile acids exhibit distinct biological effects: the tumor promoter deoxycholic acid induces apoptosis and the chemopreventive agent ursodeoxycholic acid inhibits cell proliferation. Nutr Cancer. 1998;31:111–118.
34. Garewal H, Bernstein H, Bernstein C, Sampliner R, Payne C. Reduced bile acid-induced apoptosis in 'normal' colorectal mucosa: a potential biological marker for cancer risk. Cancer Res. 1996;56:1480–1483.
35. Hirano F, Tanada H, Makino Y et al. Induction of the transcription factor AP-1 in cultured human colon adenocarcinoma cells following exposure to bile acids. Carcinogenesis. 1996;17:427–433.
36. Kanda T, Niot I, Foucauld L et al. Effect of bile on the intestinal bile-acid binding protein (I-BABP) expression. In vitro and in vivo studies. FEBS Lett. 1996;384:131–134.
37. Klinkspoor JH, Mok KS, Van Klinken BJW, Tytgat GNJ, Lee SP, Groen AK. Mucin secretion by the human colon cell line LS174T is regulated by bile salts. Glycobiology. 1999;9:13–19.
38. Li M, Vemulapalli R, Ullah A, Izu L, Duffey ME, Lance P. Downregulation of a human colonic sialyltransferase by a secondary bile acid and a phorbol ester. Am J Physiol. 1998;274: G599–G606.
39. Dawson AM, Isselbacher KJ, Bell VM. Studies on lipid metabolism in the small intestine with observations on the role of bile salts. J. Clin Invest. 1960;39:730–740.

40. Chadwick VS, Gaginella T, Carlson G, Debongnie JC, Phillips SF, Hoffman AF. Effect of molecular structure on bile acid induced alterations in absorptive function, permeability, and morphology in the perfused rat colon. J Lab Clin Med. 1979;94:661–674.
41. Breuer NF, Rampton DS, Tammar A, Murphy GM, Dowling RH. Effects of colonic perfusion with sulfated and nonsulfated bile acids on mucosal structure and function in the rat. Gastroenterology. 1983;84:969–977.
42. Milovic V, Murphy GM, Dowling RH. Deoxycholic acid (DCA), polyamines and colon cancer: low dose DCA stimulates cell proliferation and putrescine uptake in cultured Caco-2 cells. Gut. 1997;41 (Suppl 3) A251 (Abstr).
43. Peiffer LP, Peters DJ, McGarrity TJ. Differential effects of deoxycholic acid on proliferation of neoplastic and differentiated colonocytes in vitro. Dig Dis Sci. 1997;42:2234–2240.
44. Goodlad RA, Levi S, Lee CY, Mandir N, Hodgson H, Wright NA. Morphometry and cell proliferation in endoscopic biopsies: evaluation of a technique. Gastroenterology. 1991;101:1235–1241.
45. Jobson TM, Billington CK, Hall IP. Regulation of proliferation of human colonic subepithelial myofibroblasts by mediators important in intestinal inflammation. J Clin Invest. 1998;101: 2650–2657.
46. Howarth GS, Xian CJ, Read LC. Insulin-like growth factor-1 partially attenuates colonic damage in rats with experimental colitis induced by oral dextran sulphate sodium. Scand J Gastroenterol. 1998;33:180–190.
47. Riegler M, Sedivy R, Sogukoglu T et al. Effect of growth factors on epithelial restitution of human colonic mucosa in vitro. Scand J Gastroenterol. 1997;32:925–932.
48. Quadros E, Landzert NM, Le Roy S, Gasparini F, Worosila G. Colonic absorption of insulin-like growth factor 1 in vitro. Pharm Res. 1994;11:226–230.
49. Ochsenkuhn T et al. Colonic mucosal proliferation is related to serum deoxycholic acid levels. Cancer. 1999;85:1664–1669.

Section X
Chronic pancreatitis

33
Bile acids in pancreatic steatorrhoea

P.L. ZENTLER-MUNRO

INTRODUCTION

Pancreatic exocrine insufficiency is common in diseases such as chronic alcoholic pancreatitis, cystic fibrosis (CF) and haemochromatosis, and after major pancreatic resection. It is manifest most obviously as steatorrhoea, but can also cause anorexia, abdominal discomfort and social embarrassment, and can contribute to the pathogenesis of distal intestinal obstruction syndrome in CF. It leads to malabsorption of fat, fat-soluble vitamins and other micronutrients which, together with dietary deficiency, can impair growth, nutritional and pulmonary status particularly in patients with CF[1].

Pancreatic steatorrhoea often responds poorly to pancreatic enzyme replacement therapy (pancreatin). Attention has focused on improving the formulation of pancreatin so as to protect the enzymes during their passage through the stomach and accelerate their dispersal in the duodenum, and on reducing acid secretion so as to prevent their inactivation once released in the hyperacidic duodenum[2,3]. Even with optimal therapy, some patients continue to suffer severe steatorrhoea, suggesting that another pathophysiological disturbance may contribute.

Bile acids have long been known to play a crucial part in solubilizing dietary fat so as to facilitate its absorption[4]. This chapter discusses how bile acid deficiency might occur as a consequence of pancreatic exocrine insufficiency, and might contribute to the difficulty in treating pancreatic steatorrhoea.

PRINCIPLES OF FAT DIGESTION AND SOLUBILIZATION (Figure 1)

According to the classical model[5,6], fat absorption occurs in two main stages. In the first 'chemical' phase, neutral lipid (triglyceride) is hydrolysed initially by gastric lipase in the stomach to fatty acid and diglyceride, and then by the concerted action of pancreatic lipase and colipase in the duodenum to fatty acid and monoglyceride: the latter act as solutes. In the second 'physical' phase, these solutes are rendered soluble in the aqueous phase of chyme by amphipathic bile acids acting as solvents to form micelles[7] (also incorporating phospholipid and

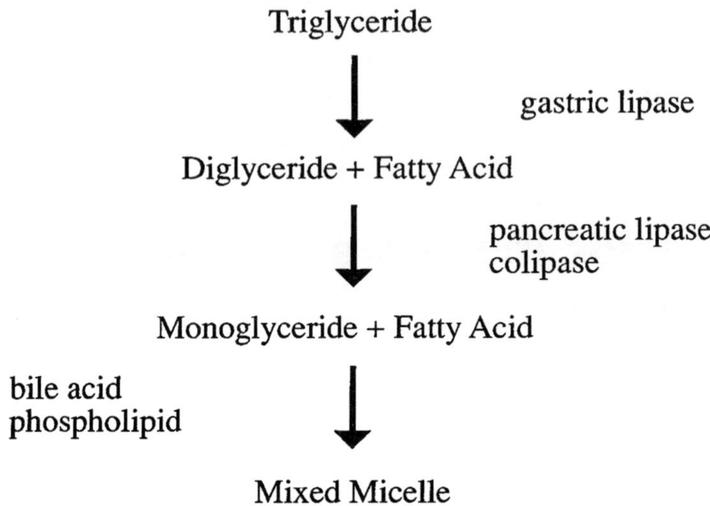

Figure 1.   Principles of fat digestion and solubilization.

cholesterol). Later studies challenging the micellar theory predicted[8] and demonstrated[9,10] other structures such as liquid crystals and liposomes (see Chapter 35). These structures can then traverse the unstirred water layer so as to present their lipid contents to the mucosal surface for absorption[4].

The process of micellar solubilization requires an adequate concentration of conjugated bile acids in the aqueous phase of duodenal chyme. The minimum concentration required to solubilize the hydrolytic products of a typical meal is known as the critical physiological concentration and is around 4 mmol/l[11]. The postprandial delivery of bile acid into the duodenum is determined largely by biliary secretion rate, and by gallbladder motility. The former is in turn determined by the integrity of enterohepatic recirculation (EHC) of bile acids, and by the liver's capacity to replace bile acid lost from the EHC[12]. The retention of bile acids in the aqueous phase depends on adequate pancreatic secretion of bicarbonate to maintain intraduodenal pH above 5 and prevent protonation and precipitation of bile acids below their pKa[13], and on adequate proteolysis to prevent binding of bile acid to undigested protein[14]. The roles of these and other processes in the pathophysiology of steatorrhoea in various diseases have been reviewed[15].

FAT DIGESTION IN PANCREATIC STEATORRHOEA (Figure 2)

The main problem in pancreatic exocrine insufficiency is, of course, an almost complete absence of pancreatic lipase and, in borderline cases, colipase[16]. An increase in gastric lipase secretion demonstrated in some, but not all, studies in alcoholic pancreatitis[17] and in CF[18] does not compensate fully for this. Pancreatic bicarbonate secretion is also greatly reduced in all forms of pancreatic exocrine insufficiency, whilst gastric acid secretion is often increased

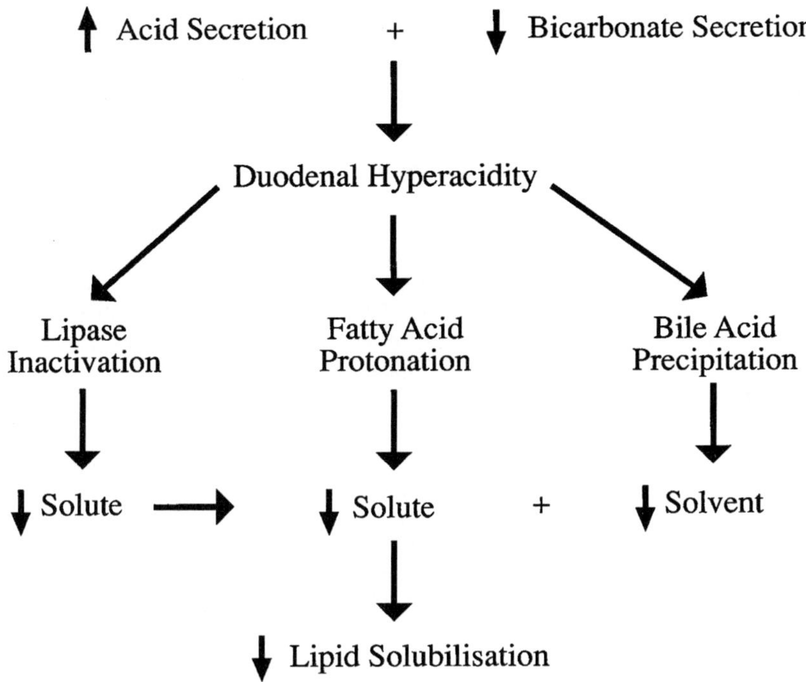

Figure 2.   pH-related disturbances in pancreatic steatorrhoea.

particularly in CF[19]. This leads to duodenal and jejunal hyperacidity in both alcoholic pancreatitis[20,21] and CF[22,23], in some patients to levels below pH 5 as seen in Zollinger-Ellison syndrome[24]. This further aggravates the primary deficiency of pancreatic lipase, since lipase (and other pancreatic hydrolytic enzymes) is irreversibly inactivated below pH 5[25]: this affects both endogenous lipase and administered lipase (in pancreatin). Enteric-coating of pancreatin cannot protect lipase once it is released in the duodenum, and it is the failure of acid suppression therapy reliably to correct steatorrhoea[3] that led to the assessment of biliary kinetics in pancreatic disease.

BILE ACID KINETICS IN PANCREATIC DISEASES

Biliary kinetics in pancreatic insufficiency have been most extensively assessed in CF[1,26]. Faecal bile acid excretion has long been known to be elevated in children with CF[27], sometimes to levels seen after ileal resection[28]. This leads to a reduction in bile acid pool size[29] and a corresponding increase in cholesterol saturation of bile[30], and is a factor contributing to the increased incidence of cholesterol gallstones seen in this disease.

The cause of this interruption in EHC of bile acids has been widely debated. The early observation that bile acid turnover could be reduced and pool-size increased by administration of pancreatin[28,29], or by substitution of dietary long-chain triglyceride with medium-chain triglyceride oil[31], suggested that faecal loss was related not to a mucosal absorption defect but to fat malabsorption. The sequestration of bile acid in an expanded oil-phase that this theory implied has not been described, although it has been proposed for cholesterol[32].

A later report that faecal bile acid excretion could be reduced by the administration of cimetidine in the absence of pancreatin[33] suggested that it might be another effect of the jejunal acidification seen in pancreatic insufficiency, as already discussed. Jejunal acidification in Zollinger-Ellison syndrome leads to precipitation of glycine-conjugated bile acids[24], and this has been confirmed in both alcoholic pancreatitis[34] and in CF[22] and is reversed by cimetidine in both diseases[34,35]. Precipitated bile acids should, however, return to the aqueous phase if pH rises further down the intestine[24]: although distal ileal pH has not been extensively investigated in these diseases, two studies have reported that hyperacidity persists[36,37] although not to levels likely to be critical in this context.

This difficulty was resolved by a careful analysis of factors influencing faecal composition in CF, which showed that faecal bile acid levels were more closely correlated with faecal nitrogen excretion than with faecal fat excretion[33]; another study showed that bile acids were sequestered in the solid phase of faeces in CF, and could be released by adding protease or by raising pH[38]. Further studies have shown that faecal bile acid loss in CF can be reduced by substitution of dietary protein with an elemental feed[39], and that bile acids bind to casein in vitro in a pH-dependent fashion[14]. It therefore appears that the increased faecal bile acid loss and reduced bile acid pool size well established in CF are related to decreased pancreatic bicarbonate and protease excretion, leading to a combination of pH-dependent bile acid precipitation and bile acid binding to undigested protein (Figure 3).

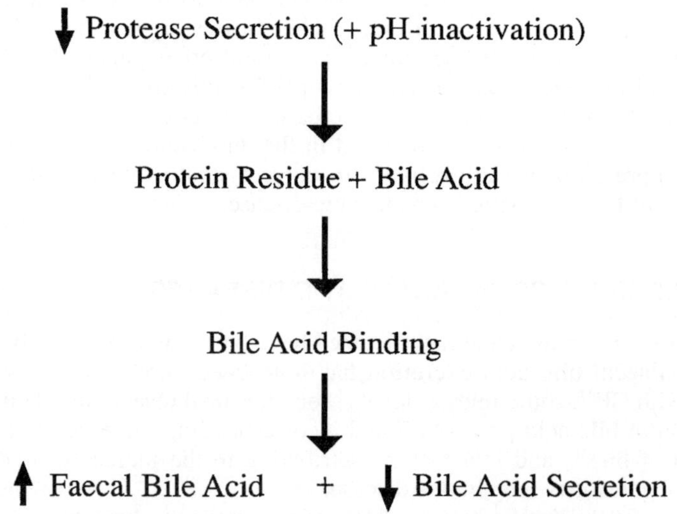

Figure 3.   Protease-related disturbances in pancreatic cholerrhoea.

The disturbance of biliary kinetics is much better established in CF than in alcoholic pancreatitis[40,41] and may be more profound, explaining the peculiarly resistant steatorrhoea in this disease. There are several potential reasons for this. The reduction in jejunal pH is probably more profound in CF, due in part to increased acid secretion as already discussed. Cholestatic liver disease is common in CF, particularly in older patients[1] (see Chapter 10), while cholestasis is not prominent in association with alcoholic pancreatitis. The effect of cholestasis on bile acid secretion has been well described in primary biliary cirrhosis[42].

In CF, bile acid secretion rates in response to maximal (hormonal) stimulation have been reported to be normal in children[43] but reduced in adults[44], perhaps due to the progression of liver disease with age. This is likely to explain the apparently paradoxical decrease in faecal bile acid excretion in CF with age[45]: increasing intrahepatic cholestasis reduces bile acid synthesis, whilst declining gallbladder motility[44] further reduces duodenal bile acid delivery and hence faecal loss, and also aggravates fat malabsorption. Adults who have benefited from recent advances in the nutritional management of CF may gain an improvement in fat absorption (perhaps due to the development of compensatory mechanisms)[1] and achieve normal weight and improved general health. A recent study of such adults[46], apparently without liver disease or symptomatic steatorrhoea, reported normal bile acid kinetics, again suggesting that the main disturbance is secondary to pancreatic and hepatic disease.

Bile acid kinetics in CF may also be disturbed as a primary result of the mucosal malfunction which affects many organs in this disease, and which could lead in the distal ileum to malabsorption of bile acid (and fat: see Chapter 34). An early study showing normal results with the [^{14}C]glycocholate breath test[47] indicated that bile acid malabsorption did not occur in CF, but this study has been criticized on methodological grounds[1]. A careful in vitro study using ileal biopsies[48] showed significantly reduced bile acid uptake, but a later in vivo study using a perfusion technique[49] did not. A recent study using the SeHCAT test showed significant impairment of bile acid absorption in about a third of patients, but was too small to distinguish convincingly between patients with and without liver disease[50].

FAT SOLUBILIZATION IN PANCREATIC STEATORRHOEA

Bile acid deficiency is likely to impair lipid solubilization only if it reduces aqueous-phase bile acid concentration below the critical physiological concentration as defined earlier. This could result from either or both of the two mechanisms already described: decreased bile acid secretion reducing total bile acid concentration in the duodenum, and reduced bicarbonate secretion and the resulting pH-dependent bile acid precipitation and binding reducing aqueous phase concentration.

Total bile acid concentration in the jejunum reflects gastroduodenal fluid secretion and transit as well as biliary bile acid delivery, and experimental values therefore depend on the meal stimulus used. Various studies have reported normal[22,43,45] or reduced[51] duodenal total bile acid concentrations, but the proportion of glycine conjugates is increased in all studies as a result of bile acid loss and the limited supply of taurine in the diet[52]. This predisposes to pH-dependent precipitation, since glycine conjugates have a pK_a around 5, whereas taurine conjugates do not precipitate above pH 2[24].

Studies in both alcoholic pancreatitis[34] and CF[22] have demonstrated that jejunal acidification leads to precipitation of glycine-conjugated bile acids and a significant reduction in aqueous phase bile acid concentration, to levels below the critical physiological concentration. In primary biliary cirrhosis[42], it is the presence of duodenal bile acid concentrations below this level (3 mmol/l) rather than pancreatic insufficiency which determines the presence of steatorrhoea, and this level is also associated with steatorrhoea rather than diarrhoea in patients with ileal resection[53]. No such relationship was sought in either of the above 'pancreatic' studies, but both demonstrated a marked positive correlation between intraluminal pH and aqueous phase lipid concentration which, in CF[22], was present even in the absence of the effect of pH on lipolysis. This study was also able to demonstrate the effect of bile acid binding to protein at pH 6, at which precipitation should not occur.

TREATMENT OF BILE ACID DEFICIENCY IN PANCREATIC STEATORRHOEA

Only studies in which the proposed deficiency in total or aqueous phase bile acid concentration is corrected can determine whether bile acid deficiency contributes critically to pancreatic steatorrhoea. Although bile acid used to be included in certain formulations of pancreatin, the species and amount of bile acid added was inappropriate and no study has shown any improvement in efficacy. Two studies have shown that oral taurine supplements increased the proportion of taurine-conjugated bile acids resistant to precipitation, and improved fat absorption modestly[54,55].

Many studies have shown that the adjunctive use of an antacid, histamine H_2 antagonist or proton pump inhibitor with pancreatin improves lipid solubilization and fat absorption[2,3], but none of these was able to separate the effect of preventing bile acid precipitation and improving bile acid conservation from the much more obvious effect of reducing acidic inactivation of administered enzymes in the stomach or duodenum. One study[35] has been able to achieve this indirectly, by showing that the administration of cimetidine alone, in the absence of endogenous or exogenous lipase, improved lipid solubilization by reducing bile acid precipitation and increasing aqueous phase bile acid concentration.

The use of natural conjugated bile acid supplements has been prevented by their susceptibility to bacterial deconjugation and pH-precipitation, and their proneness to cause secretory diarrhoea. Very recently, a novel conjugated bile acid, cholylsarcosine, has been designed to avoid these problems, and has proved effective in individual patients with ileal resection steatorrhoea (short bowel syndrome)[56]. No trial has been reported in patients with severe pancreatic steatorrhoea, for whom the drug might be very helpful.

CONCLUSION

There are several reasons to suspect that an interruption in the enterohepatic circulation of bile acids may contribute to the pathophysiology of pancreatic steatorrhoea. It is likely to result from sequestration of bile acids in the solid phase of chyme and resulting faecal loss, together with inadequate synthesis, impaired secretion in older patients and possibly mucosal malabsorption. Several studies of intraluminal processing of fat in patients with alcoholic pancreatitis and cystic fibrosis lend indirect support to this hypothesis, and a few therapeutic experiments add more direct confirmation. The development of a novel conjugated bile acid supplement may prove helpful to patients with severe pancreatic steatorrhoea. Until then, the use of an acid-suppressing drug to conserve bile acid within the enterohepatic circulation remains at least as important as the choice of pancreatin formulation in the treatment of such patients.

REFERENCES

1. Zentler-Munro PL. Cystic fibrosis – a gastroenterological cornucopia. Gut. 1987;28:1531–1547.
2. Zentler-Munro PL, Northfield TC. Pancreatic enzyme replacement – applied physiology and pharmacology. Aliment Pharmacol Ther. 1987;1:575–592.
3. Lebenthal E, Rolston DDK, Holsclaw DS. Enzyme therapy for pancreatic insufficiecy: present status and future needs. Pancreas. 1994;9:1–12.
4. Thomson ABR, Schoeller C, Keelan M, Smith L, Clandinin MT. Lipid absorption: passing through the unstirred layers, brush-border membrane, and beyond. Can J Physiol Pharmacol. 1993;71:531–555.
5. Hofmann AF, Borgström B. The intraluminal phase of fat digestion in man: the lipid content of micellar and oil phases of intestinal content obtained during fat digestion and absorption. J Clin Invest. 1964;43:247–257.
6. Borgström B. Fat digestion and absorption. In: Northfield TC, Jazrawi R, Zentler-Munro PL (eds). Bile Acids in Health and Disease. London: Kluwer Academic Publishers, 1988;217–228.
7. Mansbach CM, Cohen HRS, Leff PB. Isolation and properties of the mixed micelles present in intestinal content during fat digestion in man. J Clin Invest. 1975;56:781–791.
8. Staggers JE, Hernell O, Stafford RJ, Carey MC. Physical-chemical behavior of dietary and biliary lipids during intestinal digestion and absorption. 1. Phase behavior and aggregation states of model lipid systems patterned after aqueous duodenal contents of healthy adult human beings. Biochemistry. 1990;29:2028–2040.
9. Hernell O, Staggers JE, Carey MC. Physical-chemical behavior of dietary and biliary lipids during intestinal digestion and absorption. 2. Phase analysis and aggregation states of luminal lipids during duodenal fat digestion in healthy adult human beings. Biochemistry. 1990;29:2041–2056.
10. Fine DR, Brown C, Zentler-Munro PL, Northfield TC. The physicochemical state of lipids in postprandial chyme from humans with normal pancreatic function: a re-examination of the micellar theory. Eur J Gastroenterol Hepatol. 1992;4:903–911.
11. Badley BW, Murphy GM, Bouchier LA. Intraluminal bile salt deficiency in the pathogenesis of steatorrhoea. Lancet. 1969;2:400–402.
12. Dowling RH, Mack E, Small DM. Effects of controlled interruption of enterohepatic circulation of bile salts by biliary diversion and by ileal resection on bile salt secretion, synthesis and pool-size in Rhesus monkey. J Clin Invest. 1970;49:232–242.
13. Hofmann AF. The role of bile salts in fat absorption: the solvent properties of dilute, micellar solutions of conjugated bile salts. Biochem J. 1983;89:57–68.
14. Lanzini A, Fitzpatrick WJF, Pigozzi MG, Northfield TC. Bile acid binding to dietary casein: a study in vitro and in vivo. Clin Sci. 1987;73:343–350.
15. Zentler-Munro PL, Fine DR, Northfield TC. Fat digestion and solubilization in disease. In: Northfield TC, Jazrawi R, Zentler-Munro PL (eds). Bile Acids in Health and Disease. London: Kluwer Academic Publishers, 1988;239–252.

16. Gaskin KJ, Durie PR, Lee U, Hill R, Forstner GG. Colipase and lipase secretion in childhood-onset pancreatic insufficiency. Gastroenterology. 1984;86:1–7.
17. Moreau J, Bouisson M, Balas B et al. Gastric lipase in alcoholic pancreatitis. Comparison of secretive profiles following pentagastrin stimulation in normal adults and patients with pancreatic insufficiency. Gastroenterology. 1990;99:175–180.
18. Balasubramanian K, Zentler-Munro PL, Batten JC, Northfield TC. Increased acid-resistant lipase activity and lipolysis in pancreatic steatorrhoea due to cystic fibrosis. Pancreas. 1992;7:305–310.
19. Gregory PC. Gastrointestinal pH motility/transit and permeability in cystic fibrosis. J Pediatr Gastroenterol Nutr. 1996;23:513–523.
20. Dutta SK, Russell RM, Iber FL. Influence of exocrine pancreatic insufficiency on the intra-luminal pH of the proximal small intestine. Dig Dis Sci. 1979;24:529–534.
21. Geus WP, Eddes EH, Gielkens HAJ, Gan KH, Lamers CBHW, Masclee AAM. Post-prandial intragastric and intraduodenal acidity are increased in patients with chronic pancreatitis. Aliment Pharmacol Ther. 1999;13:937–944.
22. Zentler-Munro PL, Fitzpatrick WJF, Batten JC, Northfield TC. Effect of intrajejunal acidity on aqueous-phase bile acid and lipid concentrations in pancreatic steatorrhoea due to cystic fibrosis. Gut. 1984;25:500–507.
23. Youngberg CA, Berardi RR, Howatt WF et al. Comparison of gastrointestinal pH in cystic fibrosis and healthy subjects. Dig Dis Sci. 1987;32:472–480.
24. Go VL, Poley JR, Hofmann AF, Summerskill WH. Disturbance in fat digestion induced by acidic jejunal pH due to gastric hypersecretion in man. Gastroenterology. 1970;58:638–646.
25. Legg EF, Spencer AM. Studies on the stability of pancreatic enzymes in duodenal fluid to storage temperature and pH. Clin Chim Acta. 1975;65:175–179.
26. Isenberg JN. Cystic fibrosis: its influence on the liver, biliary tree, and bile salt metabolism. Sem Liver Dis. 1982;2:302–313.
27. Weber AM, Roy CC, Chartrand L et al. Relationship between bile acid malabsorption and pancreatic insufficiency in cystic fibrosis. Gut. 1976;17:295–299.
28. Weber AM, Roy CC, Morin CL, Lasalle R. Malabsorption of bile acids in children with cystic fibrosis. N Engl J Med. 1973;289:1001–1005.
29. Watkins JB, Tercyak AM, Szczepanik P, Klein PD. Bile salt kinetics in cystic fibrosis: influence of pancreatic enzyme replacement. Gastroenterology. 1977;73:1023–1028.
30. Roy CC, Weber AM, Morin CL et al. Abnormal biliary lipid composition in cystic fibrosis. Effect of pancreatic enzymes. N Engl J Med. 1977;297:1301–1305.
31. Smalley CA, Brown GA, Parkes ME, Tease H, Brookes V, Anderson CM. Reduction of bile acid loss in cystic fibrosis by dietary means. Arch Dis Child. 1978;53:477-482.
32. Vuoristo M, Väänänen H, Miettinen A. Cholesterol malabsorption in pancreatic insufficiency: effects of enzyme substitution. Gastroenterology. 1992;102:647–655.
33. Isenberg JN, Hendrix PY, Cox KL. Effect of short-term cimetidine administration on faecal bile acid losses in cystic fibrosis. J Pediatr Gastroenterol Nutr. 1983;2:447–451.
34. Regan PT, Malagelada JR, DiMagno EP, Go VL. Reduced intraluminal bile acid concentrations and fat maldigestion in pancreatic insufficiency: correction by treatment. Gastroenterology. 1979;77:285–289.
35. Zentler-Munro PL, Fine DR, Batten JC, Northfield TC. Effect of cimetidine on enzyme inactivation, bile acid precipitation and lipid solubilization in pancreatic steatorrhoea due to cystic fibrosis. Gut. 1985;26:892–901.
36. Gilbert J, Kelleher J, Littlewood JM, Evans DF. Ileal pH in cystic fibrosis. Scand J Gastroenterol. 1988;23(suppl 143):132–134.
37. Guarner I, Rodriguez F, Guarner F, Malagelada J-R. Fate of oral enzymes in pancreatic insufficiency. Gut. 1993;34:708–712.
38. Jonas A, Diver-Haber A. Bile acid sequestration by the solid phase of stools in cystic fibrosis patients: role of pancreatic enzymes. Dig Dis Sci. 1988;33:724–731.
39. Leroy C, Lepage G, Morin CL, Bertrand JM, Dufour-Larue O, Roy CC. Effect of dietary fat and residues on fecal loss of sterols and on their microbial degradation in cystic fibrosis. Dig Dis Sci. 1986;31:911–918.
40. Dutta SK, Anand K, Gadacz TR. Bile salt malabsorption in pancreatic insufficiency secondary to alcoholic pancreatitis. Gastroenterology. 1986;91:1243–1249.
41. Einarrson K, Angelin B, Johansson C. Biliary lipid metabolism in chronic pancreatitis: influence of steatorrhoea. Gut. 1987;28:1495–1499.

42. Ros E, García-Pugés A, Reixach M, Cusó E, Rodés J. Fat digestion and exocrine pancreatic insufficiency in primary biliary cirrhosis. Gastroenterology. 1984;87:180–187.
43. Robb TA, Davidson GP, Kirubakaran C. Conjugated bile acids in serum and secretions in response to cholecystokinin–secretion stimulation in children with cystic fibrosis. Gut. 1985;26:1246–1256.
44. Weizman Z, Durie PR, Kopelman HR, Vesely SM, Forstner GG. Bile acid secretion in cystic fibrosis: evidence for a defect unrelated to fat malabsorption. Gut. 1986;27:1043–1048.
45. Goodchild MC, Murphy GM, Howell AM, Nutter SA, Anderson CM. Aspects of bile acid metabolism in cystic fibrosis. Arch Dis Child. 1975;50:769–778.
46. Strandvik B, Einarrson K, Lindblad A, Angelin B. Bile acid kinetics and biliary lipid composition in cystic fibrosis. J Hepatol. 1996;25:43–48.
47. Roller RJ, Kern F. Minimal bile acid malabsorption and normal bile acid breath tests in cystic fibrosis and acquired pancreatic insufficiency. Gastroenterology. 1977;72:661–665.
48. Fondacaro JD, Heubi JE, Kellogg FW. Intestinal bile acid malabsorption in cystic fibrosis: a primary mucosal cell defect. Pediatr Res. 1982;16:494–498.
49. Thompson GN, Davidson GP. In vivo bile acid uptake from terminal ileum in cystic fibrosis. Pediatr Res. 1988;23:323–328.
50. O'Brien S, Mulcahy H, Fenlon H et al. Intestinal bile acid absorption in cystic fibrosis. Gut. 1993;34:1137–1141.
51. Harries JT, Muller DP, McCollum JP, Lipson A, Roma E, Norman AP. Intestinal bile salts in cystic fibrosis: studies in the patient and experimental animal. Arch Dis Child. 1979;54:19–24.
52. Thompson GN. Excessive fecal taurine loss predisposes to taurine deficiency in cystic fibrosis. J Pediatr Gastroenterol Nutr. 1988;7:214–219.
53. Poley JR, Hofmann AF. Role of fat maldigestion in pathogenesis of steatorrhoea in ileal resection. Gastroenterology. 1976;71:38–44.
54. Darling PB, Lepage E, Leroy C, Masson P, Roy C. Effect of taurine supplements on fat absorption in cyclic fibrosis. Pediatr Res.1985;19:578–582.
55. Colombo C, Arlati S, Curcio L et al. Effect of taurine supplementation on fat and bile acid absorption in patients with cystic fibrosis. Scand J Gastroenterol. 1988;23(suppl. 143), 151–156.
56. Gruy-Kapral C, Little KH, Fordtran JS, Meziere TL, Hagey LR, Hofmann AF. Conjugated bile acid replacement therapy for short-bowel syndrome. Gastroenterology. 1999;116:15–21.

34
Impaired uptake of long-chain fatty acids contributes to fat malabsorption in paediatric patients with cystic fibrosis

H.J. VERKADE, D.M. MINICH, C.M.A. BIJLEVELD,
W.M.C. van AALDEREN, F. STELLAARD, R.J. VONK,
M. LASEUR and M. KALIVIANAKIS

INTRODUCTION

In humans, under physiological conditions, dietary fat is almost completely absorbed from the intestine[1], and triacylglycerols, composed of long chain fatty acids, constitute 92–96% of dietary fat[1]. The absorption of these fats comprises several processes (Figure 1): emulsification, lipolysis, solubilization, and translocation across the intestinal mucosa. Lipolysis is mediated by enzymes originating from the gastric mucosa and the pancreas, which hydrolyse the triacylglycerols into fatty acids and 2-monoacylglycerols. These lipolytic products are then solubilized in the intestinal lumen by bile components through the formation of mixed micelles and vesicles[2–4]. The mixed micelles are not absorbed intact, but disintegrate in the unstirred water layer, and the lipolytic products translocate across the intestinal epithelium[1,5]. Finally, the absorbed fatty acids and 2-monoacylglycerols are reacylated into triacylglycerols, assembled into chylomicrons and secreted across the basolateral membrane into the lymph[1].

The proportion of dietary fat absorption is significantly decreased in several diseases such as cystic fibrosis (CF)[6,7] and other forms of pancreatic exocrine insufficiency, end-stage liver disease[5,8,9] and essential fatty acid-deficiency[10]. The symptoms of pancreatic insufficiency, such as steatorrhoea and poor growth, can be alleviated by oral supplementation with pancreatic enzymes. However, despite recent improvements in the formulation of pancreatic enzyme supplements, many patients continue to experience mild steatorrhoea[11–13], and absorb only 80–90% of their dietary fat intake. It is not yet known why this is. Therapeutic improvements in fat absorption may be of benefit for CF patients, as a positive correlation has been observed between good nutritional status and

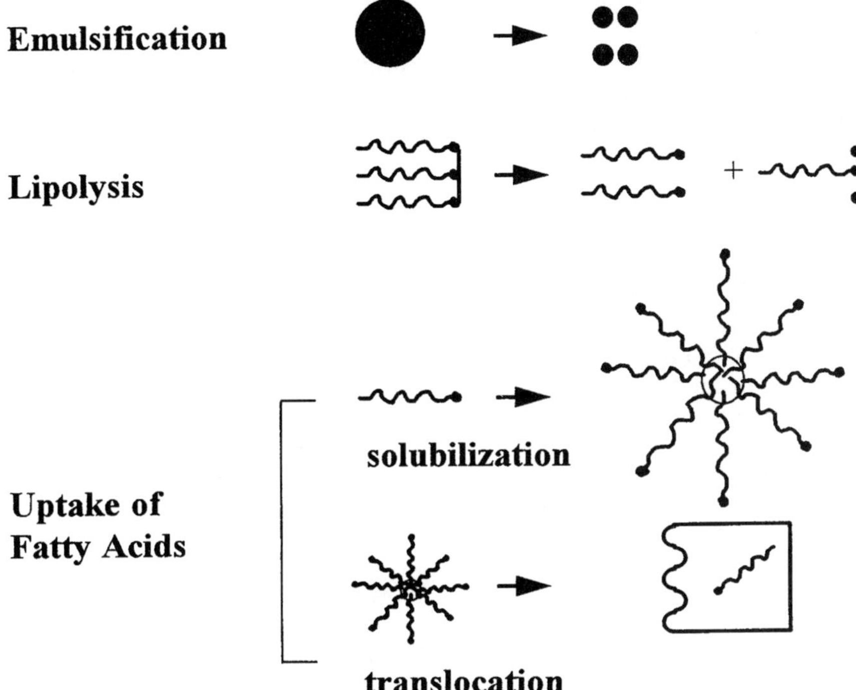

Figure 1. Physiological processes involved in fat absorption.

long-term survival and well-being of CF patients[6,14–15,25–27]. It has been demonstrated, however, that increasing the dose of pancreatic enzyme supplementation does not completely correct fat malabsorption[16], suggesting that additional factors may contribute.

An alternative explanation for continuing fat malabsorption in CF patients on pancreatic enzyme replacement therapy may involve the post-lipolytic events of the fat absorption process, leading to inefficient intestinal uptake of fatty acids[11,17,18]. Impaired fatty acid uptake in CF patients could be due to altered bile composition, decreased bile salt pool size and secretion rate, or bile salt precipitation at low intestinal pH[13,17,19–23]. Further on in the process, small bowel mucosal dysfunction or alterations in the small bowel mucus layer or mucosal function might contribute to inefficient uptake of long chain fatty acids[6,24].

The remaining fat malabsorption reflects insufficient lipolysis, due either to insufficient dosage of pancreatic enzyme replacement therapy or to adverse conditions in the intestinal lumen. Decreased pancreatic bicarbonate secretion, also due to pancreatic insufficiency, may lead to a sustained low pH in the duodenum[14], inhibiting the release of the enzymes from the acid-resistant coating of the (micro)capsules and promoting their inactivation.

The aim of the present study was to determine whether continued fat malabsorption encountered in paediatric CF patients on their habitual pancreatic enzyme replacement therapy results from insufficient lipolysis or from defective intestinal uptake of long chain fatty acids from the intestinal lumen. We chose to measure lipolysis and uptake by two independent tests in vivo. We used a previously validated method to determine lipase activity based on oral ingestion of a ^{13}C-labelled mixed triglyceride ([^{13}C]MTG: 1,3-distearoyl, 2[1-^{13}C]octanoyl glycerol) and measurement of $^{13}CO_2$ excreted in breath[28–32]. Inadequate intestinal uptake was measured by oral ingestion of a long chain fatty acid, ^{13}C-labelled linoleic acid ([^{13}C]LA)[33,34], and measurement of the concentration of [^{13}C]LA in plasma.

Fat balance studies cannot be used to assess the adequacy of these processes separately, or to determine in individual patients whether treatment should be improved by modulating diet, increasing pancreatic enzyme dose, and reducing acid secretion or supplementing bile salts. It has not yet been possible to determine whether continuing fat malabsorption in CF patients on normal doses of pancreatic enzyme is due to impaired lipolysis or reduced solubilization or uptake of long chain fatty acids.

SUBJECTS AND METHODS

Patients

The study group included 10 paediatric CF patients, three male and seven female, aged 7–18 years. The diagnosis of CF had been established by the sweat test and a DNA genotype analysis[35]. The ΔF508/ΔF508 genotype was present in six patients, and the ΔF508/other in four (subjects 1, 4, 8, 9). All patients were pancreatic insufficient and received enteric coated pancreatic enzymes. None of the patients received antacids.

Anthropometry

Anthropometric evaluation consisted of weight, height, mid arm circumference, and skinfold thickness measurements at four sites (biceps, triceps, subscapular, and suprailiac) made by one paediatrician. The Z-scores of all these anthropometric parameters were calculated based on the reference data for Dutch children described by Gerver and De Bruin[36]. The Z-score is defined as X-median/S where X is the patient's measurement, median is the median value for age and sex, and S is the standard deviation of the median. A negative value indicates a value under the median reference value.

Liver function tests

Liver function was screened by standard serum enzyme tests (γ-glutamyl transpeptidase, aspartate transaminase, and alanine transaminase) and by fasting plasma concentration of bile salt on the test day.

Diet evaluation

Intake of nutrients was calculated from 3-day consecutive food diaries by a dietitian using The Netherlands Nutrients Table 'NEVO' 1993. Intakes were

Table 1. Characteristics of cystic fibrosis patients included in the study

Patient	Sex	Age (years)	Weight (kg)	Energy (% RDA)	Carbohydrates (% energy)	Fats (% energy)	Protein (% energy)	Lipase enzymes (IU/g fat ingested)	Plasma bile salts (pmol/l)
1	F	18	55	66	52	33	15	560	13.8
2	F	18	58	104	52	31	17	710	13.5
3	M	16	53	115	48	39	13	1820	20.6
4	M	15	56	113	48	38	15	680	12.8
5	F	9	34	91	52	35	13	440	23.4
6	F	9	26	102	57	30	13	1520	13.5
7	M	8	23	110	50	37	13	830	11.8
8	F	7	27	111	52	35	13	590	18.2
9	F	7	24	92	56	32	12	860	11.6
10	F	7	23	121	54	35	11	460	30.3
Mean + SD				103 ± 16	52 ± 3	35 ± 3	14 ± 2	850 ± 460	16.6 ± 5.9

Normal range fasting plasma bile salts, 1–10 μmol/l.

expressed as the recommended dietary allowance (RDA) for weight, age and sex (Table 1).

^{13}C-labelled substrates

The mixed triglyceride (1,3-distearoyl, 2[1-^{13}C]octanoyl glycerol; S*OS) was purchased from Euriso-Top (Saint Aubin Cedex, France) and was 99% ^{13}C-enriched. ^{13}C uniformly labelled ^{13}C-LA (Campro Scientific B.V., Veenendaal, The Netherlands) had an enrichment exceeding 97% and was administered in a gelatin capsule coated with an acid-resistant layer consisting of 4.8% cellulose acetate hydrogen phthalate in acetone.

Study protocol

The study protocol was approved by the Medical Ethics Committee of the University Hospital Groningen, and included informed consent obtained from the parent and the children. The subjects were instructed to avoid consumption of naturally ^{13}C-enriched foods (e.g. corn or corn products, pineapple, cane sugar) for at least 2 days prior to the study. The [^{13}C]LA test and the [^{13}C]MTG test were performed on two subsequent days. On day 1, after an overnight fast, the patients received a capsule with [^{13}C]LA (1 mg/kg), together with their habitual breakfast (bread, butter, ham, cheese, etc.) and pancreatic enzymes. A baseline blood sample (EDTA) was collected before consumption of breakfast, every 2 h for 8 h afterwards, and at 24 h. Immediately after sampling, plasma was isolated and stored frozen (–20°C) until further analysis. On day 2, the patients received [^{13}C]MTG (4 mg/kg) mixed with their habitual breakfast and pancreatic enzymes. Breath samples were collected in duplicate at baseline and every 30 min for 6 h. After consumption of the breakfast on the first day, all faeces passed were collected for 3 days (72 h) to determine the presence of fat malabsorption. Faecal fat balance and both breath tests were performed in the same period. During the 3-day balance period, intake of nutrients was determined from food diaries. During the first 6 h of both tests, no additional food or liquids were permitted except for non-caloric drinks such as water and tea (without milk and sugar). After 6 h, patients were allowed to have their habitual lunch, including pancreatic enzymes.

Analytical techniques

Breath sample analysis

End-expiratory breath was collected via a straw into a 10 ml tube (Exetainers; Labco Limited, High Wycombe, UK), from which aliquots were taken to determine ^{13}C enrichment by means of continuous flow isotope ratio mass spectrometry (Finnigan Breath MAT, Finnigan MAT GmbH, Bremen, Germany), as described previously[29]. The ^{13}C abundance of breath CO_2 was expressed as the difference per ml from the reference standard Pee Dee Belemnite limestone (δ^{13}CPDB).

Mean values of whole body CO_2 excretion were measured by indirect calorimetry (Oxycon, model ox-4, Dräger, Breda, The Netherlands) over two separate periods of 5 min during both test days. This sampling method was compared to sampling every 30 min (results not shown). The results indicated that, under the test conditions chosen, the mean values of the CO_2 production obtained from two randomly chosen periods were within the 95% confidence interval of the mean values obtained with sampling every 30 min.

Plasma fats

Plasma fats were extracted, hydrolysed and methylated according to Lepage and Roy[37]. Resulting fatty acid methyl esters were analysed both by gas chromatography and by gas chromatography combustion isotope ratio mass spectrometry. Quantification of the resulting fatty acid methyl esters was performed with the use of heptadecanoic acid (C17:0) as an internal standard.

Faecal fats

Faecal fat was determined according to the method of Van de Kamer et al.[38] and expressed as g fat/day. The percentage of total fat absorption was calculated from the daily dietary fat intake and the daily faecal fat output and expressed as a percentage of the daily fat intake.

$$\frac{\text{fat intake (g/day)} - \text{faecal fat output (g/day)}}{\text{fat intake (g/day)}} \times 100\%$$

Plasma and faecal bile salts

Fasting and postprandial plasma bile salts were determined by an enzymatic fluorimetric assay[39]. Results were expressed as μmol/l. Faecal bile salts were extracted from an aliquot of dried homogenate of a 24 h faeces fraction[40] and fluorimetrically measured[39].

Gas liquid chromatography

Fatty acid methyl esters were separated and quantified by gas liquid chromatography on a Hewlett Packard gas chromatograph Model 5880 equipped with a CP-SIL 88 capillary column (Chrompack; 50 m × 0.32 mm) and an FID detector. The gas chromatograph oven was programmed from an initial temperature of 150°C to 240°C in two temperature steps (150°C held 5 min; 150–200°C, ramp 3°C/min held 1 min; 200–240°C, ramp 20°C/min, held 10 min). Adequate separation of linoleic acid could be achieved in this way. Quantification of the fatty acid methyl esters was done by adding heptadecanoic acid (C17:0) as internal standard.

Gas chromatography combustion isotope ratio mass spectrometry

[13]C enrichment of the palmitic acid methyl esters was determined on a gas chromatography combustion isotope ratio mass spectrometer (Delta S/GC Finnigan MAT, Bremen, Germany) equipped with an FID detector. Separation of the methyl esters was achieved on a CP-SIL 88 capillary column (Chrompack; 50 m × 0.32 mm), as described previously[34,41].

Statistics

The experimental data are reported as means ± SD. Corresponding to the literature[42–44], relationships between the percentage of total fat absorption and either plasma [^{13}C]LA concentrations or breath $^{13}CO_2$ expiration were considered exponential. All other correlations were assumed to be linear. Correlations between variables were calculated with the least squares method and are expressed as Pearson's coefficient of variation r. Differences between means were considered statistically significant at the level of $p < 0.05$.

RESULTS

Z-scores for all anthropometric parameters in CF patients were low to normal. For all parameters the 95% confidence interval did include the reference 50th centile line (Z-score 0), indicating no significant difference between our study group and the healthy reference population. Most patients had some degree of lung disease. Subjects 1 and 6–10 had normal liver biochemistry. Subject 3 was previously diagnosed as having liver cirrhosis with portal hypertension, and received ursodeoxycholic acid (750 mg/day). At the time of study, the condition of this patient had been stable for years. The bile salt concentration in plasma of this subject was in the same range as that of the other patients (Table 1). Analysis of 3-day dietary food records is shown in Table 1. In all patients approximately 50% of the energy was derived from carbohydrates, 35% from fat, and 15% from protein. Patients took pancreatic enzyme supplements in a dosage of approximately 400–1820 IU lipase/g fat ingested (Table 1).

Fat balance

Dietary intake of fat over the 3-day period ranged from 54 to 130 g/day, and the excretion of fat in faeces ranged from 5.1 to 27.8 g/day (Table 2). The percentage of total fat absorption ranged from 79 to 93% (Table 2). Under physiological conditions, healthy individuals excrete approximately 4–6 g/day of fat in the faeces[8], which generally means that over 96% of the dietary fats entering the intestinal lumen is absorbed[8]. These observations were confirmed by fat balance studies performed in our own laboratory in 13 healthy human adults (faecal fat excretion: 3.0 ± 0.9 g/day, total fat absorption: 97 ± 2%, data not shown). Despite standard pancreatic enzyme replacement therapy, faecal fat excretion in 8 out of 10 patients was > 6 g fat/day, and the percentage of total fat absorption was < 96% in all patients studied. No correlation was observed between the percentage of total fat absorption and the amount of pancreatic enzyme ingested (r = 0.12).

[^{13}C]MTG test

The baseline ^{13}C abundance in breath prior to consumption of the [^{13}C]MTG label was –23.3 ± 2.6% (range –25.5 to –17.1%). After ingestion of the [^{13}C]MTG label, different time-course patterns were observed for the excretion of ^{13}C label in breath over the 6 h study period (Figure 2A). When expressed as a

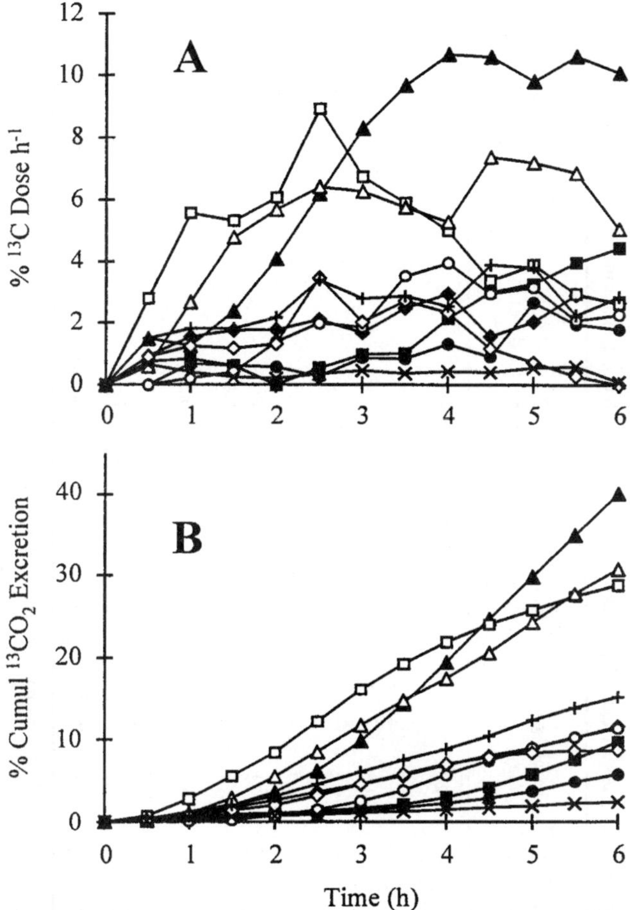

Figure 2. Time courses for the excretion of ^{13}C in breath over the 6 h study period following oral ingestion of [^{13}C]MTG (4 mg/kg) at time 0 in 10 CF patients. Each symbol represents a patient. (A) Excretion rate, (B) the cumulative $^{13}CO_2$ excretion.

proportion of administered ^{13}C, the excretion rate reached a mean maximum value of 4.9 ± 3.1%/h between 3 and 6 h after administration of the label (range 0.7–10.7%). Over the 6 h study period the cumulative excretion of ^{13}C in breath was 16.4 ± 12.5% of that administered, ranging between 2.4 and 40.2% (Figure 2B; Table 2). If defective lipolysis were responsible for the continuing fat malabsorption in CF patients, then a low percentage of fat absorption would be expected to correlate with low expiration of $^{13}CO_2$ after [^{13}C]MTG ingestion. However, no significant relationship was observed between 6 h cumulative $^{13}CO_2$ expiration and either daily faecal fat excretion (r = 0.02) or the percentage of total fat absorption (r = 0.04; Figure 3).

Table 2. Results of faecal bile salt concentrations, fat balance, [^{13}C]LA test and [^{13}C]-MTG test in the 10 cystic fibrosis patients included in the study

Patient	Faecal bile salts (mmol/kg wet weight)	Fat intake (g/day)	Faecal fat (g/day)	Total fat absorption (%)	[^{13}C]L test Plasma [^{13}C]-LA at 8 h (% dose)	[^{13}C]-MTG test Breath 6-h cumulative $^{13}CO_2$ (% dose)
1	30.2	54	4.9	91	1.5	2.4
2	10.6	85	7.0	92	1.9	9.7
3	0.7	124	14.8	88	0.9	15.1
4	8.7	133	27.8	79	0.6	5.8
5	22.1	92	9.6	90	1.3	30.8
6	20.5	66	5.1	92	2.0	11.3
7	5.3	85	6.1	93	1.3	40.2
8	6.8	93	16.7	82	0.5	28.9
9	16.1	64	9.2	86	0.5	11.5
10	16.7	88	7.1	92	1.2	8.7
Mean ± SD	13.8 ± 9.0	84 ± 22	11.1 ± 7.0	89 ± 5	1.2 ± 0.5	16.4 ± 12.5

LA, linoleic acid; MTG, mixed triglyceride. Normal range fecal bile salt: 0.1–1 mmol/kg faecal wet weight.

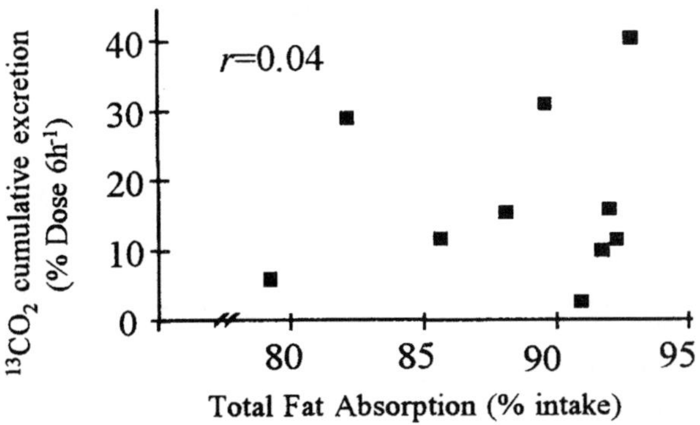

Figure 3. Relationship between the percentage of total fat absorption (72 h faecal fat balance) and the cumulative excretion of ^{13}C in breath over the 6 h study period following oral ingestion of [^{13}C]MTG (4 mg/kg) at time 0 in 10 CF patients.

[^{13}C]LA test

The baseline [^{13}C]LA abundance in plasma prior to consumption of [^{13}C]LA label was –29.1 ± 2.2% (range –32.6 to –25.5%). [^{13}C]LA concentration in plasma samples, expressed as percentage of the dose/l plasma, increased steeply after approximately 6 h (Figure 4). Peak values of [^{13}C]LA concentrations in plasma after administration occurred between 8 and 24 h. At 24 h after ingestion of the label, the enrichment of [^{13}C]LA in plasma had not yet returned to the level of baseline [^{13}C] abundance. Plasma 8 h [^{13}C]LA concentrations varied from 0.5 to 2.0% dose/l plasma (Table 2).

If defective intestinal uptake of long chain fatty acids were responsible for the continuing fat malabsorption in CF patients, then a low percentage of fat

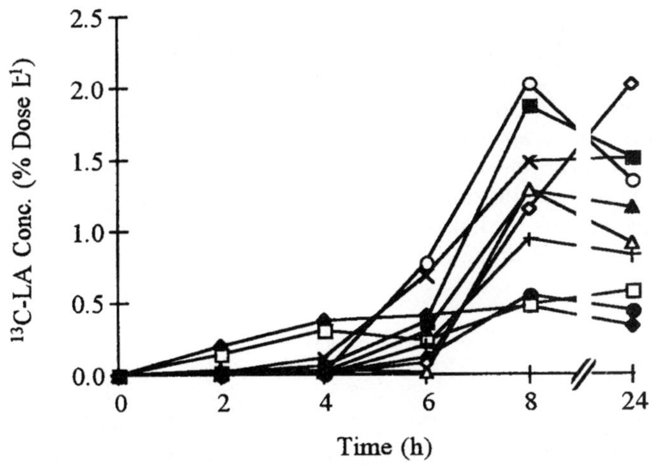

Figure 4. Time courses of [^{13}C]LA appearance in plasma of 10 CF patients after a single oral dose of [^{13}C]LA (2 mg/kg body weight) at time 0. Each symbol represents a patient.

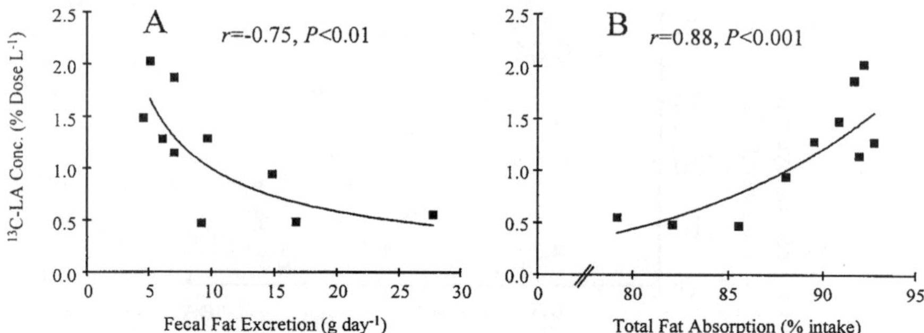

Figure 5. Relationship between the results of the 72 h faecal fat balance and the 8 h plasma [^{13}C]LA concentration after a single oral dose of [^{13}C]LA (1 mg/kg body weight) at time 0 in 10 CF patients. (A) Relationship between daily faecal fat excretion and 8 h plasma [^{13}C]LA concentration, (B) relationship between the percentage of total fat absorption and 8 h plasma [^{13}C]LA concentration.

absorption would be expected to correlate with low concentrations of [^{13}C]LA in plasma after [^{13}C]LA ingestion. Figure 5 shows the relationship between the 8 h plasma [^{13}C]LA concentrations and either faecal fat excretion or the percentage of total fat absorption. A strong, negative relationship was observed between faecal fat excretion and 8 h plasma [^{13}C]LA concentrations (Figure 5A; r = –0.75, $p < 0.01$) and, correspondingly, a strong, positive relationship was observed between the percentage of total fat absorption and 8 h plasma [^{13}C]LA concentrations (Figure 5B; r = 0.88, $p < 0.001$).

Total bile salt concentrations in plasma and faeces

Total bile salt concentrations were determined in plasma and faeces. Fasting plasma total bile salt concentrations in CF patients were high when compared with normal healthy control values and ranged from 11.6 to 30.3 μmol/l (mean 17.2 μmol/l, Table 1). Following a meal, there was no significant change in total plasma bile salts (data not shown). Faecal total bile salt concentrations in most CF patients were elevated (range 0.7–30.2; mean 13.8 mmol/kg faecal wet weight) when compared with healthy control values, indicating that they had bile salt malabsorption (Table 2). Bile salt malabsorption could result in a decreased amount of bile salts available for the formation of mixed micelles, leading to fat malabsorption. However, no significant correlation was found between percentage of dietary fat absorption and faecal bile salt concentrations (r = 0.26).

DISCUSSION

In CF patients, pancreatic enzyme replacement therapy frequently fails to restore fat absorption to normal. Our results of the 3-day fat balance confirm the presence of mild to moderate fat malabsorption (percentage of total fat absorption: 79–93%) in a group of paediatric CF patients on enzyme replacement therapy and in good clinical condition. The aim of the present study was to elucidate whether fat malabsorption in CF patients receiving habitual pancreatic enzyme replacement therapy is due to deficient lipolysis of triacylglycerols or due to impaired intestinal uptake of fatty acids.

We applied two fat substrates with different physical and chemical properties, i.e. [13C]MTG and [13C]LA. Efficient absorption of the 13C label from the mixed triglyceride is limited primarily by lipolysis[28]. After [13C]MTG ingestion, we found no relationship between recovery of $^{13}CO_2$ in breath and fat absorption coefficient, indicating that fat malabsorption in CF patients on their habitual enzyme replacement therapy is not likely to be related to defective lipolysis. The recovery of expired $^{13}CO_2$ obtained in the present study was similar to those obtained in other studies[28,30]. In healthy adults the 6 h cumulative percentage of 13C expired via the breath after ingestion of [13C]MTG varied between 23 and 52% of the dose in one study[28] and between 3 and 48% in another study[29], and in CF patients on pancreatic enzymes it varied between 0 and 45%[28,30]. In none of these studies was fat absorption related to the percentage of 13C recovered in the breath.

Efficient absorption of [13C]LA, a long chain unesterified fatty acid, differs predominantly from [13C]MTG in that it is independent of the efficacy of intestinal lipolysis (see also Figure 1), but depends on the postlipolytic events in fat absorption, solubilization and translocation across the intestinal mucosa[33,34]. The present methodology did not allow the discrimination between the solubilization or the translocation processes; therefore, these post-lipolytic events are referred to as the intestinal uptake of long chain fatty acids. Minich et al.[34] showed in a rat model for fat malabsorption (permanently interrupted enterohepatic circulation) that measuring plasma [13C]LA concentrations is a valuable method of assessing the intestinal uptake of long chain fatty acids, which correlates strongly with the efficacy of fat absorption. The [13C]LA test therefore distinguishes deficient intestinal uptake of long chain fatty acids from impaired lipolysis[34]. After ingestion of [13C]LA, a strong relationship was observed between 8 h plasma [13C]LA concentrations and total fat absorption, indicating that the observed fat malabsorption in CF patients on their habitual enzyme replacement therapy is due to defective intestinal uptake of long chain fatty acids.

As can be inferred from above, impaired intestinal uptake of long chain fatty acids may result from several processes. In the absence of adequate bicarbonate secretion, gastric acid entering the duodenum may lower intestinal pH until well into the jejunum[14]. Bile salts are readily precipitated in an acid milieu[17], and duodenal bile salt concentration may fall below the critical micellar concentration, thereby exacerbating fat malabsorption. Precipitated bile salts also appear to be lost from the enterohepatic circulation in greater quantities, thus reducing the total bile salt pool and decreasing the fraction of bile salts conjugated with glycine[23]. Intracellular events may also contribute to impaired uptake of long chain fatty acids in CF patients, e.g. due to absent fatty acid binding proteins or impaired chylomicron assembly and secretion[10]. Viscous, thick intestinal mucus, with altered physical properties, may have a deleterious effect on the thickness of the intestinal unstirred water layer, limiting translocation of long chain fatty acids across the intestinal epithelium[6,24,45.] Our data on increased faecal bile salt losses are in agreement with several other studies[19,46,47] and could be in agreement with a diminished bile salt pool in CF patients. Watkins et al.[21] showed, in a group of CF patients with normal faecal bile salt losses, that bile acid pool size nearly doubled during treatment with pancreatic enzymes. Although the present data suggest that the cause of continuing lipid malabsorption in cystic fibrosis on adequate enzyme treatment is related to insufficient long chain fatty acid uptake, they do not allow a clear identification of the specific process responsible for impaired uptake.

The [^{13}C]LA bolus was administered in an acid-resistant coated capsule, preventing the capsule from opening at a low pH environment (gastric or intestinal). In patients with a low intestinal pH due to inadequate bicarbonate secretion[14], the bioavailability of [^{13}C]LA was hypothesized to be impaired, resulting in a decreased amount of [^{13}C]LA incorporated into plasma linoleic acid. Since low intestinal pH affects uptake of long chain fatty acids, the acid-resistant capsule probably enhances the effect of the [^{13}C]LA test in correctly diagnosing solubilization disorders. The release of the substrate may be delayed in some patients, which explains the differences in timing for the offset of the individual [^{13}C]LA curves.

The study was designed such that the patients served as their own controls. Thus, in each individual patient we calculated the percentage of total fat absorption and related these results to the measurements of the [^{13}C]MTG breath test and the [^{13}C]LA test. We reasoned that these controls would be the most appropriate, given the fact that neither the optimal positive control group (pancreatic sufficient CF patients with known impaired intestinal uptake) nor the optimal negative control group (pancreatic insufficient CF patients with normal intestinal uptake) exists. The present approach allowed us to relate the results of total fat absorption to the results of lipolysis and intestinal uptake in the individual patient.

In conclusion, fat balance data indicate that, despite enzyme replacement therapy, paediatric CF patients have increased faecal fat excretion and, correspondingly, decreased percentage of fat absorption. The results of the [^{13}C]MTG test and [^{13}C]LA test indicate that continuing fat malabsorption is not likely to be due to insufficient enzyme replacement therapy, but rather due to defective intestinal uptake of long chain fatty acids. Indirect indications suggest that an increased bile salt loss leading to a diminished bile salt pool may contribute to this problem. However, preliminary studies in cystic fibrosis mouse models (*Cftr*-ΔF508/ΔF508 transgenic, *Cftr* –/–) strongly suggest that the increased loss of bile salts under cystic fibrosis conditions is independent of the presence or absence of lipid malabsorption and increased faecal lipid excretion[48]. Therapeutic attempts to normalize fat absorption in paediatric CF patients need to include a strategy to improve intestinal uptake of long chain fatty acids.

Acknowledgements

The authors thank J. Gerritsen, H. Elzinga, P.L.P. Brand, G. van Rijn and D. Theunissen for technical assistance, advice, and fruitful discussions; and the American Society for Clinical Nutrition for permission to reuse our recent data on this issue, published in the American Journal of Clinical Nutrition (1999;69:127–134).

REFERENCES

1. Carey MC, Hernell O. Digestion and absorption of fat. Semin Gastroint Dis. 1992;3:189–208.
2. Hernell O, Staggers JE, Carey MC. Physical-chemical behavior of dietary and biliary lipids during intestinal digestion and absorption. 2. Phase analysis and aggregation states of luminal lipids during duodenal fat digestion in healthy adult human beings. Biochemistry. 1990;29:2041–2056.
3. Staggers JE, Hernell O, Stafford RJ, Carey MC. Physical chemical behavior of dietary and biliary lipids during intestinal digestion and absorption. 1. Phase behavior and aggregation states of model lipid systems patterned after aqueous duodenal contents of healthy adult human beings. Biochemistry. 1990;29:2028–2040.
4. Verkade HJ, Tso P. Biophysics of intestinal luminal lipids. In: Mansbach CM, Tso P, Kuksis A (eds) Intestinal lipid metabolism. New York: Plenum Press, in press.
5. Tso P. Intestinal lipid absorption. In: Johnson LR (ed.) Physiology of the gastrointestinal tract. New York: Raven Press, 1994;1867–1907.
6. Pencharz PB, Durie PR. Nutritional management of cystic fibrosis. Annu Rev Nutr. 1993;13:111–136.
7. Shalon LB, Adelson JW. Cystic fibrosis: Gastrointestinal complications and gene therapy. Pediatr Clin North Am. 1996;43:157–196.
8. Carey MC, Small DM, Bliss CM. Lipid digestion and absorption. Annu Rev Physiol. 1983;45:651–677.
9. Porter HP, Saunders DR, Tytgat G, Brunser O, Rubin CE. Fat absorption in bile fistula. A morphological and biochemical study. Gastroenterology. 1971;60:1008–1019.
10. Minich DM, Vonk RJ, Verkade HJ. Intestinal absorption of essential fatty acids under physiological and essential fatty acid-deficient conditions. J Lipid Res. 1997;38:1709–1721.
11. Zentler-Munro PL, Fine DR, Batten JC, Northfield TC. Effect of cimetidine on enzyme inactivation, bile acid precipitation, and lipid solubilisation in pancreatic steatorrhoea due to cystic fibrosis. Gut. 1985;26:892–901.
12. Regan PT, Malagelada J-R, DiMagno EP, Go VLW. Reduced intraluminal bile acid concentrations and fat maldigestion in pancreatic insufficiency correction by treatment. Gastroenterology. 1979;77:285–289.
13. Carroccio A, Pardo F, Montalto G et al. Use of famotidine in severe exocrine pancreatic insufficiency with persistent maldigestion on enzymatic replacement therapy. A long-term study in cystic fibrosis. Dig Dis Sci. 1992;37:1441–1446.
14. Weber AM, Roy CC. Intraduodenal events in cystic fibrosis. J Pediatr Gastroenterol Nutr. 1984;8:S113–S119.
15. Robinson PJ, Smith AL, Sly PD. Duodenal pH in cystic fibrosis and its relationship to fat malabsorption. Dig. Dis Sci. 1990;35:1299–1304.
16. Robinson P, Sly P. High dose pancreatic enzymes in cystic fibrosis. Arch Dis Child. 1990;65:311–312.
17. Zentler-Munro PL, FitzPatrick WJF, Batten JC, Northfield TC. Effect of intrajejunal acidity on aqueous phase bile acid and lipid concentrations in pancreatic steatorrhoea due to cystic fibrosis. Gut. 1984;25:500–507.
18. Kalivianakis M, Verkade HJ. The mechanisms of fat malabsorption in cystic fibrosis patients. Nutrition. 1999;15:167–169.
19. O'Brien S, Mulcahy H, Fenlon H et al. intestinal bile acid malabsorption in cystic fibrosis. Gut. 1993;34:1137–1141.
20. Roy CC, Weber AM, Lepage G, Smith L, Levy E. Digestive and absorptive phase anomalies associated with the exocrine pancreatic insufficiency of cystic fibrosis. J Pediatr Gastroenterol Nutr. 1988;7 (Suppl 1):S1–S7.
21. Watkins JB, Tercyak AM, Szczepanik P, Klein PD. Bile salt kinetics in cystic fibrosis: influence of pancreatic enzyme replacement. Gastroenterology. 1977;73:1023–1028.
22. Roy CC, Weber EA, Morin CL et al. Abnormal biliary lipid composition in cystic fibrosis. Effect of pancreatic enzymes. N Engl J Med. 1977;297:1301–1305.
23. Belli DC, Levy E, Darling P, Leroy C, Lepage G. Taurine improves the absorption of a fat meal in patients with cystic fibrosis. Pediatrics 1987;80:517–523.
24. Eggermont E, De Boeck K. Small intestinal abnormalities in patients with cystic fibrosis. Eur J Pediatr. 1991;150:824–828.

25. Thomson MA, Quirk P, Swanson CE et al. Nutritional growth retardation is associated with defective lung growth in cystic fibrosis: A preventable determinant of progressive pulmonary dysfunction. Nutrition. 1995;11:350–354.
26. Macdonald A. Nutritional management of cystic fibrosis. Arch Dis Child. 1996;74:81–87.
27. Corey M, McLaughlin FJ, Williams M, Levison H. A comparison of survival, growth and pulmonary function in patients with cystic fibrosis in Boston and Toronto. J Clin Epidemiol. 1988;1:583–591.
28. Vantrappen GR, Rutgeerts PJ, Ghoos YF, Hiele MI. Mixed triglyceride breath test: a noninvasive test of pancreatic lipase activity in the duodenum. Gastroenterology. 1989;96:1126–1134.
29. Kalivianakis M, Verkade HJ, Stellaard F, Van der Werf M, Elzinga H, Vonk RJ. The ^{13}C-O mixed triglyceride breath test in healthy adults: determinants of the $^{13}CO_2$ response. Eur J Clin Invest. 1997;27:434–442.
30. Amarri S, Harding M, Coward WA, Evans TJ, Weaver LT. (13)Carbon mixed triglyceride breath test and pancreatic enzyme supplementation in cystic fibrosis. Arch Dis Child. 1997;76:349–351.
31. Swart GR, Baartman EA, Wattimena JL, Rietveld T, Overbeek SE, van den Berg JW. Evaluation studies of the ^{13}C-mixed triglyceride breath test in healthy controls and adult cystic fibrosis patients with exocrine pancreatic insufficiency. Digestion. 1997;58:415–420.
32. Kalivianakis M, Elstrodt J, Havinga R et al. Validation of the ^{13}C-mixed triglyceride breath test for the detection of intestinal lipid malabsorption. J Pediatr. 1999;135:444–450.
33. Watkins JB, Klein PD, Schoeller DA, Kirschner BS, Park R. Perman JA. Diagnosis and differentiation of fat malabsorption in children using ^{13}C-labelled lipids: trioctanoin, triolein and palmitic acid breath tests. Gastroenterology. 1982;82:911–917.
34. Minich DM, Kahvianakis M, Havinga R et al. Bile diversion in rats leads to a decreased plasma concentration of linoleic acid which is not due to decreased net intestinal absorption of dietary linoleic acid. Biochim Biophys Acta.1999;1438:111–119.
35. Kerem B-S, Rommens JM, Buchanan JA et al. Identification of the cystic fibrosis gene: genetic analysis. Science. 1987;245:1073–1080.
36. Gerver WJM, De Bruin R. Paediatric morphometrics: a reference manual. Utrecht: Bunge, 1996.
37. Lepage G, Roy CC. Direct transesterification of all classes of lipids in a one-step reaction. J Lipid Res. 1986;27:114–120.
38. van de Kamer JH, ten Bokkel Huinink H, Weyers HA. Rapid method for the determination of fat in feces. J Biol Chem. 1949;177:347–355.
39. Murphy GM, Billing BH, Baron DN. A fluorimetric and enzymatic method for the estimation of serum total bile acids. J Clin Pathol. 1990;23:594–598.
40. Kalek H-D, Stellaard F, Kruis W, Paumgartner G. Detection of increased bile acid excretion by determination of bile acid content in single stool samples. Clin Chim Acta. 1984;140:85–90.
41. Kalivianakis M, Minich DM, Bijleveld CM et al. Fat malabsorption in cystic fibrosis patients receiving enzyme replacement therapy is due to impaired intestinal uptake of long-chain fatty acids. Am J Clin Nutr. 1999;69:127–134.
42. Newcomer AD, Hofmann AF, DiMagno EP, Thomas PJ. Carlson GL. Triolein breath test: a sensitive and specific test for fat malabsorption. Gastroenterology. 1979;76:6–13.
43. Einarsson K, Bjorkhem I, Eklof R, Blomstrand R. ^{14}C-Triolein breath test as a rapid and convenient screening test for fat malabsorption. Scand J Gastroenterol. 1983;18:9–12.
44. Mills PR, Horton PW, Watkinson G. The value of the ^{14}C breath test in the assessment of fat absorption. Scand J Gastroenterol. 1979;14:913–921.
45. Smits CH, Veldman A, Verkade HJ, Beynen AC. The inhibitory effect of carboxymethylcellulose with high viscosity on lipid absorption in broiler chickens coincides with reduced bile salt concentration and raised microbial numbers in the small intestine. Poult Sci. 1998;77:1534–1539.
46. Weber AM, Roy CC, Morin CL, Lasalle R. Malabsorption of bile acid in children with cystic fibrosis. N Engl J Med. 1973;289:1001–1005.
47. Weber AM, Roy CC, Chartrand L et al. Relationship between bile acid malabsorption and pancreatic insufficiency in cystic fibrosis. Gut. 1976;17:295–299.
48. Kalivianakis M, Bronsveld I, de Jonge H et al. Increased fecal bile salt excretion is independent of the presence of dietary fat malabsorption in two mouse models for cystic fibrosis. FALK Proc. 1998;108:84.

Section XI
Concluding lecture

35
Bile acid science (cholanology) at the dawn of a new millennium: past progress and challenges for the future

A.F. HOFMANN

INTRODUCTION

The organizers of this workshop on bile acids held some 9 months before the first day of the third millennium (of the Christian calendar) have asked me to speculate about the future of cholanology (the science of bile acids) in the next century. In this chapter, I will summarize some of the achievements of bile research in the last two centuries and attempt to highlight challenges that face bile acid research in the coming century. I will make a few cautious predictions about the future, with the full realization that the record of eminent scholars and

Table 1. Judgements and predictions by experts[a]

Declaration	Declarer and Year of Declaration
"X-rays are a hoax"	Lord Kelvin, British physicist and engineer, 1900
"Everything that can be invented has been invented"	Charles Duell, Director of the US Patent Office, 1899
"I think there is a world market for about five computers"	Thomas Watson, Chairman of the IBM Corporation, 1943
"There is no reason for any individual to have a computer in the home"	Ken Olson, President of Digital Equipment Corporation, 1977
"By 1960, work will be limited to three hours a day"	John Langdon-Davies, British anthropologist and futurist
"The cloning of mammals ... is biologically impossible"	J. McGrath and D. Solter, writing in Science, 1984

[a]These and other judgements and predictions by experts can be found in Ref. 1.

entrepreneurs who have made predictions about the future is a very uneven one[1]. Table 1 lists some remarkably erroneous predictions and declarations. The field of cholanology is one of pure and applied biochemistry, and the achievements of biochemistry in the last century have been spectacular, far exceeding what anyone could have imagined 100 years ago[2,3]. Fifteen years ago, on the occasion of the sixtieth birthday of our sponsor, I attempted to summarize the current status of bile acid research and to indicate some of the areas in which there was likely to be substantial progress[4]. Eleven years ago, on the occasion of the 10th Bile Acid Meeting, a similar effort was made[5]. Let us hope that the present effort will contain no more errors than my previous endeavours. I shall limit my presentation to five main topics: bile acid chemistry; bile acid biochemistry (synthesis, conjugation, and transport); bile acids as nutritional biochemicals; bile acids as modulators of cholesterol metabolism; and bile acids as cytotoxic agents. References of journal articles that were cited on the previous reviews will be indicated occasionally by citing these reviews, rather than by citing the specific reference in order to reduce the number of citations in the bibliography.

BILE ACID CHEMISTRY

Bile acids as natural products

The chemistry of bile acids is an old field antedating modern biochemistry[6]. Elucidation of the cyclopentanoperhydrophenanthrene structure of cholesterol by Bernal in 1932 was one of the early great achievements resulting from the application of X-ray crystallography to organic molecules[4]. Using the structure established by Bernal, Rosenheim and King were able to propose the correct structure of many steroids and bile acids in a matter of months[4]. Only a few years before, Wieland and Windaus had received the Nobel prize for their remarkable studies of the chemistry of cholesterol and its metabolic products. Nonetheless, these magnificently talented chemists had to guess (and guessed wrongly) about the atomic arrangement of the steroid nucleus. Since that time, new bile alcohols and bile acids have been identified by many workers: notable contributions were made by the laboratories of the late G.A.D. Haslewood[7], T. Hoshita[8] and M. Tohma[9]. All primary bile acids and bile alcohols appear to have three features in common: they are the major end products of cholesterol metabolism; they are secreted into bile largely in conjugated form; and the conjugates are membrane-impermeable, water soluble, amphipathic molecules that have a powerful capacity to transform lamellar arrays of polar lipids into mixed micelles.

For more than a decade, I have been most fortunate to have Lee R. Hagey as a colleague in my laboratory. Dr. Hagey's doctoral thesis[10] reported the biliary bile acid (and alcohol) composition of a large number of vertebrates, based on his meticulous analyses of samples provided by the Zoological Society of San Diego. The data of Dr Hagey has shown the unique biodiversity of bile acids; Dr Hagey has also described a number of bile acids not previously reported.

Table 2. Primary bile acid structure in vertebrates: a simplified classification: default structure

Cholanoid class[a,b]	Nuclear hydroxyl groups	Side chain structure[c]	Terminal functional group[d]	Mode of conjugation
C_{27} bile alcohols	$3\alpha,7\alpha$	C8 (α,ϵ-dimethylhexanol)	C-27 = CH2OH	Sulphate
C_{27} bile acids	$3\alpha,7\alpha$	C8 (α,ϵ-dimethylhexanoic acid)	C-27 = COOH	Taurine
C_{24} bile acids	$3\alpha,7\alpha$	C5 (γ-methylbutanoic acid)	C-24 = COOH	Taurine (and congeners); glycine

[a] The subscript denotes the number of carbon atoms in the class.
[b] The A/B ring juncture is 5β (A/B *cis*) in most primary bile acids, and the default structure is defined as 5β. Exceptions are some reptilian species in which the preponderance of bile acids are in the 5α configuration (allo bile acids).
[c] In some rodent bile acids, a double bond is present between C-22 and C-23, so that the side chain has the structure of γ-methylbutenoic acid.
[d] The number indicates the carbon atom containing the terminal functional group.

With Dr Hagey, I have attempted to develop a simple classification of bile acids which would permit this area of biochemistry to be grasped easily[11]. We do not claim any originality in this work, as the principles of our classification scheme can be deduced from the writings of Haslewood[7], among others; but our approach has the benefit of simplicity. Of course, the problem with any simplifying scheme is that there are exceptions. The scheme is illustrated in Table 2.

There are three great classes of 'cholanoids' – the C_{27} alcohols, the C_{27} acids, and the C_{24} acids[11]. (Admittedly, the lamprey has C_{24} alcohols; but no other species possesses these novel bile alcohols which are eliminated via the renal system as the disulphate. In unpublished studies, we have tentatively identified (unconjugated) norcholic acid as the dominant bile acid of one deep sea fish.) Nonetheless, it is our opinion that probably more than 98% of vertebrate species will have biliary surfactants that fall into one of these three great cholanoid classes. Presumably which class of cholanoid is present in a vertebrate is determined by the evolution of peroxisomal enzymes as well as by the activity of sulphotransferases. If a bile alcohol is sulphated on the side chain, it cannot undergo oxidation to the C_{27} acid or oxidative cleavage to the C_{24} bile acid. Many species have two classes of cholanoids in their biliary surfactants, e.g. C_{27} bile alcohols and C_{24} bile acids.

We have also suggested that within each class of cholanoid it is useful to introduce the concept of a default cholanoid[11]. The default cholanoid has a hydroxy group at C-3 (from cholesterol) and at C-7 (as hydroxylation at C-7 appears to occur in virtually all cholanoids); the side chain has the structure that identifies the cholanoid class.

For the C_{24} bile acid, the default cholanoid is chenodeoxycholic acid (CDCA) in which the hydroxy groups at C-3 and at C-7 are in an α configuration. From a nomenclature point of view, it is a pity that this bile acid was not discovered first and given the name of 'cholsäure'. (Ursodeoxycholic acid (UDCA) is an exception in possessing a 7β-hydroxy group, but this is a primary bile acid only in bears and the nutria.) The default C_{27} bile alcohols and C_{27} bile acids have no accepted trivial names. Upon the three default structures are added additional hydroxy groups on the steroid nucleus, the side chain, or both. In bile alcohols, one or two additional hydroxy groups are added to the side chain, and usually only one additional hydroxy group is added to the nucleus. Since the default bile alcohol has three hydroxy groups (at C-3, C-7, and C-27), the final bile alcohol has five or six hydroxy groups). For primary C_{27} bile acids, one or two hydroxy groups are added to the side chain and seldom more than one hydroxy group is added to the nucleus. In most instances, C_{27} bile acids are tri- or tetra-hydroxy bile acids. For C_{24} bile acids, one hydroxy group may be added to the side chain and one hydroxy group may be added to the nucleus. However, usually only one additional hydroxylation occurs, with the result that most primary C_{24} bile acids are trihydroxy bile acids. Presumably what determines the site of additional hydroxylation is the specificity of microsomal hydroxylases.

The obvious challenge for the next century is to identify all sites of bile alcohol and bile acid hydroxylation. Because the default cholanoids have hydroxy groups at C-3 and C-7, one is concerned with identification of the third nuclear site of hydroxylation, as well as sites of side chain hydroxylation. Primary C_{24} bile acids with third site hydroxylations at C-1 (α and β), 2α, C-4(β), C-5(β), C-6(α and β), C-15(α), C-16(α), and C-19(β) have been identified. In the future, we are likely to find species that have other third site hydroxylation. Among C_{27} bile acids and C_{27} bile alcohols, relatively few novel sites of nuclear hydroxylation have been identified; however, little work has been done on this class of cholanoids.

There are far fewer sites for side chain hydroxylation. For C_{24} bile acids, the α hydroxy- (at C-23) and β hydroxy (at C-22) bile acids have been identified. Among the C_{27} bile acids, only C-22, C-24, and C-26 have been identified as sites of side chain hydroxylation. More work needs to be done to complete this chapter of natural product chemistry. Table 3 summarizes information that is currently available on the additional hydroxylation sites in the three cholanoid classes.

Confirmation of the structure of newly identified bile alcohols and bile acids is best done by chemical synthesis. Dr C. Cerré working in association with Dr Claudio Schteingart of our laboratory reported the synthesis of 5β hydroxy bile acids[12]. Iida and his colleagues, following up the work of the late Fred Chang, have synthesized many of the epimers of natural bile acids[13]. Tohma and his colleagues have synthesized 1β, 3α, 7α-trihydroxy-cholanoic acid[9] and 3α, 7α, 19-trihydroxy-cholanoic acid[14]; and a large variety of bile alcohols have been made in the laboratory of T. Hoshita in Hiroshima[15], as well as in that of G. Salen and A. Batta in Jersey City[16]. A challenge for the future is to prepare 3α, 7α, 16α-trihydroxy-5β-cholan-24-oic acid, a bile acid identified by Hagey as occurring in many avian species[10].

Bile acids (and alcohols) show a biodiversity in structure that is unique among small molecules in vertebrates. This biodiversity indicates that there are many biochemical solutions to the problem of eliminating cholesterol in the form of water soluble amphipathic membrane-impermeable molecules. It was the hope of G.A.D. Haslewood that bile acid biodiversity would provide useful information on evolutionary relationships[7]. At the moment, this view is not shared (or

Table 3. Primary bile acid structure in vertebrates: a simplified classification. Additional nuclear and side chain hydroxyl groups

Cholanoid class	Default nuclear hydroxyl groups[a]	Sites of additional nuclear hydroxyl groups[b]	Default side chain hydroxyl group	Sites of additional side chain hydroxyl groups[c]	Occurrence in vertebrates[c]
C_{27} bile alcohols	$3\alpha, 7\alpha$	$2\beta, 6\alpha, 12\alpha, 16\alpha$	27	24, 25, 26	Ancient mammals, amphibia, reptiles, cartilaginous fish
C_{27} bile acids	$3\alpha, 7\alpha$	$12\alpha, 16\alpha$	None	$22(S), 24(R), 25, 26$	Amphibia, reptiles, ancient birds
C_{24} bile acids	$3\alpha, 7\alpha$	$1\alpha, 1\beta, 2\alpha, 4\beta, 5(\beta), 6\alpha, 6\beta$ $15\alpha, 16\alpha, 19(\beta)$	None	$22(S), 23(R)$	Reptiles, bony fish, birds, mammals

[a] Notable exceptions include animals in which the hydroxyl group at C-7 is in a β configuration (nutria, bears) or an oxo group is present at C-7 (guinea pig). In some reptiles, a $3\alpha, 16\alpha$-dihydroxy bile acid may be a primary bile acid.

[b] In most bile alcohols and bile acids, not more than one additional nuclear hydroxyl group is present; accordingly most primary bile acids are dihydroxy (possessing the default nuclear hydroxyl groups) or trihydroxy.

[c] In most bile alcohols, one, two, or three additional hydroxyl groups may be present on the side chain. In most bile acids, either no or one additional hydroxyl group is present.

has not even been noticed) by evolutionary biologists, who believe that DNA analysis is a uniquely valuable tool for this purpose. In addition, most have never heard of bile acids and bile alcohols. Nonetheless, Dr. Hagey's studies have linked bile acid structure to evolutionary relationships in the flamingo and other wading birds[17], in the sperm whale[18], and in the Ursidae (bears)[19]. To date, this work has had little impact on the thinking of the evolutionary biologists. My prediction for the next decades is that this situation is unlikely to change unless there is independent confirmation of the relationships elucidated by such studies of bile acid structure. At its least, definition of the biliary bile acid composition of individual species may be considered to be another chapter in descriptive (phenotypic) biology, which certainly has a glorious history!

In most species, biliary bile acids and bile alcohols occur largely in con-jugated form. For C_{27} bile alcohols, conjugation is exclusively with sulphate. Such sulphate conjugation renders the compound water-soluble and capable of forming mixed micelles. For C_{27} and C_{24} bile acids, conjugation is with taurine in the majority of species[11]. A few species conjugate with derivatives of taurine (cysteinolic acid in the sea bream[20]; N-methyltaurine in some angel fish[10]), but taurine conjugation predominates. In mammals (and some species of pigeons), conjugation with glycine occurs. Conjugation with taurine or glycine lowers the pK_a of the ionizing group of the side chain, and results in the bile acid molecule being more soluble, fully ionized and membrane impermeant at the pH conditions prevailing in the biliary tract and small intestine[21].

Structure–activity relationships

General considerations

Cholanoid structure can be considered in terms of the two major functions of bile acids: elimination of cholesterol and formation of mixed micelles. For the elimination of cholesterol, the only structural requirement of the bio-transformation product is to be a substrate for the canalicular transporter and to remain unabsorbed in the biliary tract and intestine. For the formation of mixed micelles, the bile acid molecule must not only possess these properties, but must also be capable of forming mixed micelles with polar lipids. Such micelle for-mation should occur at relatively low concentration, and also be highly efficient; that is each bile acid molecule should solubilize one or more polar lipid mole-cules. For promotion of lipid absorption, there are additional requirements. First, for the accumulation of a cycling bile acid pool, an event that disassociates secretion from biosynthesis, an enterohepatic circulation is required. Second, to increase the concentration of bile acids in bile that is secreted into the intestine, concentration in the gallbladder is required. Finally, to maintain a high intralu-minal concentration, one requires molecules that are impermeable to cell mem-branes and that remain in solution in micellar form despite acidic pH, a high Na^+ concentration, and the presence of hydrophobic residues in chyme.

Nuclear biotransformations

In the conversion of cholesterol to the default cholanoids, the 3α-hydroxy group undergoes oxidation to a 3-oxo-Δ^4 intermediate, which is then reduced to give a

3α-hydroxy 5β acid. Defects in oxido-reduction in the A ring are associated with cholestatic disease, but the pathogenetic defect appears to be the inability of the canalicular transport system to transport 3β-hydroxy or 3-oxo bile acids[22]. As a result, they accumulate in the hepatocyte and cause necrosis or apoptosis. Both 3β-hydroxy and 3-oxo bile acids are water soluble, and it seems likely that the A ring changes are not required to convert cholesterol into a water soluble derivative. On the other hand, hydroxylation at C-7 is essential for water solubility, as bile acids substituted only at C-3 are quite insoluble at physiological temperatures[23].

CDCA is the predominant bile acid of several mammalian species[10]. Because the conjugates of CDCA are fully water soluble and form mixed micelles at relatively low concentrations, it seems curious that trihydroxy bile acids predominate in so many species. Trihydroxy bile acids form mixed micelles at higher concentrations and are, therefore, less potent solubilizers. We have speculated[24] that there are no functional advantages associated with the formation of trihydroxy bile acids per se. Rather, the formation of trihydroxy bile acids is useful in species possessing an anaerobic caecum in which bacterial 7-dehydroxylation occurs rapidly. If CDCA undergoes 7α-dehydroxylation it forms lithocholic acid (LCA) which is hepatotoxic whenever its proportion in biliary bile acids exceeds 10%[25]. Formation of a 3,7,X-trihydroxy bile acid prevents formation of LCA. Presumably all 3,X-dihydroxy bile acids are less toxic than LCA. Those species having considerable proportions of CDCA in biliary bile acids which also possess an anaerobic caecum have developed methods for detoxifying LCA. These include rehydroxylation to CDCA, hydroxylation at another site, to form a 3,Y-dihydroxy bile acid, and sulphation at the 3 position to form a sulphated lithocholic acid conjugate, which is rapidly eliminated from the enterohepatic circulation[24].

Extensive study of micelle formation by natural synthetic bile acids has led to the conclusion that for bile acids to form micelles at relatively low concentrations (< 10 mM), the side chain cannot be shorter than five carbon atoms, and the nuclear substituents must all be on the α face, so that the contiguous hydrophobic surface of the β face is sufficiently large to promote self-association[26]. Synthetic bile acids with hydroxy groups on the β face either have a high critical micellar concentration (CMC) or do not form micelles at all.

Little information is available on side chain structure–function relationships. The physicochemical properties of a common C_{27} bile alcohol sulphate, scymnol sulphate, have been examined and shown to differ little from those of cholyl-taurine (taurocholate)[27]. In principle C_{27} bile acids possessing a C_8 side chain should have higher critical micellization temperature (CMT, Krafft point) than C_{24} bile acids possessing a C_5 side chain; but this has not been tested. A bile acid with a low CMT is useful for species such as arctic fish whose body temperature is close to the freezing point of water. As noted above, bile acids with a side chain shorter than five carbon atoms have a CMC which is well above the concentrations that occur physiologically. Hydroxylation of the side chain at C-23 (and conjugation with taurine) was shown to result in a molecule that is more resistant to bacterial deconjugation than the corresponding bile acid lacking a C-23 hydroxy group[28].

Sulphate and taurine conjugates are fully ionized at physiological pH. When a bile alcohol sulphate undergoes deconjugation, an insoluble, membrane impermeable molecule is formed that will be promptly lost from the enterohepatic circulation[27]. However, it is not known whether deconjugation of bile alcohol sulphates occurs during small intestinal transit because little information is available on the deconjugating activity of small intestinal bacteria in species which have bile alcohol sulphates as a major biliary surfactant. Sulphatases are not present in pancreatic enzymes. Taurine- and glycine-conjugated bile acids may be termed N-acyl amidates (or aminoacyl amidates or simply amidates) to distinguish them from sulphate and glucuronide conjugates. Bile acid amidates containing glycine or taurine are resistant to pancreatic carboxypeptidases, whereas synthetically prepared amidates containing other common amino acids are rapidly cleaved[29]. Thus, conjugation of bile acids with taurine or glycine, or of bile alcohols with sulphates, results in molecules that are soluble, indigestible, and non-absorbable. Bile acid amidates differ from bile alcohol sulphates in that the unconjugated bile acid formed by bacterial deconjugation can be absorbed passively in its protonated form; if ionized, it can participate in micelle formation. In contrast, the liberated bile alcohol is poorly soluble, and is membrane impermeable. Thus, from the point of view of either conserving function or conserving the molecule, bile acid amidates are superior to bile alcohol sulphates, if subjected to bacterial deconjugation during small intestinal transit.

In summary, there is now some understanding of the biological utility of both the nuclear and side chain biotransformations that occur during bile acid synthesis and conjugation. One challenge for the next century is to define the differences in physicochemical properties between C_{27} and C_{24} bile acids (possessing the same nuclear substituents). Because the C_8 side chain is extensively branched, my prediction is that the differences will be small. The major difference is that the CMC of the C_{27} bile acids will be slightly lower and the CMT slightly higher than those of the corresponding C_{24} bile acid. Such a comparison, although desirable, is unlikely to provide major new biological insights.

BILE ACID CHEMISTRY: MIXED MICELLE FORMATION

In his elegant review of micelle formation, the late G.S. Hartley predicted that bile acid anions would self-associate to form micelles[30], a prediction confirmed repeatedly over the next five decades. The arrangement of molecules in 'simple' bile acid micelles has continued to intrigue workers, and the laboratory of Giglio and colleagues[31] has presented evidence from a variety of experimental approaches that the aggregates are helical. It seems likely that the self-association of bile acid anions to form helical aggregates is of little biological relevance, as simple micelles do not occur in vivo, except transiently or in the *mdr2* knockout mouse.

The aggregate that occurs in vivo is the mixed micelle. In bile, the mixed micelle consists of molecules of bile acids, phosphatidylcholine (PC) and cholesterol; this may be termed the biliary mixed micelle. In small intestinal contents the mixed micelle consists of molecules of bile acids, fatty acids (partially ionized) and monoglycerides; this may be termed the intestinal mixed micelle.

Definition of the molecular arrangement of the biliary and intestinal mixed micelles is a biophysical problem, and physicians in general have little biophysical training. Franz Ingelfinger arranged for Donald Small to work in the laboratory of D.G. Dervichian where they were able to define the phase equilibria of model systems simulating bile in a remarkably short time[32]. Subsequently D.M. Small spent a brief time in the laboratory of Dennis Chapman, then at Uniliver, where they obtained NMR data that were interpreted as indicating that the biliary mixed micelle was disc shaped, with the PC and cholesterol molecules arranged in a bilayer of cylindrical shape that was coated on the outside by bile acid molecules[33]. In the past decade, the validity of this view has been questioned. Hjelm et al.[34], on the basis of data obtained by small angle neutron scattering, have proposed that the solubilized lipids are not present in a bilayer arrangement (with the fatty acid chains parallel) but in a radial arrangement identical to that in a hexagonal phase of soap molecules. The bile acid molecules sit between the polar heads of the PC molecules with their hydrophilic (α) face facing the aqueous environment. The charge on the bile acid anion causes the cylinders of PC molecules to repel each other. At high bile acid/PC ratios, the shape of the aggregate approaches a sphere. Hjelm et al. extended their insightful work on the biliary mixed micelle to the intestinal mixed micelle and showed that both micelles have exactly the same structure using small angle neutron scattering[35]. If this view is correct, the major physicochemical action of bile acids is to transform an insoluble bilayer to a dispersed mixed micelle. The former array is insoluble; the mixed micelle, in contrast, is soluble and diffusible. Thus, bile acids change the arrangement of lipids from lamellar to hexagonal, and the classical McBain soap-water phase diagram (redrawn in ref. 23) is adequate to explain the actions of bile acids. Therefore, the action of bile acids in the biliary canaliculus, where they solubilize PC vesicles to form micelles, is completely similar to their action at the surface of the triglyceride droplet where they solubilize lamellar fatty acids and monoglycerides to form mixed micelles. This concept is illustrated in Figure 1.

It would appear from the above discussion that a new unifying paradigm has been discovered. The data obtained during decades of work aimed at elucidating the physical chemistry of bile have joined the data aimed at elucidating the physical chemistry of fat digestion; the physiological processes are identical from a physicochemical standpoint. The challenge for the next century is to provide a valid physical theory for the ability of bile acids to transform a lamellar phase into a cylindrical (or spherical) micellar phase. Phase equilibria for bile acid–amphiphilic lipid–water systems have been defined for relatively few bile acids, but construction of such diagrams is unlikely to provide major new biochemical insights. Probably the greatest challenge for the next decade is to communicate the advances in bile acid physical chemistry to the biochemical and biophysical community.

BILE ACID CHEMISTRY: CHEMICAL ANALYSIS

To develop and validate an analytical method, pure standards are needed. A half century ago the only bile acids that were available in high purity from biochemical supply houses were cholic acid and deoxycholic acid. Deoxycholic

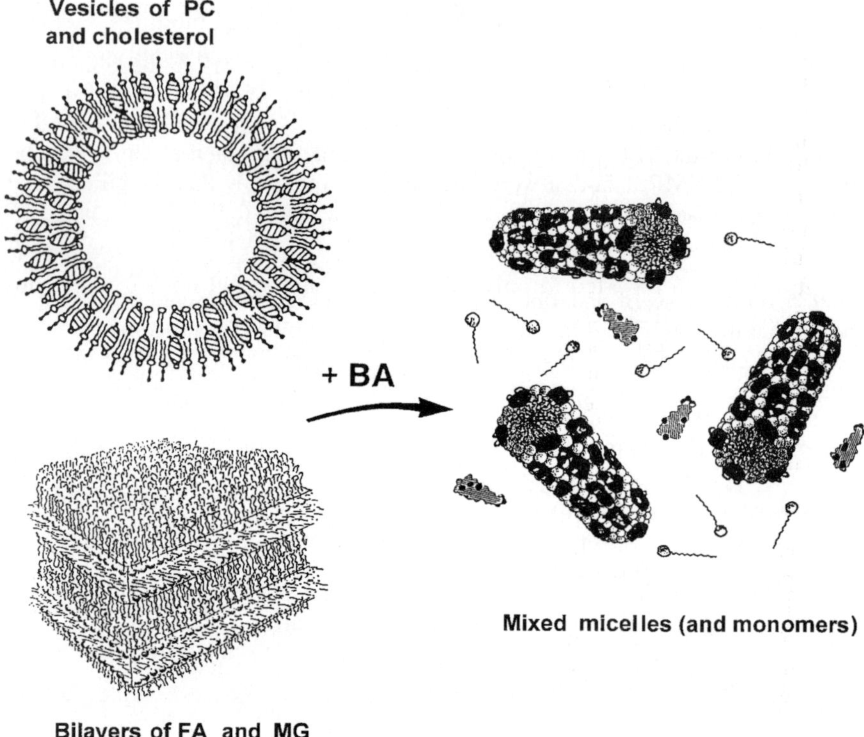

Figure 1. Conversion of phospholipid-cholesterol vesicles in the canaliculus (upper left) or fatty acid-monoglyceride lamellae in small intestinal content to mixed micelles by bile acids (BA). The mixed micelles present in canalicular bile during bile formation and in small intestinal content during fat digestion are thought to have the same molecular structure. The figure has been published previously[150].

acid was used as a precursor for the synthesis of cortisone (with a hydroxy group at C-11), but this approach was abandoned when 11-hydroxylated plant steroids were discovered that could be converted without undue difficulty to cortico-steroids[36]. Fieser's group described a synthesis of CDCA[37], but the procedure was difficult and gave low yields. The synthesis of CDCA from cholic acid was undertaken in England by Smithfield Laboratories, but few were aware of this effort. CDCA only became available as a routine laboratory chemical after it was introduced into clinical medicine for the dissolution of gallstones as a result of studies at the Mayo Clinic[38]. Of the four 3,6,7, trihydroxy epimers (α- and β-hyocholic; α- and β-muricholic), only α-hyocholic acid is readily available today, and the situation is unlikely to change in the next few decades.

Half a century ago, methods for preparing conjugated (amidated) bile acids were complex. Advances in peptide synthesis led to the introduction of the mixed carboxylic carbonic acid anhydride method which was used by Norman to describe the synthesis (and properties) of all of the common conjugated bile acids in his elegant doctoral thesis[39]. The method has been modified with newer coupling agents[40], and reasonably pure glycine and taurine amidates of the three most common natural bile acids (CA, CDCA, DCA) are commercially available. A method for eliminating surface active impurities in these compounds has recently been reported[41].

Lithocholic acid is eliminated in man predominantly as the sulphated glycine and taurine amidates. Methods for synthesizing the sulphated amidates have been reported[42]. Synthesis of the C-3 ethereal glucuronides[43] and C-24 ester glucuronides[44] has also been reported. All of these syntheses are relatively difficult, have been reported in only milligram amounts, and none of these novel conjugates is available commercially.

When the modern era of bile acid research began some 50 years ago, analytical methods for measuring bile acid concentrations were primitive. A widely used technique was based on converting bile acids to an unsaturated derivative using concentrated sulphuric acid. The principle of this technique has only recently been elucidated[45]. The last four decades have witnessed the development of extraordinarily powerful analytical techniques in organic chemistry: TLC, HPLC, GC/MS, MS/MS, and NMR. All have been applied fruitfully to bile acid analysis, and the contributions of Jan Sjövall and Ken Setchell have been particularly noteworthy[46]. TLC is a semi-quantitative technique but is rapid and simple, and plays an invaluable role in purification of labelled bile acids. The convenience of a rigid support resulted in TLC quickly replacing paper chromatography. HPLC separation of conjugated bile acids is straightforward, but the lack of UV absorbing groups in unconjugated bile acids makes measurement of a mixture of conjugated and unconjugated bile acids difficult. Laser light scattering devices offer a solution to this problem. Sjövall and his colleagues introduced several novel adsorbents that permit the rapid resolution of bile acid mixtures into well defined classes, and these are generally used for analysis of complex matrices such as urine and faeces[47]. Roda has recently reviewed available separation techniques[48].

For unconjugated bile acid mixtures, GC/MS offers excellent resolution and unequivocal identification. Introduction of cholylglycine hydrolase by Nair[49] was highly useful for C_{24} bile acids, but as yet a comparable enzyme that deconjugates C_{27} amidates has yet to be isolated. This is a task for the coming decade.

Enzymatic analysis, based on the ability of the 3-hydroxy steroid dehydrogenase isolated from *Pseudomonas testosteroni* was introduced by Talalay for steroid analysis[50] and subsequently adapted for bile acid analysis by Iwata and Yamasaki[51]. Later, individuals such as R.H. Palmer emphasized the utility of the method[52], which was modified still further by Turley and Dietschy[53]. In the original description of the methodology, the reduction of NAD was determined spectrophotometrically, a technique of limited sensitivity. The sensitivity of the method was improved by measuring the change in fluorescence caused by reduction of the NAD; this method was in turn superseded by coupling the reduction of the NAD to reduction of a tetrazolium dye[54]. The sensitivity was still further increased by developing amplification techniques and probably increased to the maximum sensitivity possible by developing a solid phase technique in which the readout involved luciferase[55]. The technique is highly useful for repetitive analyses of total bile acid concentration in bile or intestinal content, body fluids with bile acid concentrations in the millimolar range. For measurement of plasma bile acids where concentrations are in the micromolar range, the enzymatic method using reduction of a tetrazolium dye as readout is of sufficient sensitivity to detect increases in cholestatic liver disease, but not of sufficient sensitivity to detect decreases from the normal level. Here, the bioluminescence procedure has been shown to be sufficient to detect decreases in postprandial elevation caused by bile aid sequestrant ingestion[56]. There are some unidentified compounds in plasma that are measured by the enzymatic technique with the result that values obtained for plasma bile acids are erroneously high; the magnitude of the error is small[57].

Competitive binding techniques were useful historically to define the determinants of plasma bile acid levels in health[58,59], as well as to examine whether measurement of fasting state plasma bile acids provided diagnostic information that was superior to that afforded by conventional liver tests in patients with liver disease[60]. Relatively few monoclonal antibodies to bile acids have been reported, and no laboratory has reported the development of a mixture of monoclonal antibodies that would measure either total plasma bile acids (conjugated and unconjugated) or total plasma conjugated bile acids.

I conclude that the problems of measurement of bile acids in body fluids have largely been solved, at least in principle. The best method is GC/MS after chromatographic separation of classes, but such complex methodology may not always be necessary. FA BS-MS appears to be the best method for detection of inborn errors of bile acid biosynthesis. Relatively inexpensive mass spectrometers (specific ion detectors) are now available, but the FABS device is not available on these instruments. Were it to become available, relatively low cost instrumentation for the detection of inborn errors of bile acid biosynthesis would be available to major medical centres.

For measurement of bile acid monomer activity in the presence of micelles or binding molecules (for example, sequestrants or proteins), bile acid specific electrodes have been reported by several groups[61,62]. At present, such electrodes must be developed by the investigator who in turn must define their specificity and reactivity with bile acids of varying chemical structure. High concentrations of bile acids may poison such electrodes, and membranes that exclude bile acid aggregates have been developed.

The challenges in analytical methodology for the coming decades can be summarized:

(1) Development of an enzymatic method with a colorimetric readout that has an order of magnitude greater sensitivity than current methods.
(2) Development of a library of monoclonal antibodies that will permit state of the art competitive binding methods to be developed for plasma bile acid analysis.
(3) Development of inexpensive FABS/MS machines that would greatly decrease the cost of instrumentation required for the detection of inborn errors of bile acid biosynthesis.

Of these three desiderata, I think only the last is a realistic possibility. Lack of interest in the first two challenges relates to the practice and economics of clinical medicine. The clinician is not demanding measurements of plasma bile acids. His disinterest arises from his (or her) conviction that bile acid measurements will not provide cost-effective information that improves diagnosis or patient outcome. On the other hand development of low cost FABS/MS devices would have widespread applicability in paediatric centres interested in early detection of inborn errors of metabolism.

BILE ACID CHEMISTRY: RADIOACTIVE BILE ACIDS

Isotopically labelled bile acids are essential for defining pathways of bile acid metabolism and measurement of bile acid pool size and turnover rate[63]. Radioactive and stable isotopes each have their respective advantages and disadvantages[64]. For animal studies, radioactive bile acids are far more convenient. For human studies, bile acids tagged with stable isotopes permit studies without concern of radiation exposure, but measurement of isotope enrichment requires complex and expensive instrumentation. When ^{14}C became available in the 1950s, Sune Bergström, then in Lund, Sweden, quickly developed a method for the synthesis of $24\text{-}^{14}C$-tagged bile acids, and used these radiolabelled bile acids to establish many of the principles of bile acid metabolism that remain valid today[65]. Sven Lindstedt, in that group, prepared randomly labelled ^{3}H bile acids and used these to report the first values for bile acid kinetics in man[66]. Our group, working with Peter Klein, described the synthesis of $2,4\text{-}^{3}H$-labelled bile acids, but showed that some of the label was lost during enterohepatic cycling[67]. We subsequently reported the synthesis of $11,12\text{-}^{3}H$-tagged di- and monohydroxy bile acids; again, the label was imperfect in its biological behaviour[68]. Recently, we have prepared $22,23\text{-}^{3}H$ bile acids by reductive tritiation of the $\Delta^{22,23}$ derivative of the common natural bile acids. With Duane, we showed that such a label is completely stable during enterohepatic cycling in man[69]. Thus, the problem of preparing radioactively tagged bile acids appears to be solved. As yet, such $22,23\text{-}^{3}H$-tagged bile acids are not available from radiochemical supply houses, but they will be offered if demand is sufficiently great.

BILE ACID CHEMISTRY: IMPROVING NATURAL BILE ACIDS

Bile acids have had millions of years to evolve, and it is reasonable to ask whether a synthetically prepared derivative of a natural bile acid could have physicochemical or physiological properties that are superior to those of the natural bile acid.

Three types of modifications have been made and shown to have value for biological or clinical purposes. The first is to synthesize bile acids that are resistant to bacterial dehydroxylation. For unconjugated bile acids, the effort has concentrated on derivatives of UDCA with a substituent at C-7 such as a methyl group[70] or a fluoro substituent at C-6[71]. A variety of side chain modified bile acids have been prepared that are resistant to both deconjugation and dehydroxylation. These include C_{24}-sulphonates, in which the carboxyl group has been replaced by a sulphonic acid group[72,73]. It also includes C_{26} bile acids with a

β-keto group, as well as bile acids with modified side chains, for example, 22,24-cyclopropyl bile acids[74]. Proline conjugates have also been made and shown to be resistant to deconjugation–dehydroxylation[75]. Perhaps the simplest approach has been the preparation of sarcosine (N-methyl conjugates) which in animals and humans are resistant to deconjugation–dehydroxylation[76,77]. To date, only the sarcosine conjugate of cholic acid (cholylsarcosine) has been introduced into clinical studies and shown to have therapeutic value (see below).

Two approaches have been made to visualizing bile acids. For visualizing the bile acids during transport at a microscopic level, a fluorescent tag could be useful, provided the fluorescent bile acid behaved in the same manner as its corresponding untagged precursor. The smallest fluorophore that is conveniently coupled to a bile acid is the NBD group, and the laboratory of G. Kurz in Freiburg reported the synthesis and biological properties of a variety of fluorescent bile acids tagged with NBD at C-3, C-7, or C-12[78]. The synthesis of such bile acids is difficult and few other laboratories have repeated this work. Such compounds are not available commercially, and the total amount that remains today is quite small.

Coupling of fluorescein to cholyglycine was reported by Sherman and Fisher[79], who believed that the fluorescein was coupled to C-3. Subsequently, Schteingart in our laboratory showed that the fluorescein was coupled to the carboxyl group of the glycine moiety[80]. We have prepared a group of fluorescent bile acids in which the amino group of aminofluorescein is coupled to the carboxyl group of an unconjugated or glycine-amidated bile acid. Such bile acids are transported to a varying extent by hepatocyte transport systems, but not by the bile acid transport systems of the ileal enterocyte[81]. A final approach to the synthesis of fluorescent bile acids is to conjugate bile acids with lysine and couple either NBD or fluorescein to the ϵ amino group of the lysine moiety. The fluorophore thus is attached by an amino-n-butyl tether to the α-carbon atom of the glycine. Mills and his colleagues have reported the synthesis of fluorescent bile acids in which fluorescein isothiocyanate is used to couple a fluorescein moiety to the ϵ-amino group of lysine[82], and our group has reported compounds in which the NBD fluorophore is coupled similarly[81].

The future utility of these fluorescent bile acids is difficult to predict. The Birmingham group has shown that they can be used to visualize transport, and they provide a means of assessing plasma clearance of a substance with a high first pass extraction by the liver[83]. However, other dye clearance tests (ICG, BSP) are not routinely used in hepatology despite five decades of experience for a variety of reasons; it is unlikely, in my opinion, that fluorescent bile acids will offer a substantial advantage over these tests.

Our own group led by Fernando Holzinger is currently exploring the use of fluorescent bile acids to visualize the biliary tree and experimental bile leaks during laparoscopic surgery in animals. It is difficult to predict whether laparoscopic surgeons will find this method of sufficient value to incorporate it into surgical practice. It could also be used to detect liver leaks during splitting of the liver during related donor transplantation; time will tell whether rendering the biliary tree fluorescent is of practical utility.

For visualizing bile acids at the level of the whole organism, a gamma emitting bile acid has long been sought. George Boyd, now deceased, worked with his colleagues at Amersham radiochemicals to prepare SeHCAT, a homologue of cholyltaurine in which a selenium atom was inserted between the C-22 and C-23 carbons[84]. This radiolabelled bile acid has been shown to behave almost identically to cholyltaurine and has been useful for defining the kinetics of intestinal transport, ileal transport, and detecting bile acid malabsorption[85]. The isotope has been used only in animal studies in the United States because it has never been approved by the Food and Drug Administration for clinical studies despite its excellent properties.

The last class of novel bile acids to be considered has been discussed only as a possibility. This would be a dihydroxy-bile acid that was resistant to conjugation and hydroxylation in the hepatocyte. Such a compound would cycle endlessly in a cholehepatic circulation generating bile flow on each pass through the hepatocyte. The final result would be a vigorous bicarbonate choleresis[86]. We had speculated that norUDCA would behave in this manner in man, but the compound was found to be 23-ester glucuronidated, precluding cholehepatic shunting[87]. Whether such a compound can be made and whether it would have therapeutic value is unknown. The choleretic effect of bile acids is more important in man than in many animal species, as in man, bile acid independent (canalicular) bile flow is a minor component of total canalicular bile flow. Availability of a truly potent choleretic bile acid would decrease residence time of molecules in the biliary tree and might decrease the rate of bilirubin deconjugation or bacterial proliferation. The problem with a molecule that induces hypercholeresis by the cholehepatic shunt mechanism is that it would render bile supersaturated in calcium carbonate. One might also speculate that were such a mechanism to be biologically useful, it should have evolved in nature. Nonetheless, synthesis of such a molecule would seem a worthy challenge for the coming century to test whether the idea has utility. Because ester glucuronidation seems to occur to a much greater extent in humans than in rodents, screening of hypothetical compounds will have to involve human hepatocytes.

It is beyond the scope of this chapter to discuss bile acids as permeation enhancers in skin and buccal patches.

BILE ACID BIOCHEMISTRY: FROM BIOCHEMICAL PATHWAYS TO GENE CLONING TO DETECTION OF INBORN ERRORS

Konrad Bloch showed that deuterium labelled cholesterol was converted to bile acids[88], thus substantiating an idea advanced by Ruzicka some 30 years before[89]. Siegfried Thannhauser, author of the first textbook on disease of lipid metabolism, did not believe the results of the Bloch experiments because cholesterol was a flat molecule whereas bile acids had the nuclear structure of coprostanol[90]. Elucidation of the biochemical pathways of bile acid biosynthesis has been another great triumph of biochemistry, with notable contributions especially from the Karolinska group including the late Henry Danielsson[91]. Other important contributors have been Kyuichiro Okuda[92] and David Russell[93]. In the past decade, virtually all of the enzymes involved in bile acid biosynthesis have been cloned, as detailed elsewhere in this volume.

Appreciation that inborn errors of bile acid biosynthesis involving the A ring present clinically as cholestatic disease and can be treated by natural bile acid feeding is one of the great triumphs of cholanology. The challenge for the future is to screen every infant with unexplained cholestatic liver disease for a defect in bile acid biosynthesis. Eventually, prenatal screening can be done. Because of the multiple biochemical pathways by which bile acids may be biosynthesized, a defect in hydroxylation at C-27 has a more subtle clinical presentation and is often not detected until adolescence or adulthood. In principle, detection of the disease in the parent can lead to antenatal screening.

Bile acid conjugation involves at least two enzymes: a bile acid CoA synthetase and a glycine/taurine transferase. Recently, a single case of absent bile acid amidation has been identified, presenting clinically as a malabsorption syndrome (for triglyceride and fat soluble vitamins) as well as failure to thrive[94]. The principal circulating bile acid was cholic acid, which presumably was absorbed passively in the proximal small intestine. As a result, the intraluminal bile acid concentration was likely to have been below that required for micelle formation, thus precluding the absorption of fat soluble vitamins. The probability that a hepatic defect would present clinically as a malabsorption syndrome was actually predicted a decade ago[95].

Therapy with conjugated bile acids should restore lipid digestion and absorption to normal. It is curious that the affected cases do not synthesize CDCA; one possibility is that cholic acid is poorly secreted by canalicular enzymes, accumulates in the hepatocyte, and upregulates the microsomal enzyme that hydroxylates 7α-hydroxy-cholest-4-ene-3-one at C-12, the key step in cholic acid biosynthesis.

There are at least three challenges for the future. One is to clone the two or more enzymes involved in bile acid amidation in man. For all genes involved in bile acid biosynthesis and conjugation, future studies are likely to be aimed at defining what factors influence promoter activity and tissue localization of the gene. The second is to screen all infants with unexplained fat absorption by FABS/MS as this disease can be treated successfully by amidated bile acid replacement therapy. In the distant future, gene therapy may become less costly and more convenient than oral bile acid replacement therapy.

Bile acid transport

Twenty years ago, no bile acid scientist could have imagined that the transporters involved in bile acid transport in the hepatocyte and ileal enterocyte would be identified and cloned. The power of expression cloning and the PCR technique has led to identification of two bile uptake transporters on the basolateral membrane of the hepatocyte and one ATP-dependent bile acid transporter on the canalicular membrane. The contributions of Peter Meier and his colleagues Bruno Hagenbuch and Bruno Stieger have been of profound importance[96]. The story is not finished, as the canalicular membrane transporter (*spgp*) transports cholylglycine much less readily than cholyltaurine[97], whereas in the perfused liver, the two compounds are transported similarly. This discrepancy in transport rates suggests that at least one additional canalicular bile acid transporter is likely to exist.

Transporters involved in bile acid uptake and secretion across microsomal membranes are likely to be present[98], but have yet to be identified. Whether other transporters are present in the Golgi or mitochondria is unknown.

Identification of mutations in spgp as the cause of primary familial cholestasis (PFIC2) has been an exciting event in the history of paediatric cholestatic liver disease (see Chapter 8). Treatment will involve gene, hepatocyte, or liver transplantation therapy. Genetic techniques have identified another ABC type transporter as the defect in PFIC1 (Byler's disease and benign recurrent intrahepatic cholestasis), but as yet the relationship between the gene product and bile acid transport remains completely obscure[99]. Current studies focus on the up- and down-regulation of the hepatocyte transporters in experimental cholestasis[100,101].

Cloning of the apical conjugated bile acid sodium-dependent co-transporter of the ileal enterocyte in the laboratory of Paul Dawson and his colleagues was also a great advance[102]. This transporter, presently termed *abst*, is now known to be present on the apical membrane of the renal tubular epithelial cell as well as the cholangiocyte. Curiously, although bile acid malabsorption is not uncommon, identification of genetic defects in abst as a cause of such bile acid malabsorption has been difficult to obtain. Determinants of the activity of abst are poorly understood, although our group has provided evidence for negative feedback of abst activity in the guinea pig[103]. Studies in the rat suggest that there are considerable species differences in the regulation of the ileal transport mechanism[104].

Cloning of the apical sodium independent conjugated bile acid transporter that is also present in the small intestine[105] remains a challenge, although it appears to be related to the *oatp* family[106,107]. A challenge for the future is identification of the one or more basolateral transporters.

Certainly, the next few decades are going to see great advances in the understanding of the proteins involved in bile acid transport in the liver and intestine, and identification of clinical syndromes associated with their malfunction.

As yet, fluorescein-tagged antibodies to bile acid transporters have not become a part of clinical pathology. It is possible that they might provide information of diagnostic value when used to stain liver biopsies; time will tell.

BILE ACIDS AS NUTRITIONAL BIOCHEMICALS

The major functions of bile acids are the elimination of cholesterol and the promotion of lipid absorption. These may be considered opposing functions, in that elimination of cholesterol requires neither amphipathicity nor enterohepatic cycling, whereas promotion of lipid absorption requires amphipathic properties and maximal enterohepatic cycling. Elimination of cholesterol is a life-long requirement; promotion of lipid absorption is most needed during infancy when caloric requirements are highest and triglyceride has the highest proportion of dietary nutrients. From a homeostatic point of view, the regulation of the two functions also behave quite differently, at least in man. An increased cholesterol load, whether caused by excessive caloric intake, excessive cholesterol intake, or rapid weight loss, leads to relatively little increase in bile acid synthesis. On the other hand interruption of the EHC causes a marked increase in bile acid synthesis by an order of magnitude. Thus, the liver seems more concerned with nutrition than with elimination of cholesterol!

Table 4. Physiological functions of bile acids

Process	Site	Mechanism
I. Hepatobiliary		
Stimulation of bile flow	Hepatocyte	Canalicular secretion of osmotically active molecules that are impermeable to canalicular membrane
	Cholangiocyte	Potentiation of secretin-stimulated bicarbonate secretion
Stimulation of biliary phospholipid secretion	Hepatocyte	Detachment of phosphatidylcholine from canalicular membrane
	Biliary tract	Solubilization of phosphatidylcholine in mixed micelles
Feedback inhibition of bile acid and cholesterol biosynthesis	Hepatocyte	Repression of cholesterol 7α-hydroxylase
II. Intestinal		
Enhancement of lipid absorption	Small intestine	Formation of mixed micelles that promote diffusion through unstirred layer
*Cleaning of absorptive surface	Small intestine	Surface activity of bile acid anions
*Stimulation of motility; induction of defaecation	Large intestine	Neural arc
III. Whole organism		
Cholesterol elimination	Hepatocyte	Conversion to bile acids Stimulation of biliary cholesterol secretion
	Biliary tract	Solubilization of cholesterol in mixed micelles
	Intestine	Faecal excretion of cholesterol and bile acids

*Postulated, not established function.
This table has been published previously in slightly modified form[150].

Bile acids also stimulate bile flow and biliary lipid secretion in the liver. Bile flow is important in those species in which bile acid independent canalicular bile flow makes only a minor contribution to bile flow. Biliary phospholipid secretion protects the epithelium of the biliary tract from the cytotoxic effects of bile acids, and also promotes the formation of mixed micelles that solubilize biliary cholesterol. A summary of currently recognized functions of bile acids is given in Table 4.

In clinical conditions associated with interruption of the EHC, there is decreased intraluminal bile acid concentration. The effect on lipid absorption depends on the magnitude of the decrease in bile acid concentration and the area of the small intestinal epithelium. In patients with a large ileal resection, both factors contribute to the steatorrhoea that is present[108,109]. Despite recognition that bile acid deficiency occurs in patients with ileal resection and in patients with short bowel syndrome bile acid replacement therapy is not used currently in clinical gastroenterology. The reasons for this are multiple including lack of commercial availability of pure conjugated bile acids, fear that conjugated bile acid replacement will induce diarrhoea because of the secretory effects of bile acids, and finally, the widespread availability of medium chain triglycerides whose fatty acids are water soluble and therefore can be absorbed in the absence of bile acids. Together with John Fordtran and his colleagues, we have shown that conjugated bile acid replacement in a patient with short bowel syndrome can increase lipid absorption by 50% without causing an increase in diarrhoea[110]. Two types of conjugated bile acid replacement are possible. In the first, bacterial deconjugation–dehydroxylation is minimal, and a glycine- or taurine-amidated conjugated bile acid is sufficient. In principle any of the four primary bile acid amidates should work satisfactorily. In the second, bacterial deconjugation– dehydroxylation contributes to either removal of bile acids from solution or induced bile acid secretion; in such instances, the deconjugation–dehydroxylation-resistant bile acid cholylsarcosine is preferable. Obviously, cholylsarcosine can be used in all situations in which a bile acid deficiency is likely to be present, provided hepatic excretory function is normal. Whether cholylsarcosine will have clinical utility in conditions where bacterial deconjugation is considered to contribute to fat malabsorption and bacterial translocation, e.g. in cirrhosis, is under study in animals.

The challenge for the future is to define the clinical utility of conjugated bile acid replacement. It is possible that enteral feeding preparations containing long chain fatty acids and conjugated bile acids might have clinical value in some circumstances.

BILE ACIDS AS MODULATORS OF CHOLESTEROL METABOLISM

The other physiological function of bile acids is the elimination of cholesterol by conversion to a water soluble end product. In most vertebrates, including man, the end product is amphipathic and forms mixed micelles that solubilize cholesterol. In these species, bile acids promote cholesterol elimination not only by being the metabolic end product of cholesterol metabolism but also by promoting the transport of cholesterol in bile.

Defective bile acid biosynthesis leads to defective cholesterol elimination as already discussed. In principle, one would like to up-regulate bile acid biosynthesis in conditions of increased cholesterol formation, for example in obesity by direct induction of the 7α-hydroxylases involved in bile acid biosynthesis. This has not yet been accomplished but remains a challenge for the next decade. Perhaps combinatorial approaches will enable the identification of small molecules that can bind to nuclear receptors and thereby modulate the activity of these key enzymes in bile acid formation[111].

The efficient enterohepatic circulation of bile acids down-regulates bile acid formation and down-regulates cholesterol biosynthesis. The genius of Brown and Goldstein was to recognize that up-regulation of bile acid synthesis by bile acid sequestrant administration would up-regulate low density lipoprotein (LDL) receptor activity[112]. Indeed, even before Brown and Goldstein, the ability of bile acid sequestrants to lower plasma cholesterol was shown by Tennent and his colleagues at Merck who developed cholestyramine as a cholesterol lowering agent nearly 40 years ago[113]. Interruption of the EHC by cholestyramine or by ileal bypass has been shown to decrease plasma LDL cholesterol and to decrease coronary events. Nonetheless cholesytramine usage has largely been replaced by the statins because of their efficacy, convenience, and lack of side effects.

Brown and Goldstein also noted that the combination of a statin and bile acid blockers acted additively to up-regulate LDL receptors, a prediction confirmed in the clinical studies by their colleague Scott Grundy[114]. This observation has led to efforts by pharmaceutical companies to develop bile acid sequestrants with binding properties that are superior to those of cholestyramine[115]. Such agents should have less side effects because a smaller dosage is required for clinical efficacy. One new sequestrant, cholestagel, has been shown to lower LDL cholesterol in an additive manner when co-administered with the statins. Clinical trials are in progress and approval of the FDA will be sought this year.

A second approach to diminish the efficiency of bile acid absorption is to inhibit *abst*, the ileal sodium dependent bile acid transporter. Several companies have developed potent abst inhibitors[116–120]. Such agents may have a structure that does not obviously resemble a bile acid, or may be based on bile acid derivatives. Clinical testing of these agents is either occurring or is likely to occur in the near future, as animal studies have shown convincing evidence of their hypocholesterolaemic and anti-atherosclerotic properties[120]. A possible disadvantage of absorption inhibitors is that they will cause bile acid malabsorption that in turn will cause diarrhoea. If the colonic bacteria adapt to the increased load and remove bile acids from solution (by deconjugation–dehydroxylation) diarrhoea will not occur; if they do not, it is likely. Time will tell. A summary of the methods that are currently available for lowering plasma LDL cholesterol levels by up-regulating hepatocyte LDL receptor levels is given in Table 5.

The future of these statin adjuvants is difficult to predict. Statins will go off patent and become less costly. Still more potent statins may be developed. Side effects related to long-term treatment may appear. Nonetheless, my prediction is that the next two decades will see much greater interest in bile acids by the cardiovascular community which to date has had little interest in these degradation products of cholesterol.

Table 5. Methods for up-regulating LDL receptors in order to decrease plasma LDL cholesterol levels

Class of compounds	Site of action	Mechanism	Current status
Statins	Hepatocyte	Inhibition of HMG-CoA reductase	Approved throughout world
Bile acid sequestrants	Small intestinal lumen	Bile acid binding causing increased bile acid loss; up-regulation of bile acid and cholesterol synthesis	Cholestyramine and colestipol approved New sequestrants in clinical trials
Ileal bile acid transport inhibitors	Ileal enterocyte	Binding to abst; Increased bile acid loss; up-regulation of bile acid and cholesterol synthesis	Investigational; clinical trials will be initiated in 1999

BILE ACIDS AS CYTOTOXIC AGENTS

Bile acid cytotoxicity occurs when the monomeric concentration of bile acids is increased to cytotoxic levels either extracellularly or intracellularly. It does not occur in health.

Bile acid cytotoxicity was induced in intestinal perfusion studies[121,122] and bile acids are also toxic to the gastric mucosa[123]. In health, the monomeric concentration of bile acids is low in the stomach because of the paucity of duodenal gastric reflux, because glycine conjugated bile acids precipitate from solution at acidic intragastric pH, and because bile acids bind to hydrophobic residues. In the small intestine, the presence of fatty acids and monoglycerides lowers the monomeric concentration about 50%, as shown many years ago, long before bile acid toxicity was appreciated[124]. Bile acid cytotoxicity in the small intestine can also be decreased by the addition of phospholipid[125], which as fatty acids and monoglycerides, promotes cooperative mixed micelle formation. In the large intestine, bile acid cytotoxicity is prevented by deconjugation–dehydroxylation which removes bile acids from solution[126]. In the biliary tract, bile acid cytotoxicity is decreased by the presence of biliary PC which lowers the monomeric activity and surface activity of bile acids. Mucus and bicarbonate secretion might also contribute, but the simple absence of PC in bile in the *mdr2* knockout mouse is sufficient to cause a severe cholangitis[127].

Extracellular bile acid toxicity to the gastric mucosa appears to be induced by oral administration of cholylsarcosine, as evidenced by a preliminary report of nausea and vomiting in short bowel patients who received 2 g/meal and were not receiving proton pump inhibitors[128]. Bile acid cytotoxicity in the small intestine is not known to occur in disease, but can be induced experimentally by perfusion with solutions of dihydroxy-bile acids at concentrations approaching the CMC (or above), Bile acid cytotoxicity in the large intestine can occur in patients with bile acid malabsorption because of ileal resection, or induced by perfusion of dihydroxy-bile acids.

Intracellular bile acid cytotoxicity occurs when the input of bile acids into a cell occurs at a rate exceeding output and when the intracellular concentration of bile acids exceeds the binding capacity of intracellular proteins. In the hepatocyte, carrier mediated uptake of bile acids into organelles such as microsomes and the Golgi apparatus, might also cause cytotoxicity.

Uptake of conjugated bile acids by cells can only occur if a bile acid transporter is present. Therefore the only cells in which bile acid toxicity is likely to occur are the hepatocyte, the jejunal and ileal enterocyte, and the renal tubular epithelial cell. Since glycine dihydroxy conjugated bile acids can be taken up in protonated form from an acidic milieu, it remains possible that such passive uptake of conjugated bile acids could occur in the oesophageal or gastric mucosa when reflux occurs, or in the proximal small intestine in patients with gastrinoma. Such has not been shown.

The prototypic situation of intracellular toxicity is cholestatic liver disease. Bile acid cytotoxicity may be decreased by UDCA administration which decreases the cytotoxicity of the circulating bile acids and also causes some up-regulation of canalicular transporters[129]. UDCA amidates may also inhibit the uptake of cytotoxic endogenous conjugated bile acids by microsomes[98]. Remarkable antiapoptic properties of UDCA have been reported recently.[130]

Introduction of UDCA as a treatment for cholestatic liver disease has been an important advance in hepatology and has served to emphasize the cytotoxicity of bile acids. Nonetheless, it is my belief that therapeutic efforts must continue to be directed at the primary cause of the disease in PBC and PSC.

If ileal transport exceeds canalicular transport capacity, cytotoxicity of bile acids within the hepatocyte is likely to result. Historically, patients with cholestasis and pruritus were treated by biliary drainage[131,132], but this practice has been abandoned. More recently, Whitington and his colleagues have shown that partial biliary diversion decreases pruritus in some children with cholestatic liver disease[133]. The mechanism of both treatments is the same: to keep bile acids away from the active site of bile acid absorption in the ileum. Indeed, ileal bypass has recently been reported to decrease pruritus associated with cholestatic liver disease[134]. Thus, there is a good possibility that either the second generation bile acid sequestrants or bile acid resorption inhibitors will have some value in the treatment of pruritus associated with cholestatic liver disease. I also believe that the use of UDCA will decrease when more pathogenesis directed therapies become available for the treatment of cholestatic liver disease.

There are some areas of bile acid toxicity that are species specific and should be noted only briefly. Monohydroxy bile acids induce cholestasis acutely, presumably by interfering with canalicular transport. Lithocholic acid, or its precursors (CDCA and UDCA) are cytotoxic when fed chronically to species that cannot detoxify them[135]. Taurocholate is toxic when fed chronically to the guinea pig because deoxycholic and its 3-oxo derivative accumulate, and the latter is presumably poorly transported by canalicular transporters[136]. All of these bile acid-induced diseases do not appear to have any clinical relevance. Despite the many thousand patient years experience of administering CDCA and UDCA to patients, not a single case of lithocholic acid toxicity has been well documented. The human liver must have a remarkable ability to sulphate lithocholic acid.

NEW FRONTIERS OF BILE ACID ACID PHYSIOLOGY

In the last part of this essay, I will speculate bravely about some unexplored frontiers of bile acid research.

The first question is whether bile acids have as yet unidentified functions in the small intestine. Are they key determinants of the ecology of the small intestine? Bile acid diversion is associated with bacterial translocation[137–141]. This observation raises the question as to whether bile acids act synergistically with IgA to prevent bacteria from invading the epithelium by washing them off. The biological utility of having the small intestinal epithelium lavaged continuously by a detergent rich solution with a low surface tension has not been established, yet seems likely.

The second question is whether the signalling effects of bile acids are important. Bile acids mediate motilin[142] and somatostatin[143] release from the small intestine. In an intraluminal deficiency of bile acids, is the release of these hormones impaired and does this matter? By the same token, do bile acids influence intestinal motility? Promotility effects have been shown, and these can be blocked by lidocaine[144], indicating that a neural arc is involved. Bile acids lower the threshold for defaecation with rectal distension, raising the possibility that the rectum senses bile acids and that this modulates the call to defaecate. In patients with irritable bowel syndrome, perfusion of the colon with bile acid solutions induces pain; in contrast, healthy subjects do not feel pain[145]. I believe there is much to be done in the relationship between bile acids, colonic motility, colonic sensing, and induction of defaecation.

A fourth question is whether the absorption of secondary bile acids from the large intestine matters. There is a continuing throughput of dihydroxy and monohydroxy unconjugated bile acids, and there is some evidence suggesting that bile acids induce cellular proliferation[146]. After some three decades of concern and investigation, the role of bile acids in the pathogenesis of colon cancer remains completely uncertain. My own view is that deoxycholic acid is not going to play a major role in colon cancer, although it is a mild promitotic agent. There is indirect evidence that an increased input of deoxycholic acid from the colon occurs when colonic transit is sluggish, and such an increased input of deoxycholic acid causes bile to become supersaturated, increasing the likelihood of cholesterol gallstone formation[147]. Nonetheless, the sensitivity and specificity of increased biliary deoxycholic acid as a marker for cholesterol gallstones is low, indicating other factors are frequently involved.

A final question is whether bile acids interact with transcription factors in the hepatocyte, and to what extent this influences hepatocyte functions in addition to those concerned with bile acid transport and biosynthesis. Bile acids have been shown to be responsible for ductular proliferation in the bile duct ligated animals, suggesting they influence gene transcription[148].

CONCLUDING REMARKS

For someone who has been involved in bile acid research for over 40 years, it has been a very exciting time. Every biennial bile acid meeting has witnessed both basic and clinical discoveries. Initially, bile acids were thought to play a role in liver injury and their plasma levels to have diagnostic value. Then, the discovery that CDCA administration slowly dissolved gallstones caught the attention of the clinical world. In the past decade, the use of UDCA has reawakened interest in the field of bile acids, even though UDCA is palliative, not curative. Detection of inborn errors of bile acid synthesis has been followed by successful replacement therapy as well as cloning of the key enzymes. These events have been electrifying, even though the number of patients who have gained from these spectacular advances is quite small.

I have suggested that it is useful to consider bile acid therapy in the context of bile acid agonists (bile acids or bile acid derivatives that enhance the functions of bile acids) and bile acid antagonists (sequestrants or transport inhibitors)[149]. In the area of bile acid agonists, I have thought that we should distinguish displacement, where the composition but not the amount of bile acids that are cycling is changed, from replacement, where bile acids are administered in sufficient quantity to correct a deficiency. I believe that this classification continues to be valid and useful.

My prediction is that the use of bile acid agonists will increase modestly in the coming decades. In contrast, I believe that the use of bile acid antagonists will grow to a much greater extent and will eventually far exceed that of bile acid agonists. I began this essay by citing some hilariously erroneous predictions. Let us hope that I have not ended this essay by making my own.

Acknowledgements

I thank Dr Lee R. Hagey for his critique of the manuscript. The author's work is supported in part by the National Institutes of Health [DK21506) and DK37172 (PI: Dr John S. Fordtran, Baylor University Medical Center, Dallas, TX)] and a grant-in-aid from the Falk Foundation, e.V., Freiburg, Germany.

REFERENCES

1. Cerf C, Navasky V. The Experts Speak. New York: Villard, 1998:1–445.
2. Hill R, Dixon M, Gale EF et al. The Chemistry of Life. Cambridge: Cambridge University Press, 1971:1–203.
3. Fruton JS. The emergence of biochemistry. Science. 1976;192:327–334.
4. Hofmann AF. Bile acid research: some major themes during the past 60 years. In: Bianchi L, Gerok W, Popper H, eds. Trends in Hepatology. Lancaster: MTP Press, 1985:3–27.
5. Hofmann AF. Trends in bile acid research: the past and the future. In: Paumgartner G, Stiehl A, Gerok W, eds. Trends in Bile Acid Research. Boston: Kluwer Academic Publishers, 1989:19–49.
6. Sobotka H. Physiological Chemistry of Bile. Baltimore: Williams and Wilkins Company, 1937.
7. Haslewood GAD. The Biological Importance of Bile Salts. Amsterdam: North-Holland Publishing Co., 1978.
8. Hoshita T. Bile alcohols and primitive bile acids. In: Danielsson H, Sjövall J, eds. Sterols and Bile Acids. Amsterdam: Elsevier, 1985:279–302.
9. Tohma M, Mahara R, Takeshita H, Kurosawa T, Ikegawa S. Synthesis of the 1β-hydroxylated bile acids, unusual bile acids in human biological fluids. Chem Pharm Bull. 1986;34: 2890–2899.
10. Hagey LR. Bile acid biodiversity in vertebrates: chemistry and evolutionary implication. 1992 Doctoral thesis, University of California, San Diego.
11. Hofmann AF, Schteingart CD, Hagey LR. Species differences in bile acid metabolism. In: Paumgartner G, Beuers U, eds. Bile Acids in Liver Diseases. Boston: Kluwer Academic Publishers, 1995:3–30.
12. Cerré C, Hofmann AF, Schteingart CD, Jia W, Maltby D. Oxyfunctionalization of 5β-bile acids by dimethyldioxirane: hydroxylation at C-5, C-14, and C-17. Tetrahedron. 1997;53:435–446.
13. Iida T, Nambara T, Chang FC. Synthesis of uncommon bile acids. In: Hofmann AF, Paumgartner G, Stiehl A, eds. Bile Acids in Gastroenterology. Lancaster, UK: Kluwer Academic Publishers, 1995:8–26.
14. Kurosawa T, Nomura Y, Mahara R et al. Synthesis of 19-hydroxylated bile acids and identification of 3α, 7α, 12α, 19-tetrahydroxy-5β-cholan-24-oic acid in human neonatal urine. Chem Pharm Bull. 1995;43:1551–1557.
15. Une M, Hoshita T. Natural occurrence and chemical synthesis of bile alcohols, higher bile acids, and short side chain bile acids. Hiroshima J Med Sci. 1994;43:37–67.
16. Dayal B, Tint GS, Toome V, Batta AK, Shefer S, Salen G. Synthesis and structure of 26 (or 27)-nor-5β-cholestane-3α, 7α, 12α, 24S, 25ϵ-pentol isolated from the urine and feces of a patient with sitosterolemia and xanthomatosis. J Lipid Res. 1985;26:298–305.
17. Hagey LR, Schteingart CD, Ton-Nu HT, Rossi SS, Odell D, Hofmann AF. β-Phocacholic acid in bile: biochemical evidence that the flamingo is related to an ancient goose. Condor. 1990;92:593–597.
18. Hagey LR, Odell D, Rossi SS, Crombie DL, Hofmann AF. Biliary bile acid composition of the Physeteridae (sperm whales). Marine Mam Sci. 1993;9:23–33.

19. Hagey LR, Crombie DL, Espinosa E, Carey MC, Igimi H, Hofmann AF. Ursodeoxycholic acid in the Ursidae: biliary bile acids of bears, pandas, and related carnivores. J Lipid Res. 1993;34:1911–1917.

20. Une M, Goto T, Kihara K et al. Isolation and identification of bile salts conjugated with cysteinolic acid from bile of the red sea bream, *Pagrosomus major*. J Lipid Res. 1991;32:1619–1623.

21. Hofmann AF, Mysels KJ. Bile salts as biological surfactants. Colloids Surfaces. 1988;30: 145–173.

22. Stieger B, Zhang J, O'Neill B, Sjövall J, Meier PJ. Differential interaction of bile acids from patients with inborn errors of bile acid biosynthesis with hepatocellular transporters. Eur J Biochem. 1997;244:39–44.

23. Hofmann AF, Small DM. Detergent properties of bile salts: correlation with physiological function. Annu Rev Med. 1967;18:333–376.

24. Hofmann AF, Hagey LR. Bile acids and biliary disease: peaceful coexistence versus deadly warfare. In: Blum HE, Bode C, Bode JC, Sartor RB, eds. Gut and Liver. Lancaster: Kluwer Academic Publishers, 1998:85–103.

25. Schmassmann A, Hofmann AF, Angelloti MA et al. Prevention of ursodeoxycholate hepatotox-icity in the rabbit by conjugation with N-methyl amino acids. Hepatology. 1990;11:989–996.

26. Roda A, Hofmann AF, Mysels KJ. The influence of bile salt structure on self-association in aqueous solutions. J Biol Chem. 1983;258:6362–6370.

27. Goto T, Holzinger F, Hagey LR et al. Physicochemical and physiological properties of 5α-cyprinol sulfate, the biliary surfactant of the carp: why bile acids evolved from bile alcohols. Hepatology. 1997;26:295A.

28. Merrill JR, Schteingart CD, Hagey LR et al. Hepatic biotransformation in rodents and physico-chemical properties of 23(R)-hydroxychenodeoxycholic acid, a natural alpha-hydroxy bile acid. J Lipid Res 1995;37:98–112.

29. Huijghebaert SM, Hofmann AF. Pancreatic carboxypeptidase hydrolysis of bile acid-amino acid conjugates: selective resistance of glycine and taurine amidates. Gastroenterology. 1986;90:306–315.

30. Hartley GS. Aqueous solutions of paraffin chain salts. Actualities Sci Industr. 1936;1–68.

31. Campanelli AR, Candeloro De Sanctis S, Chiessi E, D'Alagni M, Giglio E, Scaramuzza L. Sodium glyco- and taurodeoxycholate: possible helical models for conjugated bile salt micelles. J Phys Chem. 1989;93:1536–1542.

32. Bourges M, Small DM, Dervichian DG. Biophysics of lipid associations. 3. The quaternary systems lecithin-bile salt-cholesterol-water. Biochim Biophys Acta. 1967;144:189–201.

33. Small DM, Penkett SA, Chapman D. Studies on simple and mixed bile salt micelles by nuclear magnetic resonance spectroscopy. Biochim Biophys Acta. 1969;176:178–189.

34. Hjelm RP, Jr, Thiyagarajan P, Alkan-Onyuksel H. Organization of phosphatidylcholine and bile salt in rodlike mixed micelles. J Phys Chem. 1992;96:8653–8661.

35. Hjelm RP, Jr, Schteingart CD, Hofmann AF, Sivia DS. Form and structure of self-assembling particles in monoolein-bile salt mixtures. J Phys Chem. 1995;99:16395–16400.

36. Djerassi C. Steroids Made It Possible. Washington: American Chemical Society, 1990:1–205.

37. Fieser LF, Rajagopolan S. Oxidation of steroids III. Selective oxidation and acylations in the bile series. J Am Chem Soc. 1949;71:3935–3938.

38. Thistle JL, Hofmann AF. Efficacy and specificity of chenodeoxycholic acid therapy for dissolving gallstones. N Engl J Med. 1973;289:655–659.

39. Norman A. Preparation of conjugated bile acids using mixed carboxylic acid anhydrides. Ark Kemi. 1955;8:331–342.

40. Tserng KY, Hachey DL, Klein PD. An improved procedure for the synthesis of glycine and taurine conjugates of bile acids. J Lipid Res. 1977;18:404–407.

41. Del Vecchio S, Ostrow JD, Mukerjee P et al. A method for the removal of surface active impurities and calcium from conjugated bile salt preparations: Comparison with silicic acid chromatography. J Lipid Res. 1995;36:2639–2650.

42. Tserng KY, Klein PD. Bile acid sulfates. III. Synthesis of 7- and 12-monosulfates of bile acids and their conjugates using a sulfur trioxide-triethylamine complex. Steroids. 1979;33:167–182.

43. Goto J, Suzaki K, Nambara T. Synthesis of 3-glucuronides of unconjugated and conjugated bile acids. Chem Pharm Bull. 1980;28:1258–1264.

44. Goto J, Murao N, Oohashi J, Igegawa. S. Synthesis of bile acid 24-acyl glucuronides. Steroids. 1998;63:180–185.

45. Fini A, Fazio G, Tonelli D, Roda A, Zuman P. Chemical properties of bile acids. V. Interaction with concentrated sulfuric acid. Farmaco. 1992;47:741–752.
46. Setchell KDR, Kritchevsky D, Nair PP (eds) The Bile Acids. Volume 4. Methods and Application. New York: Plenum Press, 1988:1–582.
47. Sjövall J, Setchell KDR. Techniques for extraction and group separation of bile acids. In: Setchell KDR, Kritchevsky D, Nair PP (eds) The Bile Acids. Volume 4. Methods and Application 1988: 1–42.
48. Roda A. Separation techniques for bile salts analyses. J Chromatography B. 1998;717: 263–278.
49. Nair PP. Enzymes in bile acid metabolism. In: Nair PP, Kritchevsky D (eds) The Bile Acids. Volume 2. Physiology and Metabolism. New York: Plenum Press, 1973:1–329.
50. Talalay P. Enzymatic analysis of steroid hormones. In: Glick D (ed). Methods of Biochemical Analysis. New York: Interscience Publishers, 1960:119–143.
51. Iwata T, Yamasaki K. Enzymatic determination and thin-layer chromatography of bile acids in blood. J Biochem. (Jpn). 1964;56:424–431.
52. Palmer RH. The enzymic assay of bile acids and related 3α-hydroxysteroids: its application to serum and other biological fluids. In: Colowick SP, Kaplan NO (eds) Methods in Cell Biology. XV. Steroids and Terpenoids. New York: Academic Press, 1969:280–288.
53. Turley SD, Dietschy JM. Re-evaluation of the 3α-hydroxysteroid dehydrogenase assay for total bile acids in bile. J Lipid Res. 1977;18:404–407.
54. Beher WT, Stradnieks S, Lin GJ. Rapid photometric determination of free and esterified 3α-hydroxy fecal bile acids. Steroids. 1983;41:729–740.
55. Roda A, Kricka LJ, DeLuca M, Hofmann AF. Bioluminescence measurement of primary bile acids using immobilized 7 alpha-hydroxysteroid dehydrogenase: application to serum bile acids. J Lipid Res. 1982;23:1354–1361.
56. Fleishaker JC, Rossi SS, Smith RB et al. The effect of colestipol dose on postprandial serum bile acid concentration: assessment by an enzymic bioluminescence procedure. Aliment Pharmacol Ther. 1990;4:623–633.
57. Rossi SS, Angellotti MA, Setchell KDR, Hofmann AF. Measurement of total fasting-state serum bile acids: comparison of a solid-phase bioluminescence enzymatic assay, a homogeneous fluorescence enzymatic assay and isotope dilution gas chromatography-mass spectrometry. Clin Chim Acta. 1991;200:63–66.
58. Schalm SW, LaRusso NF, Hofmann AF, Hoffman NE, van Berge Henegouwen GP, Korman MG. Diurnal serum levels of primary conjugated bile acids. Assessment by specific radio-immunoassays for conjugates of cholic and chenodeoxycholic acid. Gut. 1978;19:1006–1014.
59. LaRusso NF, Hoffman NE, Korman MG, Hofmann AF, Cowen AE. Determinants of fasting and postprandial serum bile acid levels in healthy man. Am J Dig Dis. 1978;23:385–391.
60. Cravetto C, Molino G, Biondi AM, Cavanna A, Avagnina P, Frediani S. Evaluation of the diagnostic value of serum bile acid in the detection and functional assessment of liver diseases. Ann Clin Biochem. 1985;22:596–605.
61. Kale KM, Cussler EL, Evans DF. Surfactant ion electrode measurements of sodium alkylsulfate and alkyltrimethylammonium bromide micellar solutions. J Solution Chem. 1982;11:581–592.
62. Moore EW, Ross JW. The surfactant electrode: a new advance for physiological and physico-chemical studies of bile salt metabolism and structure activity relationships. Gastroenterology. 1985;88:1680.
63. Hofmann AF, Hoffman NE. Measurement of bile acid kinetics by isotope dilution in man. Gastroenterology. 1974;67:314–323.
64. Hofmann AF, Klein PD. Characterization of bile acid metabolism in man using bile acids labeled with stable isotopes. In: Baillie TA (ed) Stable Isotopes. Baltimore: University Park Press, 1978:189–204.
65. Bergström S, Danielsson H, Samuelsson B. Formation and metabolism of bile acids. In: Bloch K (ed) Lipid Metabolism. New York: John Wiley and Sons, Inc. 1960:291–336.
66. Lindstedt S. The turnover of cholic acid in man. Acta Physiol Scand. 1957;40:1–9.
67. LaRusso NF, Hoffman NE, Hofmann AF. Validity of using 2,4-^{3}H-labeled bile acids to study bile acid kinetics in man. J Lab Clin Med. 1974;84:759–765.
68. Ng PY, Allan RN, Hofmann AF. Suitability of [11,12,-^{3}H$_2$]chenodeoxycholic acid and [11,12-^{3}H$_2$]lithocholic acid for isotope dilution studies of bile acid metabolism in man. J Lipid Res. 1974;18:756–758.

69. Duane WC, Schteingart CD, Ton-Nu HT, Hofmann AF. Validation of [22,23-^{3}H]-cholic acid as a stable tracer through conversion to deoxycholic acid in human subjects. J Lipid Res. 1996;37:431–436.
70. Kuroki S, Une M, Mosbach EH. Synthesis of potential cholelitholytic agents: 3α, 7α, 12α-trihydroxy-7β-methyl-5β-cholanoic acid, 3α, 12α-dihydroxy-7ϵ-methyl-5β-cholanoic acid. J Lipid Res. 1985;26:1205–1211.
71. Roda A, Pellicciari R, Polimeni C et al. Metabolism, pharmacokinetics, and activity of a new 6-fluoro analogue of ursodeoxycholic acid in rats and hamsters. Gastroenterology. 1995;108:1204–1214.
72. Mikami T, Kihira K, Ikawa S et al. Metabolism of sulfonate analogs of ursodeoxycholic acid and their effects on biliary bile acid composition in hamsters. J Lipid Res. 1993;34:429–435.
73. Schwab D, Thom H, Heinze J, Kurz G. 3α, 7α, 12α-trihydroxy-24-nor-5β-cholan-23-sulfate: synthesis and suitability for the study of cholate transport. J Lipid Res. 1996;37:1045–1056.
74. Pellicciari R, Cecchetti S, Natalini B, Roda A, Grigolo B, Fini A. Bile acids with a cyclopropyl-containing side chain. I Preparation and properties of 3α, 7β-dihydroxy-22,23-methylene-5β-cholan-24-oic acid. J Med Chem .1984;27:746–749.
75. Roda A, Cerré C, Mannetta AC, Cainelli G, Umani-Ronchi A, Panunzio M. Synthesis and physicochemical, biological, and pharmacological properties of new bile acids amidated with cyclic amino acids. J Med Chem. 1996;39:2270–2276.
76. Lillienau J, Schteingart CD, Hofmann AF. Physicochemical and physiological properties of cholylsarcosine. A potential replacement detergent for bile acid deficiency states in the small intestine. J Clin Invest. 1992;89:420–431.
77. Schmassmann A, Angellotti MA, Ton-Nu HT et al. Transport, metabolism, and effect of chronic feeding of cholylsarcosine, a conjugated bile acid resistant to deconjugation and dehydroxylation. Gastroenterology. 1990;98:163–174.
78. Schneider S, Schramm U, Schreyer A, Buscher H, Gerok W, Kurz G. Fluorescent derivatives of bile salts. I. Synthesis and properties of NBD-amino derivatives of bile salts. J Lipid Res. 1991;32:1755-1767.
79. Sherman IA, Fisher MM. Hepatic transport of fluorescent molecules: in vivo studies using intravital TV microscopy. Hepatology. 1986;6:444–449.
80. Schteingart CD, Eming S, Ton-Nu HT, Crombie DL, Hofmann AF. Synthesis, structure and transport properties of fluorescent derivatives of conjugated bile acids. In: Paumgartner G, Stiehl A, Gerok W, eds. Bile Acids and the Hepatobiliary System. Boston: Kluwer Academic Publishers, 1993:177–183.
81. Holzinger F, Schteingart CD, Ton-Nu HT et al. Fluorescent bile acid derivatives: relationship between chemical structure, hepatic- and intestinal transport. Hepatology 1997;26:1263–1271.
82. Mills CO, Rahman K, Coleman R, Elias E. Cholyl-lysylfluorescein: synthesis, biliary excretion in vivo and during single-pass perfusion of isolated perfused rat liver. Biochim Biophys Acta. 1991;1115:151–156.
83. Milkiewicz P, Baiocchi L, Mills CO et al. Plasma clearance of cholyl-lysyl-fluorescein: a pilot study in humans. J Hepatol. 1997;27:1106–1109.
84. Boyd GS, Merrick MW, Monks R, Thomas IL. Se-75-labeled bile acid analogs, new radio pharmaceuticals for investigating the enterohepatic circulation. J Nucl Med. 1981;22:720–725.
85. Hofmann AF, Bolder U. Detection of bile acid malabsorption by the SeHCAT test: principles, problems, and clinical utility. Gastroenterol Clin Biol. 1994;18:847–851.
86. Hofmann AF. The cholehepatic circulation of organic anions: a decade of progress. In: Alvaro D, Benedetti A, Strazzabosco M (eds). Vanishing Bile Duct Syndrome – Pathophysiology and Treatment. Lancaster: Kluwer Academic Publishers, 1997:90–103.
87. Zakko S, Lira M, Clerici C, Lambert K, Gurantz D, Schteingart C, Hofmann AF. Novel metabolism and hypercholeretic effect of nor-ursodeoxycholic acid in man. Gastroenterology. 1987;92:1792.
88. Bloch K, Berg BN, Rittenberg D. The biological conversion of cholesterol to cholic acid. J Biol Chem. 1943;149:511.
89. Ruzicka L. In the borderland between bioorganic chemistry and biochemistry. Annu Rev Biochem. 1973;42:1–20.
90. Thannhauser SJ. Lipidoses: Diseases of the Cellular Lipid Metabolism. New York: Oxford University Press, 1950:1–595.

91. Björkhem I. Mechanisms of bile acid biosynthesis in mammalian liver. In: Danielsson H, Sjövall J (eds) Sterols and Bile Acids. Amsterdam: Elsevier Science Publishers, 1985:231–278.
92. Noshiro M, Okuda K. Molecular cloning and sequence analysis of cDNA encoding human cholesterol 7 alpha-hydroxylase. FEBS Lett. 1990;268:137–140.
93. Jelinek DF, Andersson S, Slaughter CA, Russell DW. Cloning and regulation of cholesterol 7 alpha-hydroxylase, the rate-limiting enzyme in bile acid biosynthesis. J Biol Chem 1990;265:8190–8197.
94. Setchell KDR, Heubi JE, O'Connell NC, Hofmann AF, Lavine JE. Absence of bile acid conjugation: a new inborn error in bile acid metabolism. Hepatology. 1996;24:A977.
95 Hofmann AF, Strandvik B. Defective bile acid amidation: predicted features of a new inborn error of metabolism. Lancet. 1988;2:311–313.
96. Stieger B, Meier PJ. Bile acid and xenobiotic transporters in liver. Curr Opinion Cell Biol. 1998;10:462–467.
97. Gerloff T, Stieger B, Hagenbuch B et al. The sister of P-glycoprotein represents the canalicular bile salt. J Biol Chem. 1998;273:10046–10050.
98. Holzinger F, Schteingart CD, Ton-Nu H et al. Transport of fluorescent bile acids by the isolated perfused liver: kinetics, sequestration and mobilization. Hepatology. 1998;28:510–520.
99. Bull LN, van Eijk MJT, Pawlikowska L et al. A gene encoding a P-type ATPase mutated in two forms of hereditary cholestasis. Nature Genet. 1998;18:219–224.
100. Trauner M, Meier PJ, Boyer JL. Molecular pathogenesis of cholestasis. New Engl J Med. 1998;339:1217–1227.
101. Trauner M, Arrese M, Lee H, Boyer JL, Karpen SJ. Endotoxin downregulates rat hepatic ntcp gene expression via decreased activity of critical transcription factors. J Clin Invest. 1998;101:2092–2100.
102. Wong MH, Oelkers P, Craddock AL, Dawson PA. Expression cloning and characterization of the hamster ileal sodium-dependent bile acid transporter. J Biol Chem. 1994;269:1–8.
103. Lillienau J, Munoz J, Longmire-Cook SJ, Hagey LR, Crombie DL, Hofmann AF. Negative feedback regulation of the ileal bile acid transport system in rodents. Gastroenterology. 1993;104:38–46.
104. Arrese M, Trauner M, Sacciero RJ, Crossman MW, Shneider BL. Neither intestinal sequestration of bile acids nor common bile duct ligation modulate the expression and function of the rat ileal bile acid transporter. Hepatology. 1998;28:1081–1087.
105. Amelsberg A, Schteingart CD, Ton-Nu HT, Hofmann AF. Carrier mediated jejunal absorption of conjugated bile acids in the guinea pig. Gastroenterology. 1996;110:1098–1106.
106. Richter CP, Amelsberg A, Nitsche R, Fölsch UR. Localization of the organic anion transport polypeptide (OATP) at the brush border in human jejunum. Gastroenterology. 1999;116: A1265.
107. Amelsberg A, Jochims C, Richter CP, Nitsche R, Fölsch UR. Evidence for an anion exchange mechanism for uptake of conjugated bile acid from the rat jejunum. Am J Physiol. 1999;276: G737–G242.
108. Hofmann AF, Poley JR. Role of bile acid malabsorption in pathogenesis of diarrhea and steatorrhea in patients with ileal resection. I. Response to cholestyramine or replacement of dietary long chain triglyceride by medium chain triglyceride. Gastroenterology. 1972;62:918–934.
109. Poley JR, Hofmann AF. Role of fat maldigestion in pathogenesis of steatorrhea in ileal resection. Fat digestion after two sequential test meals with and without cholestyramine. Gastroenterology. 1976;71:38–44.
110. Gruy-Kapral C, Little KH, Fordtran JS, Meziere TL, Hagey LR, Hofmann AF. Conjugated bile acid replacement therapy for short-bowel syndrome. Gastroenterology. 1999;116:15–21.
111. Parks DJ, Blanchard SG, Bledsoe RK et al. Bile acids: natural ligands for an orphan receptor. Science. 1999;284:1365–1368.
112. Brown MS, Goldstein JL. A receptor-mediated pathway for cholesterol homeostasis. Science. 1986;232:34–47.
113. Tennent DM, Siegel H, Zanetti ME, Kuron GW, Ott WH, Wolf FJ. Plasma cholesterol lowering action of bile acid binding polymers in experimental animals. J Lipid Res. 1960;1:469–473.
114. Grundy SM, Vega GL, Bilheimer DW. Influence of combined therapy with mevinolin and interruption of bile-acid reabsorption on low density lipoproteins in heterozygous familial hypercholesterolemia. Ann Intern Med. 1985;103:339–343.
115. Mandeville WH, Arbeeny CM. Bile acid sequestrants: their use in combination with other lipid lowering agents. Drugs. 1999;2:237–242.

116. Root C, Smith CD, Winegar DA, Brieaddy LE, Lewis MC. Inhibition of ileal sodium-dependent bile acid transport by 2164U90. J Lipid Res. 1995;36:1106–1115.
117. Lewis MC, Brieaddy LE, Root C. Effects of 2164U90 on ileal bile acid absorption and serum cholesterol in rats and mice. J Lipid Res. 1995;36:1098–1105.
118. Kramer W, Wess G, Baringhaus KH et al. Design and properties of ileal bile acid transport inhibitors. In: Hofmann AF, Paumgartner G, Stiehl A, eds. Bile Acids in Gastroenterology: Basic and Clinical Advances. Boston: Kluwer Academic Publishers, 1995:205–220.
119. Hara S, Higaki J, Higashino K et al. S-8921, an ileal Na$^+$/bile acid cotransporter inhibitor decreases serum cholesterol in hamsters. Life Sci. 1997;60:365–370.
120. Higaki J, Hara S, Takasu N et al. Inhibition of ileal Na$^+$/bile acid cotransporter by S-8921 reduces serum cholesterol and prevents atherosclerosis in rabbits. Arteriosclerosis Thrombosis Biol. 1998;18:1304–1311.
121. Mekhjian HS, Phillips SF, Hofmann AF. Colonic secretion of water and electrolytes induced by bile acids: perfusion studies in man. J Clin Invest. 1971;50:1569–1577.
122. Chadwick VS, Gaginella TS, Carlson GL, Debongnie JC, Phillips SF, Hofmann AF. Effect of molecular structure on bile acid-induced alterations in absorptive function, permeability and morphology in the perfused rabbit colon. J Lab Clin Med. 1979;94:661–674.
123. Ritchie WP, Cherry KJ. Influence of hydrogen ion concentration on bile acid induced acute gastric mucosal ulcerogenesis. Ann Surg. 1979;189:637–641.
124. Hofmann AF. The function of bile salts in fat absorption: the solvent properties of dilute micellar solutions of conjugated bile salts. Biochem J. 1963;89:57–68.
125. Wingate DL, Phillips SF, Hofmann AF. Effect of glycine-conjugated bile acids with and without lecithin on water and glucose absorption in perfused human jejunum. J Clin Invest. 1973;52:1230–1236.
126. Hofmann AF, Mysels KJ. Bile acid solubility and precipitation in vitro and in vivo: the role of conjugation, pH, and Ca^{2+} ions. J Lipid Res. 1992;33:617–626.
127. Oude Elferink RP, Groen AK. The role of MDR2 p-glycoprotein in biliary lipid secretion – cross-talk between cancer research and biliary physiology. Hepatology. 1995;23:617–625.
128. Weinand I, Hofmann AF, Jordan A, Caspary FW, Stein J. Cholylsarcosine use for bile acid replacement short bowel syndrome. Gastroenterology. 1999;116:A102.
129. Beuers U, Boyer JL, Paumgartner G. Ursodeoxycholic acid in cholestasis: potential mechanisms of action and therapeutic application. Hepatology. 1998;28:1449–1453.
130. Rodrigues CMP, Fan G, Ma X, Kren BT, Steer CJ. A novel role for ursodeoxycholic acid in inhibiting apoptosis by modulating mitochondrial membrane perturbation. J Clin Invest. 1998;101:2790–2799.
131. Lake M. Nonsurgical biliary drainage. Med Clin N Am. 1935;19:677–688.
132. Varco RL. Intermittent external biliary drainage for the relief of pruritus in certain chronic disorders of the liver. Surgery. 1947;21:43–45.
133. Whitington PF, Whitington GL. Partial external diversion of bile for the treatment of intractable pruritus associated with intrahepatic cholestasis. Gastroenterology. 1988;95:130–136.
134. Hollands CM, Rivera-Pedrogo FJ, Gonzalez-Vallina R, Loret-de-Mola O, Nahmad M, Burnweit CA. Ileal exclusion for Byler's disease: an alternative surgical approach with promising early results for pruritus. J Pediatr Surg. 1998;33:220–224.
135. Tuchweber B, Weber A, Roy CC, Yousef IM. Mechanisms of experimentally induced intrahepatic cholestasis. Prog Liver Dis. 1986;8:61–78.
136. Crombie DL, Hagey LR, Lillienau J, Miyai K, Hofmann AF. Toxicity of orally administered cholyltaurine in the guinea pig: discovery of a rodent that cannot detoxify deoxycholic acid. Gastroenterology. 1992;102:A922.
137. Ding JW, Andersson R, Soltesz V, Willen R, Bengmark S. The role of bile and bile acids in bacterial translocation in obstructive jaundice in rats. Eur Surg Res. 1993;25:11–19.
138. Reynolds JV, Murchan P, Leonard N, Clarke P, Keane FB, Tanner WA. Gut barrier failure in experimental obstructive jaundice. J Surg Res. 1996;62:11–16.
139. Parks RW, Clements WD, Pope C, Halliday MI, Rowlands BJ, Diamond T. Bacterial translocation and gut microflora in obstructive jaundice. J Anat. 1996;189:561–565.
140. Cakmakci M, Tirnaksiz B, Hayran M, Belek S, Gurbuz T, Salek I. Effects of obstructive jaundice and external biliary diversion on bacterial translocation in rats. Eur J Surg. 1996;162:567–571.

141. Kalambaheti T, Cooper GN, Jackson GOF. Role of bile in non-specific defense mechanisms of the gut. Gut. 1994;35:1047–1052.
142. Hellström PM, Nilison I, Svenberg T. Role of bile in regulation of gut motility J Intern Med. 1995;237:395–402.
143. Riepl RL, Fiedler F, Kowalski C, Teufel J, Lehnert P. Exocrine pancreatic secretion and plasma levels of cholecystokinin, pancreatic polypeptide, and somatostatin after single and combined intraduodenal application of different bile salts in man. Ital J Gastroenterol. 1998;28:421–429.
144. Karlström L, Cassuto J, Jodal M, Lundgren O. Involvement of the enteric nervous system in the intestinal secretion induced by sodium deoxycholate and sodium ricinoleate. Scand J Gastroenterol. 1986;21:331–340.
145. Coremans G, Tack J, VanTrappen G, Janssens J, Annese V. Is the irritable bowel really irritable? Ital J Gastroenterol. 1991;23:39–40.
146. Milovic V, Teller I, Murphy GM, Dowling RH, Caspary WF. Physiological concentrations of deoxycholic and lithocholic acids, but not of chenodeoxycholic acid, stimulate proliferation of cultured colon cancer cells. Gastroenterology. 1999; 116:465.
147. Dowling RH, Veysey MJ, Pereira SP et al. Role of intestinal transit in the pathogenesis of gallbladder stones. Can J Gastroenterol. 1997;11:57–64.
148. Alpini G, Glaser S, Robertson W, Phinizy JL, Rodgers RE, Califiuri A. Bile acids stimulate proliferative and secretory events in large but not small cholangiocytes. Am J Physiol. 1997;36:G518–G529.
149. Hofmann AF. Bile acids as drugs: principles, mechanisms of action, and formulations. Ital J Gastroenterol. 1995;27:106–113:
150. Hofmann AF. Bile acids: their continuing importance in liver and intestinal disease. Arch Intern Med. 1999 (in press).

Index

Falk Symposium Series

43. Reutter W, Popper H, Arias IM, Heinrich PC, Keppler D, Landmann L, eds.: *Modulation of Liver Cell Expression.* Falk Symposium No. 43. 1987   ISBN: 0-85200-677-2*

44. Boyer JL, Bianchi L, eds.: *Liver Cirrhosis.* Falk Symposium No. 44. 1987
ISBN: 0-85200-993-3*

45. Paumgartner G, Stiehl A, Gerok W, eds.: *Bile Acids and the Liver.* Falk Symposium No. 45. 1987   ISBN: 0-85200-675-6*

46. Goebell H, Peskar BM, Malchow H, eds.: *Inflammatory Bowel Diseases – Basic Research & Clinical Implications.* Falk Symposium No. 46. 1988   ISBN: 0-7462-0067-6*

47. Bianchi L, Holt P, James OFW, Butler RN, eds.: *Aging in Liver and Gastrointestinal Tract.* Falk Symposium No. 47. 1988   ISBN: 0-7462-0066-8*

48. Heilmann C, ed.: *Calcium-Dependent Processes in the Liver.* Falk Symposium No. 48. 1988   ISBN: 0-7462-0075-7*

50. Singer MV, Goebell H, eds.: *Nerves and the Gastrointestinal Tract.* Falk Symposium No. 50. 1989   ISBN: 0-7462-0114-1

51. Bannasch P, Keppler D, Weber G, eds.: *Liver Cell Carcinoma.* Falk Symposium No. 51. 1989   ISBN: 0-7462-0111-7

52. Paumgartner G, Stiehl A, Gerok W, eds.: *Trends in Bile Acid Research.* Falk Symposium No. 52. 1989   ISBN: 0-7462-0112-5

53. Paumgartner G, Stiehl A, Barbara L, Roda E, eds.: *Strategies for the Treatment of Hepatobiliary Diseases.* Falk Symposium No. 53. 1990   ISBN: 0-7923-8903-4

54. Bianchi L, Gerok W, Maier K-P, Deinhardt F, eds.: *Infectious Diseases of the Liver.* Falk Symposium No. 54. 1990   ISBN: 0-7923-8902-6

55. Falk Symposium No. 55 not published

55B. Hadziselimovic F, Herzog B, Bürgin-Wolff A, eds.: *Inflammatory Bowel Disease and Coeliac Disease in Children.* International Falk Symposium. 1990 ISBN 0-7462-0125-7

56. Williams CN, eds.: *Trends in Inflammatory Bowel Disease Therapy.* Falk Symposium No. 56. 1990   ISBN: 0-7923-8952-2

57. Bock KW, Gerok W, Matern S, Schmid R, eds.: *Hepatic Metabolism and Disposition of Endo- and Xenobiotics.* Falk Symposium No. 57. 1991   ISBN: 0-7923-8953-0

58. Paumgartner G, Stiehl A, Gerok W, eds.: *Bile Acids as Therapeutic Agents: From Basic Science to Clinical Practice.* Falk Symposium No. 58. 1991   ISBN: 0-7923-8954-9

59. Halter F, Garner A, Tytgat GNJ, eds.: *Mechanisms of Peptic Ulcer Healing.* Falk Symposium No. 59. 1991   ISBN: 0-7923-8955-7

60. Goebell H, Ewe K, Malchow H, Koelbel Ch, eds.: *Inflammatory Bowel Diseases – Progress in Basic Research and Clinical Implications.* Falk Symposium No. 60. 1991
ISBN: 0-7923-8956-5

61. Falk Symposium No. 61 not published

62. Dowling RH, Folsch UR, Löser Ch, eds.: *Polyamines in the Gastrointestinal Tract.* Falk Symposium No. 62. 1992   ISBN: 0-7923-8976-X

63. Lentze MJ, Reichen J, eds.: *Paediatric Cholestasis: Novel Approaches to Treatment.* Falk Symposium No. 63. 1992   ISBN: 0-7923-8977-8

64. Demling L, Frühmorgen P, eds.: *Non-Neoplastic Diseases of the Anorectum.* Falk Symposium No. 64. 1992   ISBN: 0-7923-8979-4

64B. Gressner AM, Ramadori G, eds.: *Molecular and Cell Biology of Liver Fibrogenesis.* International Falk Symposium. 1992   ISBN: 0-7923-8980-8

*These titles were published under the MTP Press imprint.

Falk Symposium Series

65. Hadziselimovic F, Herzog B, eds.: *Inflammatory Bowel Diseases and Morbus Hirschprung*. Falk Symposium No. 65. 1992   ISBN: 0-7923-8995-6

66. Martin F, McLeod RS, Sutherland LR, Williams CN, eds.: *Trends in Inflammatory Bowel Disease Therapy*. Falk Symposium No. 66. 1993   ISBN: 0-7923-8827-5

67. Schölmerich J, Kruis W, Goebell H, Hohenberger W, Gross V, eds.: *Inflammatory Bowel Diseases – Pathophysiology as Basis of Treatment*. Falk Symposium No. 67. 1993   ISBN: 0-7923-8996-4

68. Paumgartner G, Stiehl A, Gerok W, eds.: *Bile Acids and The Hepatobiliary System: From Basic Science to Clinical Practice*. Falk Symposium No. 68. 1993   ISBN: 0-7923-8829-1

69. Schmid R, Bianchi L, Gerok W, Maier K-P, eds.: *Extrahepatic Manifestations in Liver Diseases*. Falk Symposium No. 69. 1993   ISBN: 0-7923-8821-6

70. Meyer zum Büschenfelde K-H, Hoofnagle J, Manns M, eds.: *Immunology and Liver*. Falk Symposium No. 70. 1993   ISBN: 0-7923-8830-5

71. Surrenti C, Casini A, Milani S, Pinzani M , eds.: *Fat-Storing Cells and Liver Fibrosis*. Falk Symposium No. 71. 1994   ISBN: 0-7923-8842-9

72. Rachmilewitz D, ed.: *Inflammatory Bowel Diseases – 1994*. Falk Symposium No. 72. 1994   ISBN: 0-7923-8845-3

73. Binder HJ, Cummings J, Soergel KH, eds.: *Short Chain Fatty Acids*. Falk Symposium No. 73. 1994   ISBN: 0-7923-8849-6

73B. Möllmann HW, May B, eds.: *Glucocorticoid Therapy in Chronic Inflammatory Bowel Disease: from basic principles to rational therapy*. International Falk Workshop. 1996   ISBN 0-7923-8708-2

74. Keppler D, Jungermann K, eds.: *Transport in the Liver*. Falk Symposium No. 74. 1994   ISBN: 0-7923-8858-5

74B. Stange EF, ed.: *Chronic Inflammatory Bowel Disease*. Falk Symposium. 1995   ISBN: 0-7923-8876-3

75. van Berge Henegouwen GP, van Hoek B, De Groote J, Matern S, Stockbrügger RW, eds.: *Cholestatic Liver Diseases: New Strategies for Prevention and Treatment of Hepatobiliary and Cholestatic Liver Diseases*. Falk Symposium 75. 1994.   ISBN: 0-7923-8867-4

76. Monteiro E, Tavarela Veloso F, eds.: *Inflammatory Bowel Diseases: New Insights into Mechanisms of Inflammation and Challenges in Diagnosis and Treatment*. Falk Symposium 76. 1995.   ISBN 0-7923-8884-4

77. Singer MV, Ziegler R, Rohr G, eds.: *Gastrointestinal Tract and Endocrine System*. Falk Symposium 77. 1995.   ISBN 0-7923-8877-1

78. Decker K, Gerok W, Andus T, Gross V, eds.: *Cytokines and the Liver*. Falk Symposium 78. 1995.   ISBN 0-7923-8878-X

79. Holstege A, Schölmerich J, Hahn EG, eds.: *Portal Hypertension*. Falk Symposium 79. 1995.   ISBN 0-7923-8879-8

80. Hofmann AF, Paumgartner G, Stiehl A, eds.: *Bile Acids in Gastroenterology: Basic and Clinical Aspects*. Falk Symposium 80. 1995   ISBN 0-7923-8880-1

81. Riecken EO, Stallmach A, Zeitz M, Heise W, eds.: *Malignancy and Chronic Inflammation in the Gastrointestinal Tract – New Concepts*. Falk Symposium 81. 1995   ISBN 0-7923-8889-5

82. Fleig WE, ed.: *Inflammatory Bowel Diseases: New Developments and Standards*. Falk Symposium 82. 1995   ISBN 0-7923-8890-6

Falk Symposium Series

82B.Paumgartner G, Beuers U, eds.: *Bile Acids in Liver Diseases.* International Falk Workshop. 1995   ISBN 0-7923-8891-7

83. Dobrilla G, Felder M, de Pretis G, eds.: *Advances in Hepatobiliary and Pancreatic Diseases: Special Clinical Topics.* Falk Symposium 83. 1995.   ISBN 0-7923-8892-5

84. Fromm H, Leuschner U, eds.: *Bile Acids – Cholestasis – Gallstones: Advances in Basic and Clinical Bile Acid Research.* Falk Symposium 84. 1995   ISBN 0-7923-8893-3

85. Tytgat GNJ, Bartelsman JFWM, van Deventer SJH, eds.: *Inflammatory Bowel Diseases.* Falk Symposium 85. 1995   ISBN 0-7923-8894-1

86. Berg PA, Leuschner U, eds.: *Bile Acids and Immunology.* Falk Symposium 86. 1996   ISBN 0-7923-8700-7

87. Schmid R, Bianchi L, Blum HE, Gerok W, Maier KP, Stalder GA, eds.: *Acute and Chronic Liver Diseases: Molecular Biology and Clinics.* Falk Symposium 87. 1996   ISBN 0-7923-8701-5

88. Blum HE, Wu GY, Wu CH, eds.: *Molecular Diagnosis and Gene Therapy.* Falk Symposium 88. 1996   ISBN 0-7923-8702-3

88B.Poupon RE, Reichen J, eds.: *Surrogate Markers to Assess Efficacy of TReatment in Chronic Liver Diseases.* International Falk Workshop. 1996   ISBN 0-7923-8705-8

89. Reyes HB, Leuschner U, Arias IM, eds.: *Pregnancy, Sex Hormones and the Liver.* Falk Symposium 89. 1996   ISBN 0-7923-8704-X

89B.Broelsch CE, Burdelski M, Rogiers X, eds.: *Cholestatic Liver Diseases in Children and Adults.* International Falk Workshop. 1996   ISBN 0-7923-8710-4

90. Lam S-K, Paumgartner P, Wang B, eds.: *Update on Hepatobiliary Diseases 1996.* Falk Symposium 90. 1996   ISBN 0-7923-8715-5

91. Hadziselimovic F, Herzog B, eds.: *Inflammatory Bowel Diseases and Chronic Recurrent Abdominal Pain.* Falk Symposium 91. 1996   ISBN 0-7923-8722-8

91B.Alvaro D, Benedetti A, Strazzabosco M, eds.: *Vanishing Bile Duct Syndrome – Pathophysiology and Treatment.* International Falk Workshop. 1996   ISBN 0-7923-8721-X

92. Gerok W, Loginov AS, Pokrowskij VI, eds.: *New Trends in Hepatology 1996.* Falk Symposium 92. 1997   ISBN 0-7923-8723-6

93. Paumgartner G, Stiehl A, Gerok W, eds.: *Bile Acids in Hepatobiliary Diseases – Basic Research and Clinical Application.* Falk Symposium 93. 1997   ISBN 0-7923-8725-2

94. Halter F, Winton D, Wright NA, eds.: *The Gut as a Model in Cell and Molecular Biology.* Falk Symposium 94. 1997   ISBN 0-7923-8726-0

94B.Kruse-Jarres JD, Schölmerich J, eds.: *Zinc and Diseases of the Digestive Tract.* International Falk Workshop. 1997   ISBN 0-7923-8724-4

95. Ewe K, Eckardt VF, Enck P, eds.: *Constipation and Anorectal Insufficiency.* Falk Symposium 95. 1997   ISBN 0-7923-8727-9

96. Andus T, Goebell H, Layer P, Schölmerich J, eds.: *Inflammatory Bowel Disease – from Bench to Bedside.* Falk Symposium 96. 1997   ISBN 0-7923-8728-7

97. Campieri M, Bianchi-Porro G, Fiocchi C, Schölmerich J, eds. *Clinical Challenges in Inflammatory Bowel Diseases: Diagnosis, Prognosis and Treatment.* Falk Symposium 97. 1998   ISBN 0-7923-8733-3

98. Lembcke B, Kruis W, Sartor RB, eds. *Systemic Manifestations of IBD: The Pending Challenge for Subtle Diagnosis and Treatment.* Falk Symposium 98. 1998   ISBN 0-7923-8734-1

Falk Symposium Series

99. Goebell H, Holtmann G, Talley NJ, eds. *Functional Dyspepsia and Irritable Bowel Syndrome: Concepts and Controversies.* Falk Symposium 99. 1998
ISBN 0-7923-8735-X

100. Blum HE, Bode Ch, Bode JCh, Sartor RB, eds. *Gut and the Liver.* Falk Symposium 100. 1998
ISBN 0-7923-8736-8

101. Rachmilewitz D, ed. *V International Symposium on Inflammatory Bowel Diseases.* Falk Symposium 101. 1998
ISBN 0-7923-8743-0

102. Manns MP, Boyer JL, Jansen PLM, Reichen J, eds. *Cholestatic Liver Diseases.* Falk Symposium 102. 1998
ISBN 0-7923-8746-5

102B. Manns MP, Chapman RW, Stiehl A, Wiesner R, eds. *Primary Sclerosing Cholangitis.* International Falk Workshop. 1998.
ISBN 0-7923-8745-7

103. Häussinger D, Jungermann K, eds. *Liver and Nervous System.* Falk Symposium 102. 1998
ISBN 0-7924-8742-2

103B. Häussinger D, Heinrich PC, eds. *Signalling in the Liver.* International Falk Workshop. 1998
ISBN 0-7923-8744-9

103C. Fleig W, ed. *Normal and Malignant Liver Cell Growth.* International Falk Workshop. 1998
ISBN 0-7923-8748-1

104. Stallmach A, Zeitz M, Strober W, MacDonald TT, Lochs H, eds. *Induction and Modulation of Gastrointestinal Inflammation.* Falk Symposium 104. 1998
ISBN 0-7923-8747-3

105. Emmrich J, Liebe S, Stange EF, eds. *Innovative Concepts in Inflammatory Bowel Diseases.* Falk Symposium 105. 1999
ISBN 0-7923-8749-X

106. Rutgeerts P, Colombel J-F, Hanauer SB, Schölmerich J, Tytgat GNJ, van Gossum A, eds. *Advances in Inflammatory Bowel Diseases.* Falk Symposium 106. 1999
ISBN 0-7923-8750-3

107. Špičák J, Boyer J, Gilat T, Kotrlik K, Mareček Z, Paumgartner G, eds. *Diseases of the Liver and the Bile Ducts – New Aspects and Clinical Implications.* Falk Symposium 107. 1999
ISBN 0-7923-8751-1

108. Paumgartner G, Stiehl A, Gerok W, Keppler D, Leuschner U, eds. *Bile Acids and Cholestasis.* Falk Symposium 108. 1999
ISBN 0-7923-8752-X

109. Schmiegel W, Schölmerich J, eds. *Colorectal Cancer – Molecular Mechanisms, Premalignant State and its Prevention.* Falk Symposium 109. 1999
ISBN 0-7923-8753-8

110. Domschke W, Stoll R, Brasitus TA, Kagnoff MF, eds. *Intestinal Mucosa and its Diseases – Pathophysiology and Clinics.* Falk Symposium 110. 1999
ISBN 0-7923-8754-6

110B. Northfield TC, Ahmed HA, Jazwari RP, Zentler-Munro PL, eds. *Bile Acids in Hepatobiliary Disease.* Falk Workshop. 2000
ISBN 0-7923-8755-4